AF441831

MEDICAL AND CARE COMPUNETICS 4

Studies in Health Technology and Informatics

This book series was started in 1990 to promote research conducted under the auspices of the EC programmes' Advanced Informatics in Medicine (AIM) and Biomedical and Health Research (BHR) bioengineering branch. A driving aspect of international health informatics is that telecommunication technology, rehabilitative technology, intelligent home technology and many other components are moving together and form one integrated world of information and communication media. The complete series has been accepted in Medline. Volumes from 2005 onwards are available online.

Series Editors:

Dr. J.P. Christensen, Prof. G. de Moor, Prof. A. Famili, Prof. A. Hasman, Prof. L. Hunter,
Dr. I. Iakovidis, Dr. Z. Kolitsi, Mr. O. Le Dour, Dr. A. Lymberis, Prof. P.F. Niederer,
Prof. A. Pedotti, Prof. O. Rienhoff, Prof. F.H. Roger France, Dr. N. Rossing,
Prof. N. Saranummi, Dr. E.R. Siegel, Dr. P. Wilson, Prof. E.J.S. Hovenga,
Prof. M.A. Musen and Prof. J. Mantas

Volume 127

Recently published in this series

ISSN 0926-9630

Medical and Care Compunetics 4

Edited by

Lodewijk Bos
President ICMCC

and

Bernd Blobel
eHealth Competence Center, University of Regensburg Medical Center, Germany

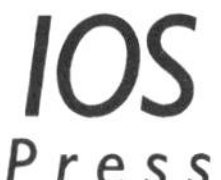

IOS *Press*

Amsterdam • Berlin • Oxford • Tokyo • Washington, DC

ISBN 978-1-58603-751-2
Library of Congress Control Number: 2007927199

Publisher
IOS Press
Nieuwe Hemweg 6B
1013 BG Amsterdam
Netherlands
fax: +31 20 687 0019
e-mail: order@iospress.nl

Distributor in the UK and Ireland
Gazelle Books Services Ltd.
White Cross Mills
Hightown
Lancaster LA1 4XS
United Kingdom
fax: +44 1524 63232
e-mail: sales@gazellebooks.co.uk

Distributor in the USA and Canada
IOS Press, Inc.
4502 Rachael Manor Drive
Fairfax, VA 22032
USA
fax: +1 703 323 3668
e-mail: iosbooks@iospress.com

LEGAL NOTICE

The publisher is not responsible for the use which might be made of the following information.

PRINTED IN THE NETHERLANDS

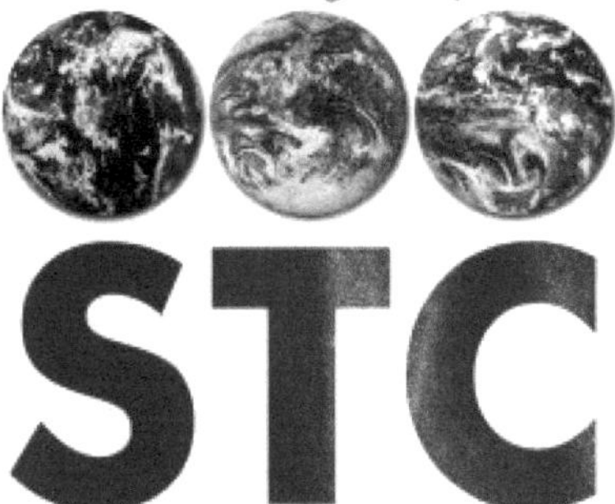

Scientific Technologies Corporation
STC

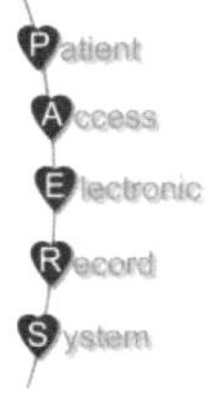

Patient
Access
Electronic
Record
System

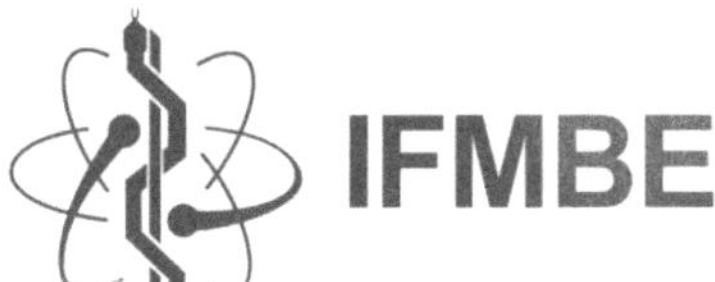

IFMBE

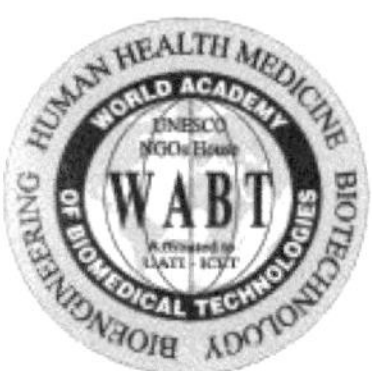

WORLD ACADEMY
UNESCO
NGOs House
WABT
HUMAN HEALTH MEDICINE
BIOTECHNOLOGY
BIOENGINEERING
OF BIOMEDICAL TECHNOLOGIES

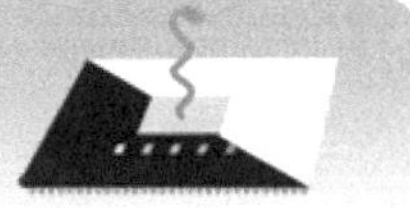

ICMCC
The international council on medical & care compunetics

Medical and Care Compunetics 4
L. Bos and B. Blobel (Eds.)
IOS Press, 2007

vii

Preface

This book accompanies the fourth annual ICMCC Event.

In the past 12 months the role of ICMCC with regards to patient-related ICT has become obvious with the start of the Record Access Portal. It is our goal to come forward with a recommendation to the WHO on Record Access. This recommendation will therefore be one of the leading issues of the Round Table on the Responsibility Shift from Doctor to Patient.

The 2007 ICMCC Event deals with the following subjects:

- EHR and Record Access;
- Digital Homecare;
- Behavioral compunetics;
- The Paradigm Change Challenge towards Personal Health.

This last session has been organized by Prof. Dr. Bernd Blobel from the eHealth Competence Center (University of Regensburg Medical Center, Germany) jointly with the European Federation for Medical Informatics (EFMI) Working Groups "Electronic Health Records (EHR)" and "Security, Safety and Ethics (SSE)".

Due to personal circumstances this book has really been a group effort and I therefore would like to thank by name all members of the scientific board: Bernd Blobel, Denis Carroll, Brian Fisher, Richard Fitton, Chris Flim, Hermie Hermens, Peter Pharow, Denis Protti, Laura Roa and Kanagasingam Yogesan.

On behalf of the ICMCC Foundation board I wish to thank the STC, PAERS, IF-MBE and the WABT-ICET-UNESCO for their support to make this conference possible.

Finally I would like to thank all the authors who have contributed to making the fourth ICMCC Event into an interesting and challenging conference.

Lodewijk Bos
Event chair

Board Lists

Council Board

Drs Lodewijk Bos, president, The Netherlands
Robert von Hinke Kessler (vice-president, treasurer, secretary general),
    The Netherlands
Denis Carroll (vice-president), Westminster University, UK
Dr. Andy Marsh (vice-president), VMWSolutions, UK
Prof. Brian O'Connell (vice-president), Central Connecticut State University, USA
Michael L. Popovich (vice-president), Scientific Technologies Corporation, USA
Prof. Kanagasingam Yogesan (vice-president), Centre of Excellence in e-Medicine,
    Australia

2007 Scientific Committee

Drs Lodewijk Bos, president of ICMCC, The Netherlands (Event Chair)
Prof. Dr. Bernd Blobel, eHealth Competence Center, University Regensburg, Germany
Mr. Denis Carroll, University of Westminster, UK
Dr. Brian Fisher, GP, Director PAERS, UK
Dr. Richard Fitton, GP, UK
Drs. Chris Flim, Promotor and co-producer of Dutch Record Access initiatives,
    Netherlands
Prof. Hermie Hermens, University of Twente, Roessingh Research & Development,
    Netherlands
Dr. Peter Pharow, eHealth Competence Center, University Regensburg, Germany
Prof. Denis Protti, University of Victoria, Canada
Prof. Laura Roa, Biomedical Engineering Program, University of Sevilla, Spain
Prof. Kanagasingam Yogesan, Centre of Excellence in e-Medicine, Australia

ICMCC Advisory Board

Dr. Rajeev Bali, Coventry University, UK
Drs Iddo Bante, CTIT/TKT, Business Director, The Netherlands
Prof. Dr. Bernd Blobel, Associate Professor, Head, eHealth Competence Center,
    University of Regensburg Medical Center, Germany
Prof. Peter Brett, Aston University, Birmingham, UK
Dr. Ir Adrie Dumay, TNO, The Netherlands
M. Chris Gibbons, MD, MPH, Associate Director, Johns Hopkins Urban Health
    Institute (UHI), President-elect International Society of Urban Health, Baltimore,
    USA

Brian Manning, University of Westminster, UK
Prof. Dr. Joachim Nagel, University of Stuttgart, President IUPESM, Germany
Prof. Neill Piland, Idaho State University, USA
Prof. Laura Roa, Biomedical Engineering Program, University of Sevilla, Spain
Prof. Joseph Tritto, World Academy of Biomedical Technologies, UNESCO, France

Contents

Keynotes

Medical and Care Compunetics 4
L. Bos and B. Blobel (Eds.)
IOS Press, 2007

Medical and Care Compunetics the Future of Patient-Related ICT

Drs Lodewijk BOS[1]
President ICMCC

Abstract. This article deals with the role of compunetics in the future of patient-related ICT. Information supply, knowledge centers, gathering of personal and secondary data, the role of patient and professional networks, e-learning are the topics covered here.

Introduction

Compunetics deals with ICT, Information, Communication and Technology. The word Compunetics is derived from the combination of Computing and Networking [1] but the new term allowed including social aspects, becoming "computing and social and technical networking". [2]. Now, three years after the introduction of the word, it can be defined as the field concerned with the social, societal and ethical implications of computing and networking (**COMPU**ting & **N**etworking, its **EThIC**s and Social/ societal implications). The concept of compunetics was first applied in the area of medicine and care by ICMCC (the International Council on Medical & Care Compunetics) and is quickly gaining ground. [47,17] A logical consequence of this concept is the now emerging field of behavioral compunetics.

1. Information

Information is the core of our modern society, as it is the basic ingredient of the knowledge society. It can be defined as: "data that have been organized and communicated" (Quote from Marc Porat). [3] "In the early nineties, under the aegis of the United States National Information Infrastructure, the Internet facilitated the creation of an "information-for-all" environment. Despite the unstructured nature of its existence, the Internet has seen an unprecedented global growth in its role as a promoter of information solutions to the citizens of the world" wrote one of the ICMCC founder fathers Swamy Laxminarayan [4]. Information should be made available in as broad a way as possible to the citizen as well as the professional. In health, for both target groups the largest network in the world, the World Wide Web, will be the source of information in the future. However, there is a problem with the web.

- In the day of books and classical libraries, you knew where to find your information, in what specific book, on what specific shelf.

---

[1] ICMCC, Stationsstraat 38, 3511 EG Utrecht.
www.icmcc.org, lobos@icmcc.org.

- There were, and are, ways – standards – how to find information in libraries even if you didn't know in advance what you were looking for. If you had trouble finding it, there was always someone who could point out a starting point or who would mention a recent addition to the material of your subject. And afterwards you would remember where that information was physically stored.
- If you had doubts about the reliability of the information that same person, the librarian, could help you, from his experience and knowledge.

We all have had numerous moments of frustration when discovering that you could not repeat the steps you took on the internet that caused you to stumble upon certain information and therefore the information was lost to you. Since a while, we see all kinds of web facilities coming up to bookmark that information and annotate it. We have to learn to create our own librarian.

In our days, information is available in abundance. Through publications, research communities, international projects, more and more people have access to information. Especially in the health area there is a need for it. "The number of U.S. adults who have ever gone online to look for health or medical information has increased to approximately 117 million, up from about 111 million last year (2004) [...] Almost six in 10 (58%) say that they have looked for information about health topics often (25%) or sometimes (33%), an increase of eight percentage points from 2004 (50%)." [5]

"In 2005, the criteria perceived as the most important indicators of quality and usefulness for health Web sites among non-professional and professional groups of users: (1) availability of information, (2) ease of finding information/navigation, (3) trustworthiness/credibility and (4) accuracy of information. Both non-professional and professional users, in Europe and the USA, favor academic/university sites (89.4%, n=1403) and sites sponsored by medical journals (88.9%, n=1394), closely followed by government agencies (86.1%, n=1395). We have also observed that a significant number of Web users, about 25% of a sample of 1,386 persons from all over the world, lack confidence in sites sponsored by pharmaceutical manufacturers and commercial, mainstream media organizations." [6]

Research has taught us that information on the internet is often biased or plain simply wrong. [7] Most people have no way to recognize this. In a qualitative study, using focus groups, the researchers concluded: "The results showed that there was a range of search and appraisal skills among participants, with many reporting a limited awareness of how they found and evaluated Internet-based information on medicines. Poor interpretation of written information on medicines has been shown to lead to anxiety and poor compliance to therapy. This issue is more important for Internet-based information since it is not subject to quality control and standardization as is written information on medicines. Therefore, there is a need for promoting consumer search and appraisal skills when using this information. Educating consumers in how to find and interpret Internet-based information on medicines may help them use their medicines in a safer and more-effective way." [8] As all the information is freely available, the internet information supply might be seen as one of the leading problems in patient safety in the coming decade. It is relatively easy to find agreements or standards on any other aspect of patient safety; it will be hard, maybe even impossible to do so for the web, although there are a number of initiatives for quality labelling. [9–11] "Regulation does not seem like the right strategy for improving the quality of health information on the internet. Other approaches, such as educating the producers of this content, look like a better long term bet. However, such initiatives should not hinder the evolution of communities, resources, and processes that are improving healthcare outcomes." [12]

2. Knowledge Centre

With the right of the individual to be informed a whole new problem emerges related to those who are involved in decision making processes concerning the individual. For with the empowerment of the individual, the classical way of decision making will disappear and the individual, the citizen, the consumer, the patient will either want to know on which information decisions are based and might want to verify that information, or will posses knowledge exceeding that of the decision maker, in casu the caregiver (a growing phenomenon in the medical world called "expert patient"). This is a double edged sword, for it means that the information and knowledge accessible to the decision maker should be made available to the individual and the decision maker should be able to quickly acquire the information and knowledge that he seems to lack. However, "[i]f we assume that about 1% of the new literature added every year is of relevance to a healthcare stakeholder, then it would still take a stakeholder 10 years (reading an average of one article a day) to be updated with the healthcare advances of 1 year." [13]

On the other side, "[b]roadly speaking, the patient's perspective of healthcare knowledge sharing aims to educate and empower patients [...] to understand their health condition and to self-manage their healthcare process. This aim is pursued by facilitating the provision of online patient-specific healthcare knowledge [...] in a proactive and timely manner through patient education and support programs." [14]

And that is where knowledge centres based on the principle of compunetics will play an essential role.

There are ways to organise knowledge in a central semi-controlled, nevertheless open way, a knowledge centre. Avoiding the reinvention of the wheel as well as redundancy of science, research and experience, is a key argument in favour of those centres. We should develop the wheel, not reinvent it time and again due to the fact that we don't know what knowledge and information is available. An inventory, a knowledge centre, could not only help to save billions of dollars a year by avoiding redundancy, could not only be an important source of knowledge to professionals, caregivers and policy makers, it could also be the basic information needed to assist in building new infrastructures.

Davenport et al. define knowledge as "a fluid mix of framed experience, values, contextual information, and expert insight that provides a framework for evaluating and incorporating new experiences and information. It originates and is applied in the minds of knowers. In organizations, it often becomes embedded not only in documents or repositories but also in organizational routines, process, practices, and norms" [15]. In this paper a shorter definition is used: Knowledge is information combined with experience. That is why best practices (evidence-based medicine) have become such an important concept in the informational health society. And we have to bring those together. "At an individual level [evidence-based medicine] is a way of helping health practitioners who are overwhelmed with the information explosion." [16] But not only best practices; failures and disappointments are often more important in the learning process. They should be included as well, if only to avoid that others have to go through the same experience.

Knowledge centres should be about knowledge sharing, between individuals, providers, professionals and projects. Therefore, it will be necessary to start knowledge centres that will focus on the inventory of a particular field and that will help to identify gaps in research and development and will stimulate or even initiate work to fill those gaps. As described above, especially in medicine and care such centres will be of extreme importance. These will be centres of sustainable knowledge of benefit on strategy and policy level as well as on the personal level of the individual. Knowledge centres will also be able to stimulate research in areas that lack sufficient attention, at the same time, as an independent institute, bringing global coordination in ongoing work like (bio)medical technology, disease surveillance and bioterrorism.

In the near future, many facets of (bio)medical technology and their products will get closer to the citizen, causing his interest in the matter to grow. A knowledge centre will also be a citizen portal of access to global knowledge, thus helping him to make informed decisions about his health and well-being. This possibility to control decisions that impact an individual's life is called empowerment.

"Applied compunetics to support the public health mission of disease mitigation offers system users an opportunity to have the right tools at the right time in which to make the right decisions. Preparedness for disease outbreaks will, in part, be a function of rapid detection and action. Rapid detection equates to identifying indicators that an outbreak is likely. Build the right public health electronic environment and the technologist will be as valuable as the first responder to mitigating disease impacts." [17]

"Computing and high speed communications are not only enabling governmental and secular institutions around the world at an unprecedented rate; the combination of these two synergistic technologies is even transforming the way we think of humanity and human potential. They are unveiling deep structure in the behavioral and social sciences that may forever alter the way we look at our selves and interact with others. These new technologies and methodologies are fundamentally changing the way we are approaching the prevention and management of large-scale social crisis." [18]

A small example of such a knowledge center is the portal on Record Access created on the ICMCC website. This portal is the first in its kind, where most of the (scientific) information on the access of patients to their electronic health records is gathered [19]. Discussion platforms are being created to enable exchange of ideas and experiences, also between the professionals and the consumers. Other examples could be the areas of assistive technology and digital homecare.

3. Networks

The internet is not only the leading source of information, it is also becoming one of the leading communication tools, especially in its capacity as facilitator of networks. In the concept of compunetics social, societal and ethical implications play a key role. Networks are a major example of the social and societal aspects. "The extraordinary value of [ICTs] lies not only in the information that can now be exchanged but also in their ability to bring people together to build and shape partnerships and a joint programme of action, enabling more informed decision-making and more cost-effective use of resources." [20]

Communication (and therefore networking) is an essential element in the knowledge society. In medicine and care this means communication between researchers and their tools, between caregivers and their tools, between all those tools, but above all between any of the aforementioned and the patient and between patients.

Of growing importance on the internet are networks of patients, often called support groups.

"Rather than worrying about "the quality of medical content" on the Internet, as many medical professionals do, patients figured out that the most effective strategy was to organize social networks focusing on specific healthcare issues. The power of these healthcare-oriented social networks can be quite phenomenal. Having good "medical content" may well be useful, but being able to tap into the expertise of hundreds or thousands of e-patients around the globe is considerably more powerful. The amazing thing is that patients figured this out a long time ago, while most healthcare professionals still don't really get it." [21]

"The patients who produce these sites certainly don't know everything a physician might know, but they don't need to. Good clinicians must have an in-depth working knowledge of the ills they see frequently and must know at least a little about hundreds of conditions they rarely or never see. Online self-helpers, on the other hand will typically know only about their own disease, but some will have an impressive and up-to-date knowledge of the best sources, centers, treatments, research, and specialists for this condition. A smart, motivated, and experienced self-helper with hemophilia, narcolepsy, hemochromatosis or any number of rare genetic conditions may well know more about current research and treatments for their disease than their own primary practitioner. And when it comes to aspects illness that some clinicians may consider secondary-e.g., practical coping tips and the psychological and social aspects of living with the condition-some experienced self-helpers can provide other patients with particularly helpful advice. The things clinicians know and the things self-helpers know can complement each other in some interesting and useful ways." [22]

Also the caregiver might benefit from social networks. "Knowledge sharing through discussion forums has both a problem-solving aspect and learning aspect to it, because observing practitioners not only learn about a potential solution to a atypical clinical problem, but, as the discussion unfolds, they also observe the tacit problem-solving strategy and reasoning methods employed by specialist practitioners. […] Sharing the tacit knowledge of healthcare experts, via socialization, can assist fellow practitioners in terms of providing them practical insights into what solution will work, why it will work, and how to make it work." [14] A very recent example is the Ask Dr. Wiki site opened in March 2007. [23]

The interaction between the networks of these two groups, patients and caregivers is becoming more important.

"These online community networks do not replace traditional research channels or the healthcare process, including doctors visits, but they do augment it and improve it by leveraging the organizational, analytic, and communicative ability of a few to inform, support, and guide many. Although online patient networks are run by patients for patients, we think that if providers are integrated into these networks, quality can be improved and errors reduced. Healthcare professionals can seed the communities with quality scientific information, which will augment the experiences being shared." [24]

Not only do these groups provide exchange of information between participants, they can also be assistant in research. "The prospect of research-oriented online support groups offers a number of appealing scenarios. Patient groups could design and conduct their own studies, collecting their own data, analyzing their results, and publishing their results. They could provide researchers with access to perfectly targeted study populations at little or no cost. But whatever role they play, once they become active players in medical research, patient groups will demand a voice in deciding what should be studied and how that research will be conducted. And while such e-patient initiatives may encounter some resistance, in the end it seems likely that the financially-strapped medical research establishment will come to consider such e-patient research an offer it can't afford to refuse." [25] A recent example is a project from the Kennedy Krieger Institute, started in April 2007. "IAN, the Interactive Autism Network, is an innovative online project designed to accelerate the pace of autism research by linking researchers and families." [26]

The exchange of experience will not only play an essential role in decision making, it will also help to overcome health inequalities.

4. Data

The term "data" is commonly used to indicate the basic elements for scientific research. In the context of this paper on medical and care compunetics we look at two different sets of data: personal and secondary.

4.1. Personal Data

For the patient to have access to the appropriate information to make informed decisions, access to his personal health information is elementary. Record Access (RA) is an essential part of patient empowerment also because it enables the patient to have control over his treatments. The Electronic Health Record (EHR) will be the central container of data about a specific patient. A number of different names are circulating to indicate the various elements of the EHR, namely the EMR (Electronic Medical Record), PHR (Personal Health Record), CCR (Continuity of Care Record) [27]. Discussions are ongoing about the differences between these terminologies and how the various elements can or should be combined. [28]

In this paper the EHR is seen as the final storage of all information concerning the patient:

- medical and care information;
- monitoring data from external sources;
- personal input from the patient.

In my view, all medical and care data concerning a person should be gathered in one "document" that should be, in principle, fully accessible to the individual (examples of exceptions are young children and mentally incapacitated persons). Caregivers and other persons of his choice should also have access; whether third party access should be full depends on the indication of the owner of the record and the role of the caregiver.

"The benefits of RA appear to be substantial. Patients describe improved trust in their doctors, improved confidence in their clinicians, and they feel more informed and in control of their condition and its management. There is some evidence for improved health practices by patients – for example, improved compliance in heart failure. In general, patients are keen on RA in principle and in practice. Additional advantages of RA include that it can be used to reduce recording errors and thus increase patient safety, and that patients looking up information in their records can save time for practices." [29]

4.1.1. Medical and Care Information

All information concerning the individual's health, condition and treatment should be included in the EHR. This will help to build an overview of on-going treatments and exams, avoid duplication of exams – because they are requested by a different doctor or institution – and will also be a tool in helping to avoid medication errors/interactions. It will also create a personal health history from which both patient and caregiver can benefit. Care related information (e.g. information from nurses, physiotherapists) should be included in the EHR as well to complete the patient's medical picture.

"Over time these may join up to provide a "clinical pathway" highlighting the journey a patient makes as they move from one stage of management to another." [30]

Communication between doctors and patient as well as between doctors should also be part of the EHR. "Many physicians who began exchanging email with their patients because of repeated requests from patients have become active promoters of doctor-patient email because of its benefits for physicians and provider organizations." [31]

4.1.2. Monitoring Data from External Sources

With the growing development of digital homecare and other ways of monitoring and tele-medicine, the data gathered by these procedures will also have to be included in the EHR. It can be discussed in which form this should be done, like weekly summaries or development curves.

"Today, with the huge amounts of medical data and information and the growing number of medical information systems, there is an increasing need for medical information that is complete, homogeneous, precise, updated, reliable and accessible at the point of care. Information based on the historical medical data of the patient collected in real time from all relevant internal and external sources can be the basis for an optimal decision-making process. This information is essential to insure the quality of the medical care process and healthcare service and it needs to be provided effectively and efficiently utilizing all the sophisticated techniques for collecting, browsing and presenting data that today's information technology has to offer." [32]

Integration and interoperability are key issues to achieve the gathering and storage of these data. "Interoperability implies a number of different concepts, e.g. functional interoperability and internetworking, semantic interoperability and application gateways. Health information integration (eHealth) established a demand for interoperability between clinical and healthcare-related stakeholders, systems and processes or workflows. Domain-specific communication and interoperability standards are well established, but have to be supplemented for trans-domain use." [33]

4.1.3. Personal Input from the Patient

Patients should be encouraged to input their own health observations. Personal habits, use of over-the-counter drugs, sleeping problems, alcohol and recreational drug use but also work or relationship related stress are some examples of what could be included.

"Illness narratives refer to the reflective and insightful autobiographical accounts of illness. They are not merely chronicles of events but can also provide valuable insights in how patienthood, brought upon by the assaults of illness, is experienced as a disruption of selfhood. [...] Stories have a recuperative role and can be used to recuperate persons, relationships, and communities. [...] Narratives shared over a prolonged time allow strong bonds to be formed, engendering trust and effective care." [34]

"Accessing medical records has also shown improvements on patients' education, a better knowledge of the disease and more participation in their health treatment. Improvements on adherence made patients more careful in following medical recommendations and provided for self-empowerment. It allowed them more autonomy and self-efficacy by increasing a sense of ownership to their medical records. [...] The access to medical records helps correcting errors and omissions but patients can also make unauthorized additions or deletions." [35] Nevertheless, patients should be able to point out possible errors in the record and request for correction.

To be able to provide the patient with optimal information about his condition the data in the EHR should be linked to independent and accurate information on the internet. From there the patient should be able to make further searches to information. This is where knowledge centres can play a major role.

4.2. Secondary Data

Secondary data are data derived from other data sets.

Data gathered anonymously from the **EHR**s, medical, personal as well as from digital monitoring, can be used for research purposes e.g. for epidemic and pandemic surveillances. Other data to be used are:

- Pharmaceutical and Over-the-Counter Sales
- Hospital Emergency Department and Emergency Medical Services Encounter Data
- General Information "Hot Lines"
- School and Work Absenteeism
- Animal Disease Reporting
- Medical Examiner Reports
- Hospital Discharge Data [36]

"Healthcare at the moment is a reactive process; we should be turning it round to proactive productive testing to prevent people from being ill. We could get a much better profile for diseases and use predictive profiles to help or to warn people in advance. [...] People must realise we are what we eat and breathe." (quote from Prof. Michel Thick) [37]

Another aspect is that the use of these data "is expected to streamline patient check-in, provide up-to-date health information, support referrals among providers, facilitate parent access to immunization and other records, automate patient appointment reminders and promote access to preventative health information." [38] Use of these data can "enable health risk assessment, determine an individual's baseline susceptibility to disease, their current health status and current risks for major, chronic or uniquely inherited diseases. [...] the individual and their provider should develop a strategic health plan to mitigate risk and track health status in order to determine if any particular diseases are developing." [39]

"A major attraction of the [EHR] is the potential that it creates for conducting re-cords-based clinical research, epidemiological studies and quality monitoring on very large data sets. However, it is in breach of European privacy standards to use data in this way originally collected for the purpose of providing healthcare to the individual. This could be achieved by incorporating into the information charter references to use personal health records without patient's explicit consent for the purpose of clinical audit, performance review, research, epidemiology and other activities deemed neces-sary for provision of high quality healthcare. It will also be necessary to identify under what circumstances the patient's consent would be sought." [40]

"In today's global community the ability to prepare for a disease outbreak in order to mitigate the public health, social, and economic impacts on a community depends upon data to support the decision and response process. Data can come from a variety of sources. These sources not only include the medical and health care community, but also geographic, demographic, and socio-economic data. The ability to capture and utilise the data effectively from these types of data sources can mean the difference between a manageable disease outbreak that represents little or no threat to a commu-nity and one that causes a significant social and economic impact." [17]

"[I]n the case of the US population (compared to the rest of the world) this society is much more "transient" or mobile. As people move seeking better job-opportunities, the associated consequence is that the individuals will be seeking care in the new loca-tions which generates having scattered medical records. Not having the complete pic-ture is a problem that not only can generate "medical errors", but does not allow those caring for the individual to have the information needed to do to risk assessment / man-agement, prevention, and disease management. In the future as we evolve our system more into the phase of prevention, the "total picture" will be even more critical since genetic information could be associated with environmental data for example (i.e. qual-ity of air, water, etc.)" [18]

Another aspect of gathering secondary data is **social networking analysis**. On the level of healthcare professionals knowledge flows and knowledge gaps in healthcare providers can be identified by social network analysis which can also examine different types of knowledge applies by healthcare professionals. [41] It would be interesting to see if these procedures could also be used for patient networks.

A third aspect would be the analysis of the way health information sites are being used, e.g. using **click-through analysis**. It could be a tool to provide information to the patient in a more efficient and consistent way as it would give indications of the infor-mation needs of the patient. A study analyzing how users interact with the list of ranked results (i.e. the "results page" for short) from the Google search engine and how their behaviour can be interpreted as relevance judgments shows "that users make in-formed decisions among the abstracts they observe and that clicks reflect relevance judgments. However, we show that clicking decisions are biased in at least two ways. First, we show that there is a "trust bias" which leads to more clicks on links ranked highly by Google, even if those abstracts are less relevant than other abstracts the user viewed. Second, there is a "quality bias": the users' clicking decision is not only influ-enced by the relevance of the clicked link, but also by the overall quality of the other abstracts in the ranking. This shows that clicks have to be interpreted relative to the order of presentation and relative to the other abstracts." [42]

Data sets should be linked to provide a maximum effect. This is where interopera-bility plays a key role.

"Surveillance systems reduce the risk to public health from dangers such as communicable diseases, hazardous or unsafe foods, terrorism and other catastrophes. In such emergencies it is absolutely necessary to alert both clinicians and consumers quickly. By knitting together a unified network of surveillance systems from hospital organisations, physician practices, public health agencies and other sources of incoming data on medical threats, public health professionals will have the relevant information they need to react early or issue preventive measures. The only way to create such a network is to make all the data-collection systems interoperable." [43]

As Allwes and Popovich argue in their article about orphan diseases "ACC, in and of itself, doesn't have the large numbers of affected individuals to be sway policy and industry to stop and take notice. However, if taken in whole with the rest of the orphan diseases, there is a strength that all orphan diseases can draw from. Disease processes can be explored for generalization, drug development can be based on the uniqueness of orphan diseases, and patient participation can be capitalised through a common area of shared knowledge." [44]

5. e-Learning

As knowledge should be used to create knowledge, knowledge centres should become the basis for the development of e-learning programs, on different levels and not only for professionals. "One of the essences of the knowledge society is the ability to learn [...] based on the concept that we learn how to learn. Education must no longer be seen as a period of learning limited in time but as a process to be pursued throughout one's existence." [3] "Knowledge sharing [...] is not just an activity, but in itself is a knowledge resource." [14]

For the professional the classical master/apprentice relationship has modified and partially disappeared, as information as well as knowledge has become more openly available. In earlier days, the master taught his apprentice his skills, according to prescribed procedures, and within the confines of his trade or trade group. Building knowledge societies should involve not only promoting, wherever appropriate, distance education but also developing the capacity for learning and continuous discovery. [3]

Education is one of the most important tools for empowerment. With the internet and its accessibility, the concept of education has changed. Having a basic education means that you have the means and know-how to satisfy your curiosity and know how to get answers to questions. The internet enables people to find answers, often in abundance and mostly in an unstructured way. In principle, we have learned how to learn.

Basic in the educational discussion, also because of the important role of it in the UN Millennium goals, should be the issue of the responsibility of the "user" (i.e. the one who is learning). The need of people to be informed can not be structured in the way we used to do it in previous times. The acquirement of knowledge will become more and more personalised. Therefore education, beyond the classical schooling (up to the level of universities), will loose its directional structure, i.e. from a certain point onwards it will be a person's private decision to continue his education, either through specified programs or by just looking for answers to specific questions, always assisted through networks of discussion and exchange. E-Learning could be an important tool in achieving this new education paradigm. Projects like the UNESCO Avicenna Virtual Campus [45] have shown that students do benefit immensely from this form of education. For the individual consumer, knowledge centres can be the point of reference for (exchange of) information and experience.

To promote e-learning we will also have to use economical arguments, like the fact that people can study when and where they wish, so there are less costs involved locating and transporting people to fixed locations. The overhead costs for e-learning will be considerably lower. The downside is, that you will have to trust the user's sense of responsibility because you lack the possibility to control it the way it was done at any educational institution. Another negative aspect might be the, lack of, social interaction (see also [46]); however, the growth of networks and communities on the internet seems to offer a strong counter balance. This is one of the key elements of the compunetics concept.

The third aspect in the definition of compunetics is the ethical implications of ICT. E-learning, as well as patient networks can be important tools in tackling the problems of health inequality. "[E]ffectively addressing inequalities will require innovative collaborative approaches that address patient factors, provider factors, healthcare system factors and relevant environmental factors. While the magnitude of quality and inequality problems combined with the relative failure of past efforts to improve these inequalities represent daunting challenges, recent and impending advances in information technology and compunetics offer significant opportunities for improvement the provision of high quality medical care and the reduction in inequalities. If governments and healthcare systems are to reap the maximum potential the field of compunetics has to offer, more work will need to be done in several key areas." [47]

Illiteracy is an important aspect of the health inequality. "Language barriers and illiteracy have been identified as common obstacles to ICT access. The convergence of voice, video and images, and the increasing variety of languages available on the Internet means that the importance of this obstacle may be diminishing. However, text-based rather than voice protocols still remain the most widely-used Internet applications, so basic literacy is still considered an important determinant of access." [20] Part of this can be corrected due to the recent technological developments which enable sites like YouTube. Here you can provide people with information by image and speech, not requiring trained reading abilities. An example is the collection of small EHR information clips put on YouTube by Dr. Hannan Amir. [48] Another example are the patient information videos produced by Nobel Films in The Netherlands. [49]

Especially in health and care illiteracy is a serious problem, influencing aspects like dosing levels of prescribed medications; immunization requirements and schedules; disease symptoms or warning signs; treatment or therapy instructions. [50]

"[H]ealthcare organizations can take a number of steps to enhance patients' understanding of health information. These steps include replacing complicated medical words with plain language and writing information at an appropriate reading level. In addition, more and more organizations are turning toward resources that support visual learning, including diagrams, illustrations, videos, and animations that deliver important information in formats most patients can comprehend." [51]

One of the first and essential steps in the development and acceptance of patient e-learning in health has been the development of information on prescription as introduced by Healthwise. [52] In a recent white paper Don Kemper pointed out the "three rules for a consumer-based health care transformation": the rules of

- self-care – help people do as much for themselves as they can;
- guidelines – help people ask for the care they need. Give them tools to understand the evidence-based guidelines;

- veto – help people say "no" to care they don't need. Give them a sense of their autonomy. [53]

As stated before, finding the correct information is a problem on the internet. "While we are beginning to expect that the information we need will be instantly available, we want individual specific information to only be available to those that have a right to see that data." [54] Information on prescription is part of the solution. We should be looking at developing ways to use the data in the EHR to function as the basis for a personalized search engine.

Prescribed information can and should be extended by visual tools. "Eventually, as patients begin to have online access to their electronic health records, the doctor could even "prescribe" visual health information for the patient to review, which would be waiting when the patient logged on. This would not only provide a documented record that information was recommended to the patient, but would also capture data regarding which information was actually viewed by the patient." [51]

"People with low health literacy will have difficulty learning information from many written patient education materials because these tend to require higher reading proficiency than many patients possess. They may have difficulty reading medical forms and medication labels, and difficulty with taking their medications correctly. Although health literacy can affect all social classes, it more commonly affects elderly, low income, and minority patients. Low literate patients with chronic physical and mental diseases have been found to be less likely to improve their health." [55] Unfortunately almost all research done into the use of pictograms in patient information has been in relation to medication information. A good example of a more general site working with pictograms, although still in its construction stage, is Foldercare. [56]

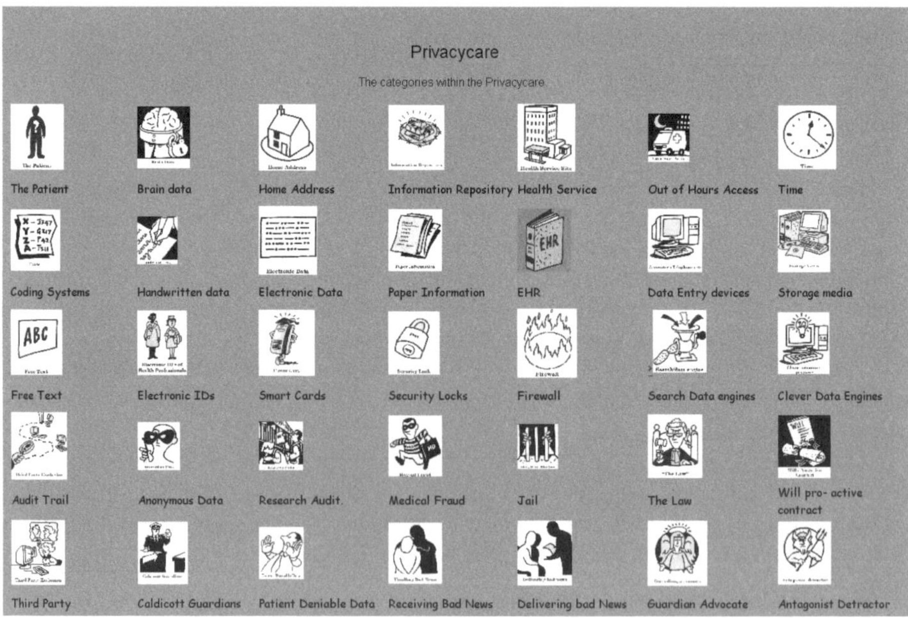

Figure 1. Page from Foldercare website.

Another step should be the standardization of terminology. "Language is not used uniformly in medicine. Clinicians often use different phrases to mean the same thing or the same phrase to mean different things. Standardisation, using a concept-based clinical terminology, largely resolves this situation by creating a common platform for practitioners to deliver enhanced patient care while allowing a basis for comparison and communication. Relevant clinical information concerning a citizen will need to be consolidated from many different clinicians and from different care settings to ensure that the citizen's care is coordinated and continuous. The variety and diversity of health information technology currently employed within and across care settings presents an added problem which is overcome by using a standardized clinical terminology to enable system interoperability, i.e. the ability for unambiguous data to be exchanged between systems, regardless of the technology used. Without such standardisation, specially built interfaces and other workarounds become necessary, creating the potential for errors, costly additional administration and compromising the care of citizens." [57] With a global terminology standard it will be much easier to implement the use of plain, national, languages for the benefit of the individual.

Health inequalities are especially obvious in the fields of urban and rural health. In these areas compunetics, both medical and care and behavioural, should and could play an important role.

Conclusion

Through compunetics, the gathering of knowledge, information and (social) data will be the basis to making health and care delivery more efficient for the professionals, to help build new infrastructures, even to confront the consequences of a disaster, be it man made or natural. It will also help patients to make better informed decisions. Knowledge centres can function as information containers providing better overview of and access to knowledge, causing a positive economic benefit, and bringing awareness about the necessary changes in infrastructure and education. Organizations like ICMCC can build the bridge between patients and professionals by creating these knowledge centres and stimulate the use of compunetics.

References

Last access to all internet links on April 10, 2007

[1] Bos L. et al. (eds.), *Medical and Care Compunetics 1*, IOS Press, 2004.
[2] Chaussalet T., Bos L., ICMCC special issue, *International Journal of Medical Informatics*, 75, 2006.
[3] *Building Knowledge societies*, Item 8.1 of the provisional agenda, UNESCO 164th Executive Board Meeting, 2002.
[4] Laxminarayan S., Foreword, in: Clinical Knowledge Management, Opportunities and challenges, R. Bali, 2005.
[5] Krane D., Number of "Cyberchondriacs" – U.S. Adults Who Go Online for Health Information – Increases to Estimated 117 Million. *Harris Interactive, HealthCare News*, 2005, Vol. Issue 8, http://www.harrisinteractive.com/news/newsletters/healthnews/HI_HealthCareNews2005Vol5_Iss08.pdf
[6] *9th "Health on the Net Survey of Health and Medical Internet Use"* – http://www.hon.ch/Survey/Survey2005/res.html.
[7] Ferguson T., From patients to end users, *BMJ* 2002; 324: 555–556, http://bmj.bmjjournals.com/cgi/content/full/324/7337/555.

[8] Peterson G., Aslani P., Williams K.A., How do Consumers Search for and Appraise Information on Medicines on the Internet? A Qualitative Study Using Focus Groups, *J. Med. Internet. Res.* 2003; 5(4):e33, http://www.jmir.org/2003/4/e33/.

[9] Mayer M.A., Karkaletsis V., Stamatakis K., Leis A., Villarroel D., Thomeczek C., Labsky M., López-Ostenero F., Honkela, T., MedIEQ – Qualisty Labelling of Medical Content Using Multilingual Information Extraction, in: *Medical and Care Compunetics 3*, L. Bos et al. (eds.), 2006, pp. 183–190.

[10] Health on the Net Foundation, http://www.hon.ch/.

[11] QMIC, http://www.qmic.nl/qmic/home.do.

[12] Purcell G.P., Wilson P., Delamoth T., The quality of health information on the internet, *BMJ* 2002; 324:557–558, http://bmj.bmjjournals.com/cgi/content/full/324/7337/557.

[13] Dwivedi, A.N., Bali, R.K. Naguib R.N.G., Building New Healthcare Management Paradigms: A Case for Healthcare Knowledge Management, in: *Healthcare Knowledge Management*, Bali et al. (eds.), 2007; pp. 3–10.

[14] Abidi S.S.R., Healthcare Knowledge Sharing: Purpose, Practices, and Prospects, in: *Healthcare Knowledge Management*, Bali et al. (eds.), 2007; pp. 67–86.

[15] Davenport T.H. and. Prusak L., *Working Knowledge: How Organizations Manage What They Know.* Harvard Business School Press, Boston, MA, 1998.

[16] Fennerssy G., Burstein, F., Role of Information professionals as Intermediaries for Knowledge Management in Evidence-Based Healthcare, *Healthcare Knowledge Management*, Bali et al. (eds.), 2007; pp. 28–40.

[17] Popovich M.L. and Watkins T., Applied Medical & Care Computnetics to Public Health Disease Surveillance and Management: Leveraging External Data Sources – A Key to Public Health Preparedness, in: *Medical and Care Compunetics 3*, L. Bos et al. (Eds.), 2006 pp. 151–161.

[18] Kun L., The Use of Technology to Transform the Home into a Safe-Haven, in: L. Bos et al., Medical and Care Compunetics 4, 2007.

[19] http://recordaccess.icmcc.org.

[20] Dzenowagis, J., Connecting for Health – Global Vision, Local Insight, *Report for the World Summit on the Information Society,* WHO 2005, http://www.who.int/kms/resources/WSISReport_Connecting_for_Health.pdf.

[21] Ferguson, T., Medical Knowledge as a Social Process: An Interview with John Lester, The Ferguson Report, Number 9, September 2002, http://www.fergusonreport.com/articles/fr00902.htm.

[22] Ferguson T., Can Useful and Reliable Online Health Resources be Produced by 'Medically Unqualified' Persons?, The Ferguson Report, Number 5, July 1999, http://www.fergusonreport.com/articles/fr079902.htm.

[23] www.askdrwiki.com.

[24] Lester J., Prady S., Finegan Y., Hoch D., How Online Patient Networks Can Enhance Quality and Reduce Errors, *Patient Safety & Quality Healthcare*, 2004, http://www.psqh.com/octdec04/lesterfineganhoch.html.

[25] Ferguson, T., e-Patients as Medical Researchers, The Ferguson Report, Number 9, September 2002, http://www.fergusonreport.com/articles/fr00903.htm.

[26] http://www.ianproject.org/.

[27] See: http://www.propractica.com/definitions.htm.

[28] For an overview of the discussion see the EHR definitions page of the ICMCC RA portal http://recordaccess.icmcc.org.

[29] Fischer B., Fitton R., Poirier, C., Stables D., Patient Record Access – The Time Has Come, in: *Medical and Care Compunetics 3*, L. Bos et al. (eds.), 2006, pp. 162–167.

[30] Hannan A., Webber F., Towards a Partnership of Trust, in: *Medical and care Compunetics 4*, L. Bos et al. (eds.), 2007.

[31] Ferguson T., Online patient-helpers and physicians working together: a new partnership for high quality health care, *BMJ* 2000; 321:1129–1132, http://www.bmj.com/cgi/content/full/321/7269/1129.

[32] Shabtai I., Leshno M., Blondheim O., Kornbluth J., The Value of Information for Decision-Making in the Healthcare Environment, in *Medical and Care Compunetics*, L. Bos et al. (eds.), 2007.

[33] Norgall T., Blobel B., Pharow P., Personal Health – the Future Care Paradigm, in: *Medical and Care Compunetics 3*, L. Bos et al. (eds.), 2006, pp. 299–306.

[34] Lee C.K., Foo S., Narratives in Healtcare, in: *Healthcare Knowledge Management*, Bali et al. (eds.), 2007; pp 130–141.

[35] Ferreira A., Correia A., Silva A., Corte A., Pinto A., Saavedra A., Pereira A.L., Pereira A.F., Cruz-Correia R., Antunes L.F., Why facilitate patient access to medical records, in: *Medical and Care Compunetics 4*, L. Bos et al. (eds.), 2007.

[36] Popovich M.L., Daub E.M., White Paper: *Concept for an Integrated Bio-Intelligence Network by 2010*, Scientific Technologies Corporation, 2002.

[37] Data from half a million patients to aid research, *E-Health Insider*, March 29, 2007, http://www.e-health-insider.com/news/item.cfm?ID=2578.

[38] Western Governor's Report, WGA, 1999, http://www.westgov.org/wga/publicat/newsltr/7-99web.htm.

[39] Snyderman R., Yoediono Z., Prospective care: a personalized, preventative approach to medicine, in: *Pharmacogenomics* 2006, 7(1), 509, http://faculty.fuqua.duke.edu/~mluce/hlthmgmt491/Snyderman%20Yoediono%20Pharmacogenomics%202006%20Jan.pdf.

[40] Bassinder J., Bali R.K., Naguib R., Knowledge Management and Electronic Care Records: incorporating social, legal and ethical issues, in: *Medical and Care Compunetics 3*, L. Bos et al. (eds.), 2006, pp. 221–227.

[41] Liebowitz J., The Hidden Power of Social Networks and Knowledge Sharing in Healthcare, in: *Healthcare Knowledge Management*, Bali et al. (eds.), 2007; pp. 104–111.

[42] Joachims T., Granka L., Pan B., Hembrooke H., Gay, G., Accurately Interpreting Clickthrough Data as Implicit Feedback, *SIGIR'05*, August 15–19, 2005, http://www.cs.cornell.edu/People/tj/publications/joachims_etal_05a.pdf.

[43] Office of the National Coordinator for Health Information Technology (ONC), *Goals of Strategic Framework*, United States Department of Health & Human Services, http://www.hhs.gov/healthit/goals.html.

[44] Allwes D., Popovich, M.L., Empowering Patients and Researchers through a Common Health Information Registry: A Case Example of Adrenocortical Carcinoma Patients and Researchers, in: *Medical & Care Compunetics 4*, L. Bos et al. (eds.), 2007.

[45] http://avicenna.unesco.org/.

[46] Kay P., *Online Training and e-Learning*, March 8, 2007, http://www.ukbusinesstraining.co.uk/articles/online_training.php.

[47] Gibbons M.C., Health Inequalities and Emerging Themes in Compunetics, in: *Medical and Care Compunetics 3*, L. Bos et al. (eds.), IOSPress, 2006, pp. 62–69.

[48] http://www.youtube.com/watch?v=LW4OcgVyB4w.

[49] http://www.depatientmaghetzeggen.nl/dp_main.html (site in Dutch).

[50] Taleff A.E., Sehgal V., Cook-Palmer A., Tackling Health Literacy, *Patient Safety & Quality Healthcare*, 2006, http://www.psqh.com/julaug06/tackling.html.

[51] Nienkamp M., Visual Learning Tools Overcome Health Illiteracy, *Patient Safety & Quality Healthcare*, 2006, http://www.psqh.com/julaug06/visual.html.

[52] Kemper D., Mettler M., *Information Therapy*, Healthwise, 2002.

[53] Kemper D., The Healthwise® Ix® Solution, 2007, http://www.healthwise.org/f_white_papers.aspx.

[54] Maloney D.L., *Card Technology in Healthcare*, CardTech/SecurTech 2001, http://www1.va.gov/card/docs/CardCT2001c_DM.doc.

[55] Hill L.H., and Roslan M.M., Using Visual Concept Mapping to Communicate Medication Inofrmation to Chronic Disease Patients with Low Health Literacy, in: *Concept Maps: Theory, Methodology, Technology*, Proc. of the First Int. Conference on Concept Mapping, A.J. Cañas, J.D. Novak, F.M. González (Eds.), Pamplona, Spain 2004, http://cmc.ihmc.us/papers/cmc2004-077.pdf.

[56] www.foldercare.co.uk.

[57] Donnelly K., SNOMED-CT: *The Advanced Terminology and Coding System for eHealth*, in: Medical and Care Compunetics 3, L. Bos et al. (eds.), 2006, pp. 279–290.

Medical and Care Compunetics 4
L. Bos and B. Blobel (Eds.)
IOS Press, 2007

The Use of Technology to Transform the Home into a Safe-Haven

Luis Kun[1]
Senior Research Professor of Homeland Security at the IRM College of the National Defense University; Fort McNair, Washington DC, 20319 – email: l.kun@ieee.org

Abstract. On June 14, 2006 three reports were published by the Institute of Medicine (IOM) in regards to "THE FUTURE OF EMERGENCY CARE IN THE UNITED STATES HEALTH SYSTEM". The three combined reports: Hospital-Based Emergency Care at the Breaking Point, Emergency Medical Services at the Crossroads and Emergency Care for Children Growing Pains, are a clear reflection of the state we currently face, even without a major disaster. Some key findings drawn from all three reports showed that the emergency care system is ill-prepared to handle a major one. For example, many of the 41 million citizens who do not have medical insurance end up using the Emergency Departments (ED) as their source of "regular" care and many of these EDs are at or over capacity, there is little surge capacity for a major event, whether it takes the form of a natural disaster, disease outbreak, or terrorist attack. If we had during the major disaster event, a "contagion" element, i.e. pandemic flu, then the problem would be even more complicated, since the "regular" hospital patient population would need to be isolated from these patients. If we add to this equation the length of time involved in the "current" process of vaccine creation and production (i.e. the volume of vaccines that would be required to be provided to the citizens of the world), the scenario does not look to promising. A new model is needed then to address these requirements. In the developed world we have a number of devices (e.g., radio, TV, Computers, telephones, mobile devices, etc.) and infrastructure (e.g., cable, wireless networks, etc.) that are already supplying the homes and the individuals with a large number of independent applications and different types of information. These stovepipes or independently developed family that include: tele-banking, Telehealth, tele-education, e-commerce, entertainment on demand, etc. when "connected" as an integrated set, may provide an ideal environment, where families may stay at home for a long period of time (quarantine) and would have all the mechanisms in place for getting food and water from supermarkets, drugs from the pharmacy, the children would be able to go to school from home (in turn their school grounds may become temporary hospitals), adults could telecommute to work and minor conditions could be consulted and treated through these systems (with the help of a Telehealth platform that would include electronic health records), etc.

1. Introduction and Discussion

Multiple "Pandemic-Flu" strategy-related documents have been produced at different levels and by different stakeholders in the last couple of years. The Department of Health and Human Services (DHHS)(0), the World Health Organization (0), the White House / Homeland Security Council (0, 0) and other Federal Departments (0, 0). Many

---

[1] Disclaimer: The views expressed in this paper are those of the author and do not reflect the official policy or position of the National Defense University, the Department of Defense, or the U.S. Government.

private as well as public businesses have realized the importance of having a Continuity of Operations Plan and have embarked on that task (0). Last year the IOM published a study on June 14, 2006 in regards to "The Future of Emergency Care in the United States Health System" (0). With the purpose of creating a vision for the future of emergency care, the committee published a series of three reports that looked at hospital-based emergency and trauma care, at pre-hospital emergency medical services (EMS), and at the special challenge of providing emergency care for children. The outcome were three volumes of the report entitled:

1. Hospital-Based Emergency Care: At the Breaking Point,
2. Emergency Medical Services At the Crossroads and
3. Emergency Care for Children: Growing Pains.

The principal topics addressed included: Overcrowding, Fragmentation and lack of coordination between: health care, public health and public safety; Shortage of specialists; Lack of Disaster Preparedness and the Shortcomings in Pediatric Emergency Care.

Some of the key findings drawn from all three reports could be summarized in a sentence: "The emergency care system is ill-prepared to handle a major disaster". Many EDs and trauma centers are overcrowded, and with many EDs at or over capacity, there is little surge capacity for a major event, whether it takes the form of a natural disaster, disease outbreak, or terrorist attack. There are in addition a large number of issues that are related to the problem but they will not be addressed here. For example:

4. EMS received only 4 percent of Department of Homeland Security first responder funding in 2002 and 2003;
5. Emergency Medical Technicians in non-fire based services have received an average of less than one hour of training in disaster response;
6. Both hospital and EMS personnel lack personal protective equipment needed to effectively respond to chemical, biological, or nuclear threats.

Overcrowding. (Drawn from *Hospital-Based Emergency Care: At the Breaking Point*) Critical specialists are often unavailable to provide emergency and trauma care. Three quarters of hospitals report difficulty finding specialists to take emergency and trauma calls. Key specialties are in short supply. On-call specialists often treat emergency patients without compensation due to high levels of uninsurance. These specialists also face higher medical liability exposure than those who do not provide on-call coverage. Demand for emergency care has been growing fast emergency department (ED) visits grew by 26 percent between 1993 and 2003, but over the same period, the number of EDs declined by 425, and the number of hospital beds declined by 198,000. ED crowding is a hospital-wide problem—patients back up in the ED because they can not get admitted to inpatient beds. As a result, patients are often "boarded"—held in the ED until an inpatient bed becomes available—for 48 hours or more. Also, ambulances are frequently diverted from overcrowded EDs to other hospitals that may be farther away and may not have the optimal services. In 2003, ambulances were diverted 501,000 times—an average of once every minute.

EMS and EDs are not well equipped to handle pediatric care. (Drawn from *Emergency Care for Children: Growing Pains.)* Most children receive emergency care in general (not children's) hospitals, which are less likely to have pediatric expertise, equipment, and policies in place for the care of children. Although children make up 27 percent of all ED visits, only 6 percent of EDs in the U.S. have all of the necessary supplies for pediatric emergencies. Many drugs and medical devices have not been adequately tested on, or dosed properly for, children. While children have increased vulnerability to disasters—for example, children have less fluid reserve, which leads to rapid dehydration—disaster planning has largely overlooked their needs.

Emergency care is highly fragmented. (Drawn from *Emergency Medical Services At the Crossroads*) Cities and regions are often served by multiple 9-1-1 call centers. Emergency Medical Services (EMS) agencies do not effectively coordinate EMS services with EDs and trauma centers. As a result, the regional flow of patients is poorly managed, leaving some EDs empty and others overcrowded. EMS does not communicate effectively with public safety agencies and public health departments— they often operate on different radio frequencies and lack common procedures for emergencies. There are no nationwide standards for the training and certification of EMS personnel. Federal responsibility for oversight of the emergency and trauma care system is scattered across multiple agencies

If in addition to all these issues we reflect that in a "normal / average" year 36.000 Americans die from the "regular" flu and over 200.000 end up hospitalized. That there are less than 6000 hospitals in the US and less than a thousand of them have more than 1000 beds. That despite of a pandemic occurring, people will not stop having other health related illnesses and performed procedures (i.e., heart attacks / open heart surgery or angioplasty, colonoscopy / polyp removal, pacemaker implants, dialysis, etc.) and or accidents that will require hospitalization (i.e., broken hips / hip replacement. knee surgery, etc.). We can safely assume as a result of these reports, that the current EMS / ED environment today in the US can not handle a major disaster. An alternative solution needs to be sought.

From the perspective of the Computer based Patient Record (CPR) and the transformation of paper to electronic health records (EHR) and its advantages a lot has been written and debated for at least the past twenty years. It has been my personal experience that in the case of the US population (compared to the rest of the world) this society is much more "transient" or mobile. As people move seeking better job-opportunities, the associated consequence is that the individuals will be seeking care in the new locations which generates having scattered medical records. Not having the complete picture is a problem that not only can generate "medical errors", but does not allow those caring for the individual to have the information needed to do to risk assessment / management, prevention, and disease management. In the future as we evolve our system more into the phase of prevention, the "total picture" will be even more critical since genetic information could be associated with environmental data for example (i.e. quality of air, water, etc.)

In "Redefining Health Care," Michael Porter, (0), states: "Today, medical records are scattered. There are separate records at individual physician offices and at various treatment facilities. Specialists usually send summaries to the patient's primary care provider or family physician, not the full record of their care. Records are not kept in a form that is easy to integrate. Current proposals for records management aim to facilitate requests for records, when needed, from the various providers (the so-called pointer system). However, this approach is cumbersome, technologically questionable, and inherently costly. Patients need to have ownership of their own medical records. They need a secure, complete personal medical record that is all in one trusted place (though there is no need for everyone's records to be in the same place)."

Dr. Yasnoff made a presentation entitled: "A Feasible Path to Sustainable Community Health Information Infrastructure", in which he developed the concept of a "Health Record Bank" (0). This concept is one that synergizes well with the concepts presented in this paper. While a patient is at home and he may be visited (via a Telehealth infrastructure) the information could be "accessed from the bank" and after the encounter is completed, the new information could be incorporated into that record and "deposited in the bank" again.

During a special briefing in the US Senate (March 21, 2007) Dr. McDonald (0) President of Global Health Initiatives Inc and the coordinator of the National Disaster Risk Communication Initiative (NDRCI) spoke of a rapidly growing National Testbeds for Community Preparedness and Resilience. Some of the key focus areas include: Anticipatory Science Base - Prospective Best Practices; Situational Awareness - Common Operating Picture; Strategic Action in Mission Critical Gaps and Intelligent Social Networks - Smart Swarms. His group works at the Community level and can generate online multi-user environment for exercises and games (e.g. National Capital Region Pan-Flu Exercise). Their communities are Global, and promote Real-time data and transparent disease surveillance to address the needs of vulnerable communities. Some mission critical gaps for Pandemic Preparedness & Response include: environmental scan, Disaster Knowledge Management System, Community Resilience Networks, multi-level triage systems, risk communication repository, social distance management, models of psychosocial dimensions, social network models, Standard Pandemic Flu Plans, training modules for responders, Pandefender game to educate the public, exercises of pandemic flu preparedness, improving preparedness, providing situational awareness, engaging intelligent social networks and contributing to a breakthrough in public health and community resilience.

In the past few years, human societies have been confronted with challenges that have created demands for significantly enhancing communications for disaster preparedness and response. The threat of mounting natural disasters, terrorist attacks, and global change combined with massive growth in communication capabilities are fundamentally altering human potential and in so doing rapidly transforming functional life capacity and cultures. One of the requirements then is for the individual family in having a constant "virtual connection" with their "community" to generate an informational awareness.

Computing and high speed communications are not only enabling governmental and secular institutions around the world at an unprecedented rate; the combination of these two synergistic technologies is even transforming the way we think of humanity and human potential. They are unveiling deep structure in the behavioral and social sciences that may forever alter the way we look at our selves and interact with others. These new technologies and methodologies are fundamentally changing the way we are approaching the prevention and management of large-scale social crisis. The DKMS Resilience Network is architected to do both with great efficiency. It is designed to significantly reduce the cost of enabling rapid and broad development of H5N1 preparedness and business continuity through viral-like spread of memetic messages, algorithms, principles, protocols, and interoperable systems. Once enabled for H5N1, the Disaster Knowledge Management System Resilience Network is architected to be able to be rapidly repurposed as an all hazards knowledge management infrastructure of great flexibility and broad utility at a fraction of the cost of any other methodology.

Focusing on the mitigation to a pandemic requires certain understanding of the process. For example the fact that it occurs in a series of 2 or 3 waves requires a very different response and protection that if it happened just once. At the citizen level (as well as at the business level) as the outbreak spreads from a locality, to a region, to a national and later to an international dimension, new failures of the supply/demand chain will occur. The specific mutation of the HN51 virus that will create a pandemic, can not be predicted therefore the vaccine that will be needed to mitigate or prevent it can not be predicted either. On the other hand the current process of vaccine production is inadequate and can not be relied upon for such an event. The need to shorten the current 6.5 to 8 month cycle required to produce a vaccine (by using eggs) needs to be replaced by a new methodology and will not be discussed here. The mass production of the found vaccine, and its distribution will not be discussed either.

Many steps can be taken by authorities to strengthen collaborative preparedness activities which could include simulations and decision modeling exercises among local, national, and international partners and particularly including the interdependent parties. These could include for example exercises where local, state, federal authorities would be working a simulation with the pharmaceutical companies (suppliers) and the (agencies) distributors of the vaccines. These exercises could also help improve governmental ability to provide timely, clear and effective information, while improving the education of first-responders. While others, e.g. Department of Homeland Security (DHS), Department of Defense (DOD), Department of Education (DE), etc,, may look on ways to increase the surge capacity in healthcare services. Imagine schools' gymnasiums becoming temporary hospitals with "isolation" beds provided by DOD. Schools should probably be closed since children become the source of infection to the rest of the family members, however the children could continue to go to school via distance learning (DL). People can be encouraged of maintaining basic supplies at home but sooner or later they will ran out, therefore the need is to have the ability to get food and water through sound communications. Adults should have the ability to telecommute / "work from home", thus avoiding contact with infected people or spreading themselves the disease if they are already sick. Meanwhile the question should be raised in terms of what can or should we do at the personal level through our homes and its current infrastructure. While schools and business explore the possibility of "distance learning" and "working-from-home" for some schools / businesses respectively thus, reducing the potential for infection and spread.

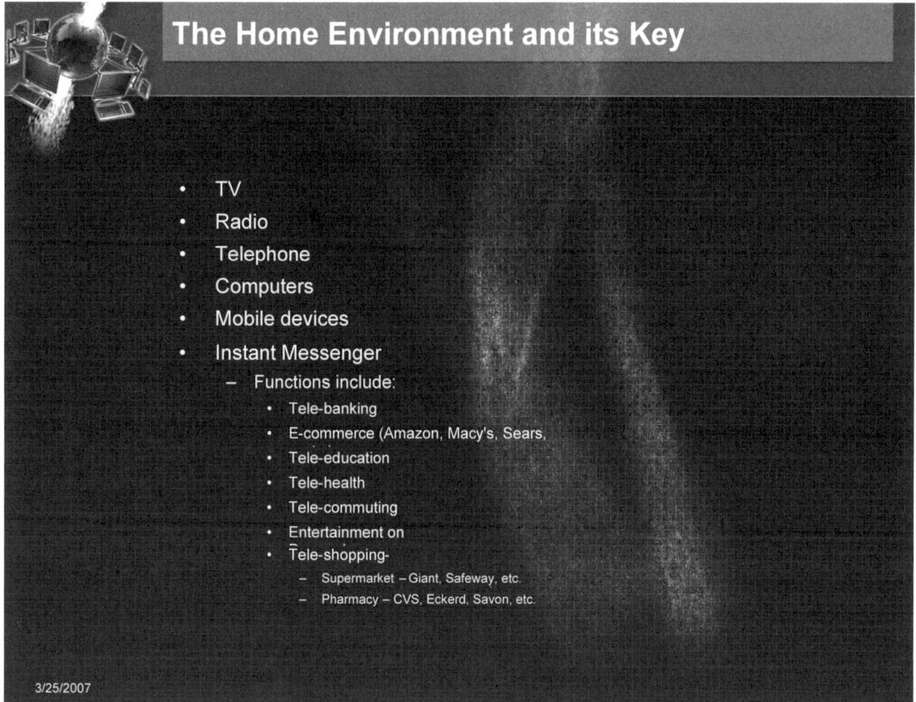

Figure 1. A list of technologies and or applications that are available in the home environment.

Discussion

In figure 1 the home environment and its key IT assets are shown. The reader can see a list of devices and technologies available to the homes of the developed nations and of those that have the resources to buy them, anywhere else. There is also a list of functions that are available through the use of this environment. Some technologies such as television are owned by 98% of the general public. This fact makes this device a preferable "route" to reach millions of people. Imagine for example if just by adding a wireless keyboard a some small circuit people would be able to convert the TV into a "bidirectional" device, where information could be both sent and received by the user.

From a functionality perspective if we think about Telehealth services, figure 2 shows a few environments depicted by circles, which enable a number of situations that may not be currently addressed. For example beyond the regular maintenance or consultations with a health care provider there maybe requests for medications refills in which case the physicians office may contact electronically the patient's pharmacy system. In other cases the patient may initiate this process and at the same time could make requests of food and water to the family's supermarket of choice also electronically. In case of an emergency, i.e. pandemic flu, there may be some additional services that can be provided to the family including special directions / permission for accessing a special unit that may provide a respirator or any other special need outside the home.

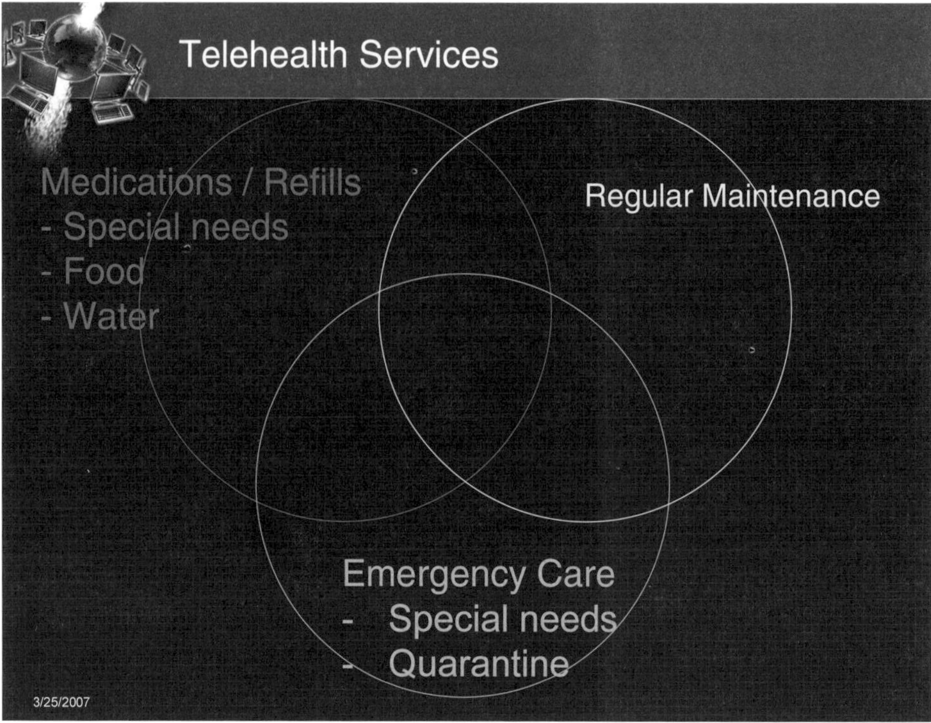

Figure 2. Telehealth Services could include: Regular maintenance, Medication Refills, Consultations, and Emergency Care related special needs.

As the family members have telehealth encounters with their respective health providers (from home), it is crucial to update the patients' records, so that others including the patient are aware in the future of all the actions taken. Yasnoff's model of a Health Record Bank is shown in figure 3 and it is a concept that fits very well with these scenarios. All these transactions between patient and providers not only are recorded and "deposited" in the Bank, but assure the continuity that is required for a lifetime longitudinal record. Figure 4 shows the many different transactions that occur from the home and where this "Health Record Bank "fits" within the vision.

The final piece of this model is the connection between that individual / family with the rest of his/her community which is shown both in figure 4 and in more detail in figure 5. The Community Health and Emergency Management System provides through the Disaster Knowledge Management System (DKMS) a Resilience Network a wealth of authoritative and reliable information for all those involved. It becomes part of the de-facto infrastructure that can help the communities involved and its citizens better define assets, liabilities, capabilities and requirements.

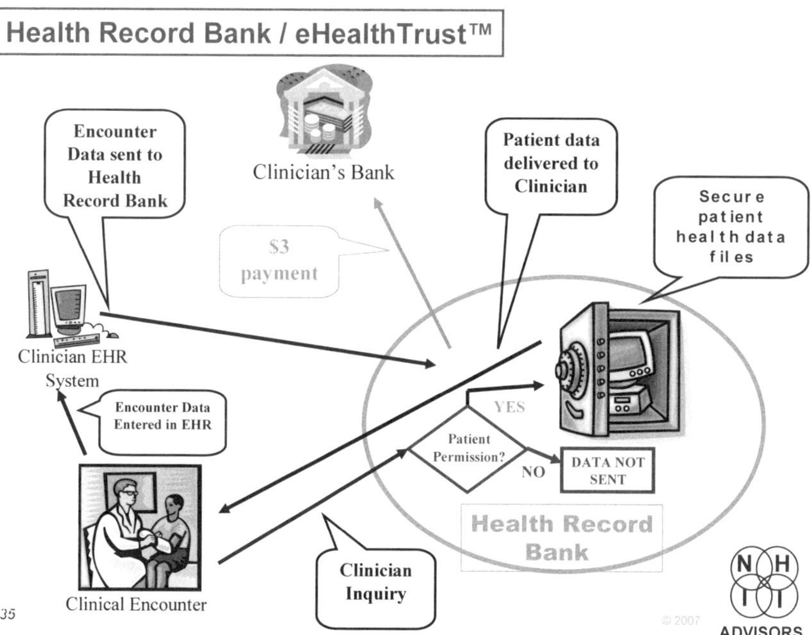

Figure 3. Health-related encounters and transactions between patient, health care provider and the Health Record Bank. Source NHII Advisors. Used with permission of the author.

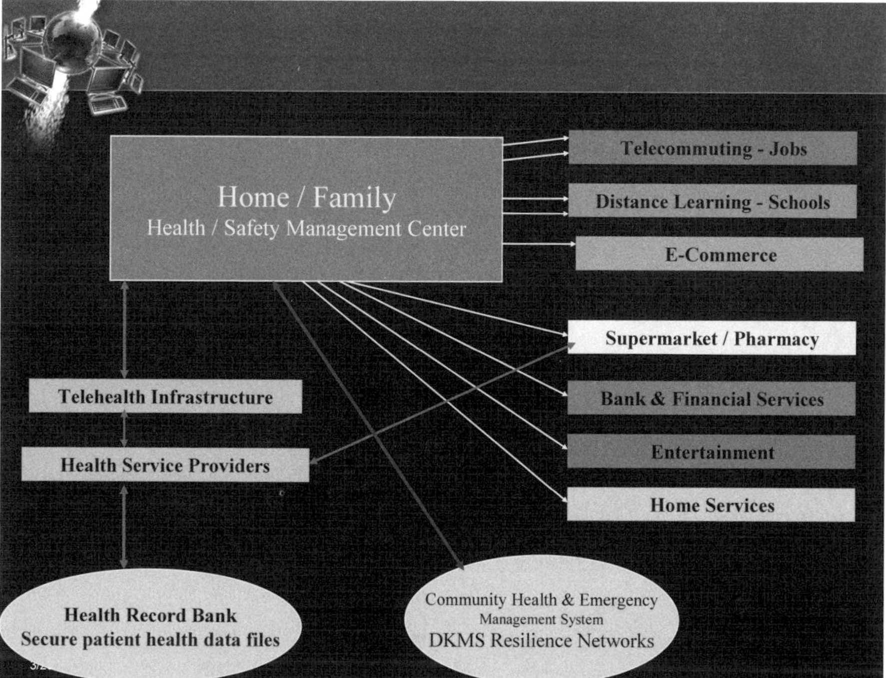

Figure 4. Many of the services that can be provided to the home environment will require the ability to save all the home-health related activity into the "Health Record Bank"

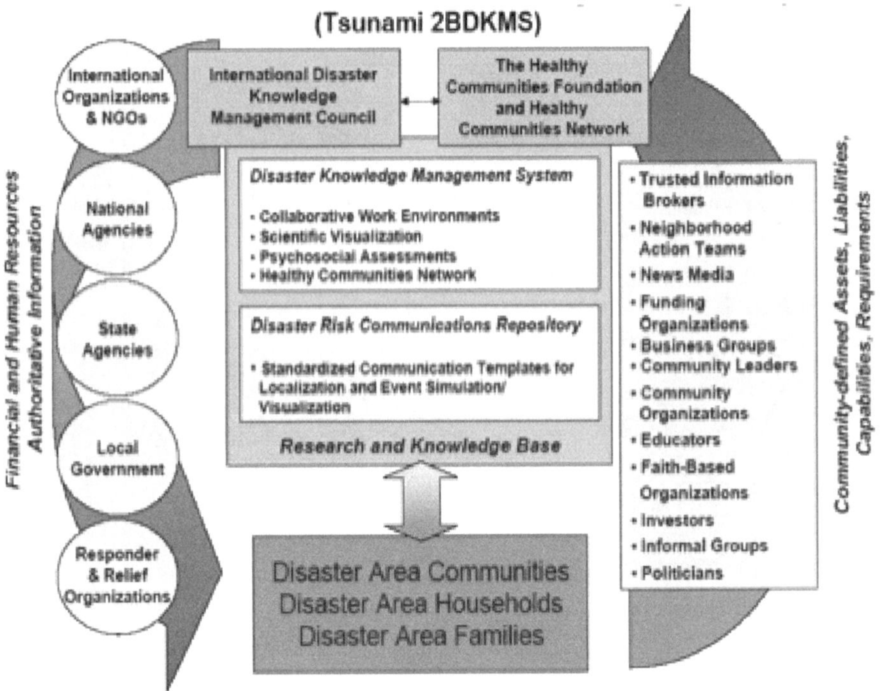

Figure 5. Disaster Knowledge Management System (DKMS) Resilience Network. With permission from Global Health Initiatives, Inc.

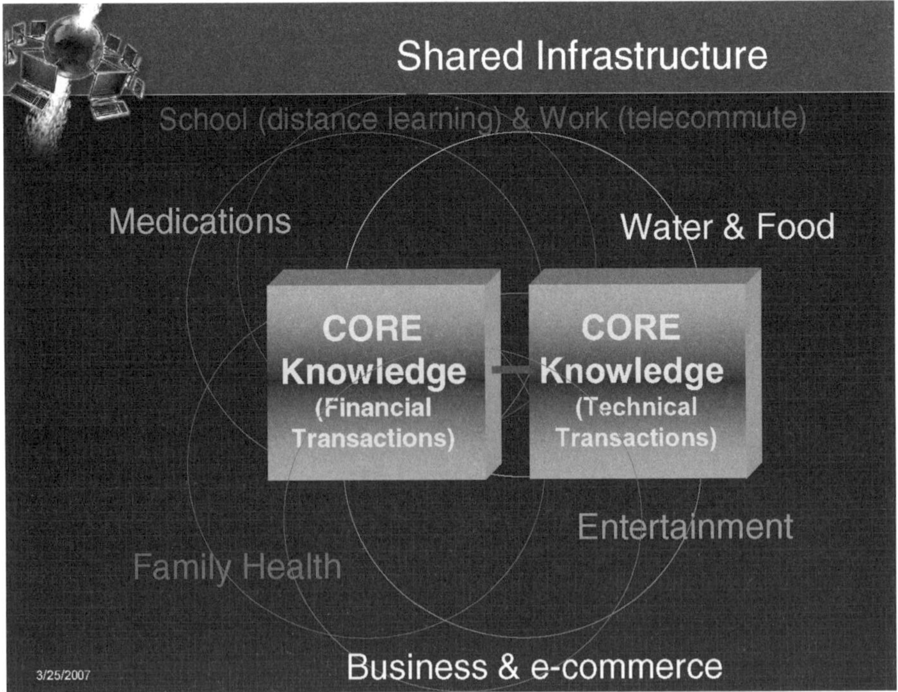

Figure 6. Shared "home-infrastructure" to multiple and distinct applications that share certain common "financial" and "technical" transaction-elements.

Critical infrastructure protection (CIP) activities are intended to enhance the cyber and physical security of both the public and private infrastructures that are essential to national security, national economic security, and national public health and safety. The Cybersecurity aspects of Public Health and the Health Care sector for example are very critical to this home-shared- application-infrastructure. There are a number of "core knowledge" functions that are critical from both a financial and a technical transaction (see figure 6) perspective that need to be present and that require careful consideration.

REFERENCES

[1] HHS Pandemic Influenza Plan, US Department of Health and Human Services, November 2005.
[2] WHO global influenza preparedness plan 2005.
[3] National Strategy for Pandemic Influenza, Homeland Security Council, White House, November 2005.
[4] National Strategy for Pandemic Influenza, Implementation Plan, Homeland Security Council, White House, May 2006.
[5] Pandemic Planning Report, US Department of Agriculture, June 2006.
[6] Human Capital Planning for Pandemic Influenza, Information for Departments and Agencies, U.S. Office of Personnel Management, July 2006.
[7] PREPARING FOR A PANDEMIC INFLUENZA - A PRIMER FOR GOVERNORS AND SENIOR STATE OFFICIALS, National Governors Association (NGA) November 2006.
[8] Fiberlink - Communications White Paper: "PLANNING FOR A PANDEMIC: TURNING OFFICE WORKERS INTO MOBILE WORKERS FOR BUSINESS CONTINUITY", February 2007.
[9] IOM's COMMITTEE ON THE FECUSHS: "THE FUTURE OF EMERGENCY CARE IN THE UNITED STATES HEALTH SYSTEM", June 14, 2006.
[10] Porter, Michael: "Redefining Health Care: Creating Value-Based Competition on Results,"; page 272, Harvard Business School Press Book, May 26, 2006.
[11] Yasnoff, William: "A Feasible Path to Sustainable Community Health Information Infrastructure", Presentation to the IEEE-USA Medical Technology Policy Committee, January 19, 2007, Washington DC.
[12] McDonald, Michael, briefing of the Capitol Hill "Steering Committee on Telehealth and Healthcare Informatics" focused on HIT and Natural Disasters. Wednesday, March 21st, 2007: HIT for Disasters and Avian Flu. Russell Senate Office Building. Washington DC.
[13] Kun- Critical Infrastructure for Emergency and Disaster Management: *"The Home Environment"*, IEEE-SSIT - ISTAS'06, New York, June ,9th, 2006.
[14] Hammond, Ed: The Mechanics of Information Exchange and Interoperability. http://www.tkgnet.net/conference/summer2005/presentations/Ed_Hammond.pdf
[15] "Interoperability for the National Health Information Network" (NHIN)- IEEE-USA Medical Technology Policy Committee – Interoperability White Paper – November 2005 http://www.ieeeusa.org/volunteers/committees/mtpc/documents/InteroperabilityLetter.doc
[16] Telemedicine and Homecare for the Elderly with Chronic Diseases Legislation HR1101 – March 97 – Balanced Act of 1997 – Diabetes.
[17] Shea, S. et al.: A Randomized Trial Comparing Telemedicine Case Management with Usual Care in Older, Ethnically Diverse, Medically Underserved Patients with Diabetes Mellitus" JAMIA; 13:40-51, 2006. http://www.j-amia.org/cgi/content/abstract/13/1/40
[18] Cafazzo, Joseph: "The Telemanagement of Diabetes Through the Use of Bluetooth-Enabled Mobile Phones." University Health Network, 2006 http://www.atmeda.org/Forum2006/JCafazzo_Presentation_ DiabetesTelemanagement.pdf

EHR and Record Access

Medical and Care Compunetics 4
L. Bos and B. Blobel (Eds.)
IOS Press, 2007

Advantage Technology, Equitable Usage of Available Resources and Infrastructure and Effective Practice Management – Key to Quality Healthcare Delivery in India

*H.R.SINGH and V.R.SINGH**
Biomedical Measurements and Standards Group
National Physical Laboratory New Delhi110012, India
**Fellow IEEE and Distinguished Professor-AICTE, NPL, India*
*(*also corresponding author)*
hrst_52@rediffmail.com & vrsingh@yahoo.com

Abstract: The impact of technological advancement and the widespread availability of resources and their utilization, to meet the health care requirements of the community, an important fundamental need of the human being. After food and shelter is discussed. Some of the most sought criteria relating to the technology selection and the practice management are devised and proposed for their implementation to achieve quality health, particularly in the rural areas. An insight into the government policies, programs and as a result, the impact on the ultimate goal of achieving the desired health care, mainly during the last two decades is covered here. A model of health care for remote areas is proposed here to assist in the improvement of the conditions of better health care and better quality of life of the human being.

Keywords: Health care, bio-medical developments, practice management, biotelemetry.

1. Introduction

Human civilization has always been greatly affected or rather each evolution made in human society has been inseparably related to the new developments in science and technology [1]. There have been a significant technological advancement and tremendous growth of application oriented products and infrastructure in the field of telecommunication, medical biotechnology and information science. These developments are likely to play a significant role to meet the growing demand of facilities and services in healthcare sector especially in rural areas. India being the highly populated country with geographically dispersed population comprising with high percentage of children, women and aged population, needs quality based and cost effective means of healthcare programs on a much larger scale, employing the technological outbreak and resource utilization judiciously. The estimated population projections as per age group are depicted [2] in Table 1. The figures in the graph show that there is going to be quite a substantial growth in the total population during the next two decades. However, during the same period a marginal decline in the population of the people of age group varying between 0-15 years is noticed. The population of the people between age group 15-64 years and above is steadily growing and contributing to the overall population growth.

Table 1: Population Projections (in millions)

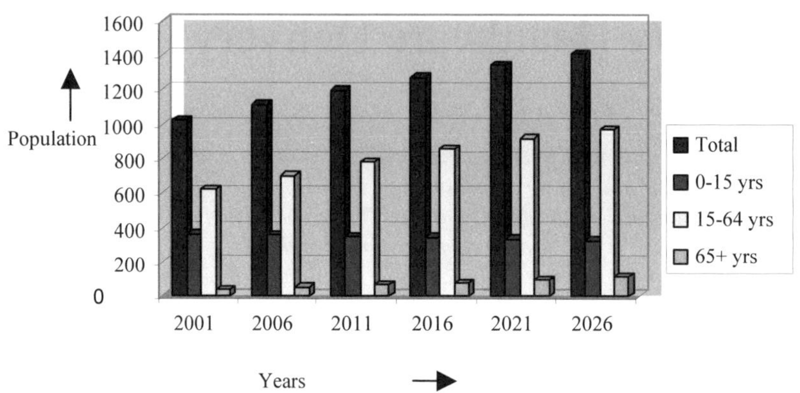

In view of the alarming population explosion expected in next two decades, Government of India, to augment health services in rural areas of the country, has conceptualized a National Rural Health Mission [2] and initiated a number of healthcare schemes by proposing a huge expenditure in health sector from existing 0.9 percent to 2-3 percent of GDP. The last two decades, as a result of this, have witnessed remarkable improvements [2] in all the important health indicators as shown in Table 2.

Table 2: Selected Health Indicators					
(Person years)					
S No	**Parameters**	**1951**	**1981**	**1991**	**Current level**
1.	Crude Birth Rate (per 1000 Population)	40.8	33.9	29.5	25.0 (2002)
2.	Crude Death Rate (per 1000 Population)	25.1	12.5	9.8	8.1 (2002)
3.	Total Fertility Rate (TFR) (per woman)	6.0	4.5	3.6	3.1 (2001)
4.	Maternal Mortality Rate (MMR) (per 100,000 live births	NA	NA	437 (1992-93)	407 (1998) 301 (2005-2006)
5.	Infant Mortality Rate (IMR) (per 1000 live births)	146 (1951-61)	110	80 58(2006)	63 (2002)

6.	Child (0-4 years) Mortality Rate, per 1000 children	57.3 (1972)	41.2	26.5	19.3 (2001)
7.	Couple Protection Rate (percent)	10.4 (1971)	22.8	44.1	48.2(1998-99) NFHS
8.	Life Expectancy at Birth Male	37.2	54.1	59.7 (1991-95)	63.9 (2001-06)
	Female	36.2	54.7	60.9	66.9 (2001-06)

*NFHS: National Family Health survey

The availability of need based technology at the doorstep and most importantly the culture conducive to its use for better and affordable health services, makes this program more widespread and people oriented. New developments in instrumentation, measuring instruments, biotelemetry and diagnostic tools, both hardware and web based make it suitable for patient monitoring, tele-consulting and even converting hospitals into a complete telematic process. The system provides linkages to the patients, practitioners, specialists and peripheral health service providers connecting each other by information exchanges sharing assistance and even cross fertilization of ideas employing bio-telemetry [3]. The advent of personnel computers and its growing usage, internet and web-based provisions [4], link established using phone lines, DSL, Cable, ISDN and satellite technology are some of the few support provisions that arc essentially required for remote connectivity, care delivery and for service providers education. Having a broad network of internet options, the financial and organizational aspects of technology adoption, implementation, maintenance and their sustainability for rural healthcare are becoming more easily manageable.

Information communication technology [5] (ICT) and evolution of telemedicine services [6] for deploying in far reaching areas, uneven terrain and the places and masses, which have been totally inaccessible so far, are playing significant role in creation of employment opportunities, improving social aspect of education and delivery of better healthcare. Health as defined by ICMR (Indian Council of Medical Research) in Indian context is primarily a social science with technology as a support, not in reverse [7]. Apart from these high technological development to be used as a supportive tool to spread the healthcare network on wider scale, equally important is to promote highly affordable, effective and trusted, the use and practice of our old traditional alternative approaches [7] of Ayurveda, Homeopathy and Unani medicine in parallel. Keeping the modality of aspect in view, the following considerations need to be addressed in technology choice, their adoption and implementation strategy

- Creating a vision and planning for highly suitable, need based, result oriented scheme for Health Information Technology [8].
- Right choice of technology for defined task keeping in view the – aspects of its long term sustainability.
- Its cost effectiveness and managing the funds for investments, revenue enhancements and productivity gains.
- Building partners to share the responsibilities for effective implementations and smooth running.

2. Technologies and Resources and their Equitable Usage

Although the information and communication technology [5] has been undoubtedly the most accepted and highly trusted technology, but the role of several other support services and technologies like emergent of internet, personnel computers, web cameras, imaging and scanning etc. is also not ruled out in providing and improving quality of care delivery in far remote areas. Bio-nanotechnology, development of new biomedical sensors [9] and materials have its own role to play in developing smart card for holding enormous amount of data information in as minimum as possible space. The new development in electro-medical instrumentation, devices for data analyses and processing, substantial growth of imaging and scanning equipments have made it possible to display, process and detect the audio-video clippings of certain kind of diseases. For tumors in kidney, lever and other cardio-vascular problems, it is now possible to see it in real time with more clarity and better diagnosis and detection level, the root cause of the problems. Technology developments in digital stethoscope, X-rays, high resolution cameras, ultrasound ECG cameras, data compression techniques, high resolution scanners and data scrambling [10] devices ensure the confidentiality and data security of the network. High speed data transmission through telemetry not only help interconnecting several hospitals with each other for better interaction among the specialists, service providers and patients, but also helps in the diagnosis in pediatric cardiology and in radiology by transmitting digital medical images. Specialists can view in real time and conduct a diagnostic examination at the bed side itself in a distant place. Image transmission [10] is done by capturing ultrasound images electronically with higher resolution and transfers them over computer networks for doctor's review and recommendations.

Technology, as already said exists for developing patient information smart cards with built in microchips containing identification information, vaccination and medical history including that is inherited. The use of such card will obtain the immediate attention of the paramedical staff equipped with all emergency care including immediate access to medical alert patient data base on arriving at the hospital during emergency. However, security and confidentiality of information marked on smart card and their unauthorized use are still a major concern. Data compression algorithms [11] to reduce redundancy in stored or communicated data is required for image transmission with better quality and occupying lesser storage space. The data compression technique may help greatly in reducing size of the data to be transmitted on the network through radio telemetry for applications in remote areas. The zoom effect for highlighting a portion of interest of the image to emphasize the desired location for better understanding and easy detection of the default makes it further attractive to be used as biomedical tool in delivering the desired health care. Encryption algorithms [10] ensure the security of data in special cases if required and system can encrypt interchanged data using Blowfish Cipher Algorithm [10], [12]. The communication between the telemedicine and the base unit is always made through the ID number using the encrypted messages and other relevant details of the patient are never mentioned.

Keeping in view the limitations and disadvantages of earth based technology particularly related to care delivery system deeper into highly uneven and hilly terrain, satellite technology [13],[14] could serve as an alternative in terms of cost and with much larger coverage effectively, safely and in near real time. Multi channel bio-telemetry, development of high data density acoustics, bio-technology and ground breaking development in internet facility, wireless technology and mobiles are few more advantages that add to its already existed multifold advantages for better healthcare to the distant community. Plans and strategies to introduce the concept of health robot [15] to conquer the tyranny of distance by activating the device through voice commands for desired operations is another added advantage in the technology up-gradation. Advanced computational intelligence and development of DNA based computers allow faster and accurate diagnosis of special kind of viruses. Today the technology exists for remote fetal monitoring allowing obstetricians to use their Personal Digital Assistant (PDA's) to remotely access fetal heart tracing, maternal contraction pattern and other critical real time data, transmitted directly from hospital's labor and delivery unit.

The role of voice activated devices [15] have also been undoubtedly great in activating devices according to voice commands as per requirements and need of doctors/specialists by sitting at a distant place far from place of operation. It is now possible to deliver healthcare services with high degree of reliability and safety in health hazardous and infected areas or in a situation where providing health services normally are difficult and risky by employing biotelemetry for transmission of speech signals. The use of Independent Component Analysis [16] (ICA) based algorithms, to remove the noise and other artifacts from the contaminated ECG signals, before it is transmitted over the network to distant places for the convenience of the specialists to have a quick look and suggest remedial measures have now become a practice. In order to make best use of the expertise, experiences and huge infrastructures available with the national laboratories and other R&D institutions maintaining national standards of vital parameters related to biomedical instrumentations, it is proposed to transmit these signals to the hospitals, specialists and service providers in rural areas to calibrate their instruments before they are actually put to use. Video conferencing [17] a two way interactive communication between the patients, specialists and any other associated with the program could be another major application of biotelemetry for establishing a live demonstration of the activities going on in real time at both the end. This will provide to the patient, a level of satisfaction and confidence having talked to the specialist live, about their problems and to the specialist, a better means of understanding and detecting correctly about the disease and prescription.

3. Practice Management in Health Services

Healthcare to any group, community or any country has always been a priority and the funds, program implementation and management are also largely a responsibility of Govt of India, unlike many other countries have to follow slightly a different approach to promote and spread the fruits of technological revolutions in rural healthcare, keeping in view its vast boundaries, different weather conditions, in-equality/disparity in socio-economic conditions and scattered population. Although there has been a substantial growth of investments by private participation [18] in terms of quality and volume of healthcare services, but they are mostly affluent centered, and the urban poor and people belonging to remote locations are still struggling hard to get their dues as far as their healthcare needs are concerned. Some of the issues that need to be emphasized for achieving targeted results timely and effectively by putting best management skills, professional involvement and proper investments are as follows.

- Development of health information exchanges [19] connecting three or more with each other and equipped with all modern gadgets and infrastructures. The attachment of reference laboratories, imaging centers, pharmacies and other healthcare providers and traders to these exchanges will produce better results.

- Provision of high speed internet link, providing the experts and specialists performing micro-surgery operations and telecasting it in real time to a place far from the activity centre.
- Creation of home monitoring provisions in homes. Establishing tale-health kiosks in service centers, churches, schools and community centers, malls and other places of public gathering to help creating new innovative program to improve healthcare and create awareness in the community to be more careful and vigil towards their healthcare needs.
- Emphasis on community based health scheme, planning and organizing support for development of healthcare delivery system to meet current and future needs of the people. Generate healthcare program and regulate health plans supplemental nutrition program for women, infants and children (WIC). Publishing multidisciplinary medical bulletins, with information on medical topics concerning healthcare initiatives.
- Disease management of chronic illness such as diabetics, chronic disease etc.
- Establishment of web based information system at state, district and block level with fast connectivity to collect, evaluate, monitor and exchange data on demand.
- Prepare action plan to aid and advise state and district program manager in all matters of information management and build an information culture.
- Ensuring downward information flow for management decision.
- Use innovations to enhance the reach of healthcare.
- Slot for technology update for introducing new developments in the existing program towards quality improvements.
- Medical record digitization and creation of data bank of the facts and information related to a particular disease for quick reference in emergency situations by the doctor and specialists.
- Creation of a board of specialists, doctors, service providers and participation from govt. sector for periodic monitoring, evaluation and suggesting unbiased opinion for quality improvement.
- Design and device of innovative program, activities and ideas to make people feel connected with technology.
- Data access security restricted to doctors, specialists and patient by introducing computer generated identification number code.
- Promotion of practice productivity and development of disease based software program to help maintain a disease data bank of clinical information.
- Mobilize healthcare professionals with the new development in technology or provision for technology up-gradation as and when takes place.
- Executing plans for sharing of existing resources, infrastructure, expertise, knowledge base and experiences of the institutes, hospitals, specialists or anyone associated with healthcare program. Laboratory, clinic, service providers, doctors, specialists, patients, insurance companies, clinical information store and any other should be technologically linked with each other.
- Diseases based specialists and hospitals should be properly tagged and interconnected through e-clinic with the online appointment of specialists.

- Interactive – Remote Patient Care
- Promoting special schemes for old age people, children, women, handicapped and most under privileged persons for their healthcare needs on priority basis.
- Community involvement, community participation self reliance and self determination are other vital parameters for such program to get through.
- Dedicated network back up power circuits with advanced fire fighting capabilities.

4. Government Policies, Programs and Participation by Private Sector – Facts and Figures

The setting up of National Rural Health Mission (NRHM) [2] to cover up the whole country with special focus on eighteen states having week socio-demographic indicators or primary health infrastructures would prove to be a milestone in quality healthcare delivery, it is presumed. The primary responsibilities of the mission would be to raise the public expenditures, increase investment in the control of communicable diseases, ensure healthcare for the poor through health insurance schemes, improving availability of life saving drugs and other healthcare measures at reasonable cost. After independence, another major step towards self reliance in science, agriculture, health sector and education has been the introduction of the concept of five year growth plan to handle each sector independently with the targeted money assigned to reform the particular sector. To health sector, the Govt. of India projected a number of hospitals and dispensaries in rural areas for dealing independently with health related needs [20-21] as shown in Table 3.

Table 3: Progress in establishing healthcare centers in Indian rural areas (1951-2006)				
		1950-1951	1991-1992	2005-2006
1.	No. of Medical Colleges	30	146	242
2.	No. of Dental Colleges			
	BDS	4	57	205
	MDS	+	23	67
3.	No. of Colleges of ISM &H	1.4.1999	1.4.2003	1.4.2005
	Ayurvedic	167	209	219
	Unani	37	36	37
	Siddha	2	6	6
	Homoeopathy	116	180	178
		1952	1982	2005
4.	No. of Hospitals (as on 1st January)	2694	6804	7008
5.	No. of Beds (all types) (as on 1st January)	117178	569495	469672

6.	Beds per lakh population	32	83	89
		1967	1991	2004
7.	No. of Sub-Centers	17521	130984	142655
8.	No. of Primary Health Centers	4793	20139	23109
9.	No. of Community Health Centers	-	2070	3222
		1951	1991	2005
10.	No. of Allopathic Doctors Registered with Medical Council of India (As on 31st December)	618	3936	7675
11.	No. of Doctors per lakh Population	17 (in 1951)	47 (in 1991)	70 (in 2004)
12.	No. of Dentist Registered with Dental Council of India (As on 31st December)	3290	10751	55344
		1951	1991	2004
13.	No. of Dentist per million Population	9	13	45
		1951	1991	2004 (As on 31.3.2004)
14.	No. of Registered General Nursing Midwife with Nursing Council of India (As on 31st December)	16550	340208	865135
		1950-51	1990-1991	2004-05
15.	Gross National Product (Rest. In Cr.)			
	At current prices	255	5365	23241
	At 1993-94 prices	3687	7321	12416
		1951-56 (1st Plan)	1997-2002 (IX Plan)	2002-2007 (X Plan)
17.	Plan Outlay (Rest. In Cr.)			
	Total	65.3	35204.95	58920.3
	Health	65.2	19818.40	31020.3
	Family Welfare	0.1	15120.20	27125.0
	ISM&H	-	266.35	775.0
			1985-1986	1989-1990
18.	Per Capita Expenditure on Health & Family Welfare & Water Supply & Sanitation (Rest.)		55.06	83.03

However, the progress of these schemes was greatly affected either by the non-availability of the qualified staff or by those, who are not willing to serve in rural areas due to various personal reasons. This short fall of doctors and other paramedical staff during the plan (1995 – 2000) is shown [21] in Table 4.

Table 4 : Healthcare during the Tenth Plan (1995-2000): health manpower in primary healthcare centers					
Staff Position	Required Clinicians	Sanctioned Clinicians	In-Place Clinicians (serving)	Gap, required & in-place	Gap, sanctioned & in-place
Doctors in PHC	25663	29702	22506	3157	7196
Specialists in CHC	22348	6579	3741	18607	2838
Nursing Staff in SC	134108	87504	73327	60781	14177
Lab. Technicians in PHC	27936	15865	12709	15227	3156
Specialists in PPC	3100	--	--	--	--

CHC: Community healthcare; PHC: Primary healthcare; PPC: Private and public centers; SC: Secondary care

Govt. of India is likely to introduce a novel initiative for the first time ever to routinely screen the school children for various health complications that leads to more serious diseases later on. Starting from January 2007, a pilot project at national level, regional cells in six states and six regional resource centers to control, monitor and collecting information on actual burden of the dieses like cardio-vascular and diabetics has been proposed with an investment of Rest. 1680 core [22]. The scheme would focus mainly on risk factor prevention and detection, management of emergencies due to Cads, training and orientation of healthcare providers at all levels, standardization of treatment guidelines, promotion of healthy living and eating habits [21].

The Govt. has also taken up the reproduction and child health program for achieving population stabilization by introducing several family planning measures especially in high fertility states. An ambitious plan to control the healthcare activities at district level by highly trained personnel such as IIM graduate supported by a chartered accountant (CA) is also underway. However, the implementation of various population control measures, have not been up-to the level of desired satisfaction and require a lot more to be done to match this demand. To fill the gap, govt. has initiated a number of measures to attract the involvement of private institutions in healthcare by encouraging them to invest in this much needed social welfare program. As a result, the past two decades have seen a large number of entrepreneurs from the medical fraternity setting up a chain of world class medical institutions, diagnostic centers and healthcare outlets to deliver quality services in rural areas by tapping the use of vast technological developments and resources in healthcare sector. The All India Institute of Medical Sciences, The Apollo Group, The Forties Hospitals, The Escorts Hospitals, The MS Swami Nathan Foundation and recently introduced The Bill Gates Foundation including several others smaller partners are doing significant work in this area by establishing more comprehensive service facilities across the country. To further strengthen this sector as a major source of revenue earner, govt. is also keeping its eye open to enter in international market by encouraging medical tourism for foreign visitors especially in rural areas. The Apollo group, the Max Healthcare, another leading healthcare agency, Lockhart and the Escort etc as a part of their growth strategy [18] are eyeing markets in several parts of the world through tie- ups with insurance providers to cover-up the interests of the foreigners coming to India. Govt. has also started programs with several smaller healthcare providers to promote medical tourism in India on a very large scale which according to a study conducted by Confederation of Indian Industry [18] shows a potential market of US$ 2 billion by 2012. The study also shows that the total healthcare market could rise from US$22.2 billion currently to US$ 50 billion by 2012, considering India the biggest Medicare hub in the region. For accreditation of hospitals and healthcare service providers, the govt. has set up the National Accreditation Board and Healthcare Providers (NABH) [18].

5. Bottlenecks achieving desired healthcare mark

Financial implications have always been a great hindrance in execution of any community based program. Unfortunately, the participation of private sector in healthcare delivery in urban and remote areas has been very poor in the beginning and govt. has to bear this huge investment alone to meet the healthcare demand of the community. Apart from the govt. efforts, the socio-economic conditions, the education, social and cultural background, their reluctance to adopt family planning measures and lack of other welfare education have been other great problems to get them the full advantage of healthcare program in rural areas. Shortage of trained professionals as already indicated above, specialists and volunteers can also be termed another major concern. There are certain untapped places in far remote areas, where govt. has made substantial investment on health schemes and provided proper health care facilities, but few doctors are not willing to accept the assignment in these rural hospitals. These problems may probably be overcome by providing basic amenities required for doctors and their families other than the healthcare facilities for community. It should also be a mandatory condition for each major hospital to adopt hundred villages around it and provide healthcare needs to them in rural areas. A tenure internship program in community healthcare practices for each medical graduate must be exercised before they pass out their degrees. Abuse of alcohol and use of smokeless tobacco, apart from their poor social and economic background, have been a major hurdle in solving of their healthcare problems. Accelerated urbanization, increase in number of vehicles and inadequate and highly deplorable conditions of roads and highways is the main cause of alarming increase in the rate of accidental injuries in India. High mortality rate amongst those with multi-system injuries are due to lack of pre hospital care and inadequate critical care. It is estimated that mortality in serious injuries is six times worse in India compared to any developed country. Inadequate number of ambulances and ambulance personals with certified formal training and dismal conditions of trauma management, particularly in rural areas are other considerations that need to be properly addressed. Do we need a rural health cadre [23] for further improving the delivery in India, is still a topic of intense debate.

Besides above, there are several other factors that require due attention before the start of healthcare program, these includes arrangement of providing drinking water on community basis, easy access to food retailers for fresh fruits and vegetables to avoid water borne and diet linked diseases. Tuberculosis, respiratory infections, asthma and certain other kind of infections arising out of poor quality of housing, seasonal and part time work such as in agriculture and various cottage industries are other associated concerns to be looked into, apart from other work related stress and risk in rural areas.

6. Conclusion

An overview of technologies available, the selection of appropriate technology to meet the growing need of better healthcare delivery in rural areas, its implementation and effective management to provide affordable and need based services to the community have been given. The advantages of having such a vast network of technology of telemetry for interlinking patients and rural medical health providers with the doctors, specialists and professional service providers in urban areas or in a hospital are widely discussed. Various options including new developments in imaging, scanning, zooming affect to highlight the required portion of the image, bandwidth compression for reducing the burden of high storage area with same quality of image capturing and data encryption for network security are specially highlighted in the discussion. Several issues and bottleneck parameters that raise hindrances to effectively dealing with the situation in providing better health services in rural areas have been pin pointed for further improvement. The importance of private participation in rural healthcare mission have its own role to play and is discussed with reference to their much better conditions in terms of infrastructure and economic conditions with solid back up of highly qualified and experienced doctors and specialists. The medical tourism and its potential in terms of revenue earnings boot the healthcare industry, making it as the largest service sector in the economy. It is concluded, that the technology and the optimal use of facilities and resources with effective practice management and strong willpower to do good for the rural and deprived peoples are essential tools to serve the people for their healthcare needs.

7. Acknowledgements

The authors are grateful to the Director, National Physical Laboratory, New Delhi, India for the support in the present work.

8. References

[1]. "Popularizing Scientific Knowledge, Promoting Social Development: http://english.people.com.cn

[2]. Government of India, Population and RCH: overview http://www.indianngos.com/issue/population/overview.htm

[3]. J. Hanley, "Uses of telemetry in healthcare," Biotelemetry 1990; 15:196 - 198.

[4]. A.E. Cragsman, C.R. Doran, and S.C. Simmons, "Internet & world-Wide-Web Technologies for Medical date Management and Remote Access to clinical Expertise," Aviate. Space Environ. Med. 70(2):185-190, 1999.

[5]. Fran Torso and Jane Metzger, "Rural Healthcare Delivery: Connecting Communities through Technologies" A Report   Available:chcf.org/documents/hospitals/RuralHealthCareDelivery.pdf

[6]. M. Moore, "The Evolution of Telemedicine," Future Generation Computer System. 15(2): 245-254, 1999.

[7]. Nosier H. Anita, "Alternative Approaches to Delivery of Medical Technology for   Rural Health" Current Science, vol.87, no.7, Oct. 2004.

[8].   N.H.Lovell and B.G. Celler, "Information Technology in Primary Healthcare" Int. J. Med. Inform., 55(1):9-22, 1999.

[9].   "Biomedical Sensors & telemetry for Remote Monitoring of Patients," May8, 2001. http://www.nttc.edu/telemed/bmfact.html

[10]. E. Kyriacou, S.Pavlopoulos, "Multipurpose Healthcare Telemedicine System with Mobile Communication Support Link," Biomedical Engineering on Line 2003, 2:7 http://www.biomedical-engineering-online.com/content/2/1/7

[11]. K.Sayood, "Introduction to Data compression," Morgan Kaufmann Publishers, Inc. 1996, 27 - 54

[12]. B. Schneier, "Applied Cryptography" John Wiley & sons 1996,336 - 339

[13]. J. Chouinard, "Satellite Contributions to Telemedicine," Canadian CME   Experiences .Can. Med.Assoc.J.128:850-855, 1983.

[14]. H. Murakami, K. Shimizu, "Telemedicine Using Mobile Satellite Communication,"   IEEE Trans. Biomed. Eng. 41(5):488-497, 1994.

[15]. H.R. Singh, A.M Ansari and S.S. Agrawal, "Design and Development of Voice/Tele-operated Intelligent Mobile   Robot," Proceedings of IEEE Tencon-97 International Conference on Speech and Image Processing, Vol.1 pp 177-180, Dec.97.

[16]. Gracee Agrawal, Manju Singh, V.R Singh and H.R Singh, "Applications of Independent Component Analysis for removing Artifacts and noise from Biomedical Signals using Mat lab," Proceedings AdMet-06, New Delhi India.

[17]. P.W. Callas, M.A. Ricci, and M.P. Caputo, "Improve Rural provider Access to Continuing Medical Education through Interactive Video-conferencing", Telemedicine J. e-Health 6(4):393-399, 2000.

[18]. IBEF, Healthcare Sector http://www.ibef.org/industry/healthcare.aspx

[19]. N.A. Brown, "The Telemedicine Information Exchange-An Online Resource," Compute Bio. Med. 28(5):509-518, 1998.

[20]. "Ministry of Health," Govt. of India, DGHS   http://www.moh.nic.in

[21]. K. Singh, "Biotelemetry: Could Technological Developments Assist Healthcare in Rural India," The International Electronic journal of Rural and Remote Health Research, Education, Practice and policy, ISSN 1445-6054

[22]. "School Kids to be Tested for Heart Disease, diabetes," The Times of India, Publications, page14, December 13, 2006.

[23]. "Do We Need a Rural Health Cadre," The Times of India, page18, Sunday, December 24, 2006.

Medical and Care Compunetics 4
L. Bos and B. Blobel (Eds.)
IOS Press, 2007

Primary healthcare information system – development and deployment issues

Ranko STEVANOVIC[a], Vinko KOJUNDZIC[b], Galibedin GALIJASEVIC[c]
[a] *Croatian National Institute of Public Health, Croatia*
[b] *Maticnjak Ltd, Croatia*
[c] *ABA informatika Ltd, Croatia*

Abstract. Croatian national primary healthcare ICT Implementation strategy is determined by Croatian national health strategy and plan, Croatian ICT development strategy for 21st century, and requirements specifications for the heath information system. National primary healthcare ICT implementation strategy components are accented: purpose of the ICT implementation strategy, information principles, need and ICT enablement in domains of patients, healthcare professionals, policy-makers and managers and public. Based on the determinants, three organizational levels have been established – government, ministerial and project levels. General architecture of Croatian primary healthcare information system and its implementation as well as national ICT environmental accelerations for national primary healthcare ICT environmental accelerators for health ICT implementations are presented.

Keywords. health ICT implementation strategy, healthcare functional requirements, healthcare standards, electronic health record, integrated healthcare, agent based software technology, healthcare computer, communication network, healthcare implementation.

Introduction

Conceptual design of national healthcare information system has been based on international documents:

- eEurope Action Plans: 2000, 2002, 2005;
- EU eHealth Strategy;
- The eEurope Smart Card (eESC) initiative;
- Selected National eHealth Strategies (GB, USA).

1. Project organization and management

1.1. Preparatory stage of the project, process of procurement and in the PHIS[1] pilot

Government level: Government Steering Committee for Internet Infrastructure Development – responsible for strategic ICT policy and infrastructure decision making;

---

[1] PHIS = Primary Healthcare Information System

Health Information System Expert Group – Advisory group of experts in the fields of medicine and health as well as ICT.

Ministerial Level: Advisory teams to Minister of health (representatives from Hospitals, Institute for public health, Institute for health insurance, Faculty of Medicine, Chambers of Health). Regulatory bodies for public procurement for the health ICT projects.

Pilot project Levels: Primary healthcare team and selected implementation team representatives in Pilot project.

1.2. The implementation stage of the project Primary health information system

Ministerial Level: During the implementation stage of the project there are two bodies: Supervisory board and Project Management Unit. Supervisory board has a task of business sponsorship of the project and supervising completion of project milestones. It is consisted of highest officials from Ministry of Health and Social Welfare, Croatian Institute for Health Insurance, Central State Administrative Office for e-Croatia and high level representative from suppliers of the PHIS. Project Management Unit (PMU)[2] has a task of operational management of PHIS implementation. Its head is assistant minister and members are representatives on the operational level from Ministry, Croatian Institute for Health Insurance, Croatian National Institute for Public Health and suppliers. PMU and its members are free to use outside experts opinions.

2. The Requirements and Functional Specifications

2.1. National Requirements

The strategic national requirement for the NHIS is to enable necessary data for preparing reform of health system.

The strategic information system requirements are:

- to ensure patients can be confident that professionals in the national health system caring for them have reliable and rapid access, 24 hours a day, to the relevant personal, medical and health information necessary to support their care;
- to eliminate unnecessary travel and delay for patients by providing remote on-line access to services, specialists and care, wherever practicable;
- to provide access for patients to accredited, independent, multimedia background information and advice about their condition and to provide every health care professional with on-line access to the latest local guidance and national evidence on treatment, and the information they need to evaluate the effectiveness of their work and to support their professional development;
- to ensure the availability of accurate information for managers and planners to support local Health Improvement Programs and the National Framework for Assessing Performance;

---

[2] PMU = Project Management Unit

- to provide fast, convenient access for the public to accredited multimedia advice on lifestyle and health, and information to support public involvement in, and understanding of, local and national health service policy development.

The specific targets are:
- reaching agreement with the professions on the security of electronic systems and networks carrying patient-identifiable clinical information;
- developing and implementing a first generation of person-based Electronic Health Records, providing the basis of lifelong core clinical information with electronic transfer of patient records between GPs;
- implementing comprehensive integrated clinical systems to support the joint needs of GPs and the extended primary care team, either in GP practices or in wider consortia (eg, Primary Care Groups);
- connecting all GP practices to NHS Virtual Private Network (NHS VPN);
- providing 24 hour emergency care access to relevant information from patient records;
- using NHS VPN for appointment booking, referrals, discharge information, radiology and laboratory requests and results in all parts of the country;
- the development and implementation of a clear policy on standards in areas such as information management, data structures and contents, and telecommunication, with the backing and participation of all key stakeholders;
- community prescribing with electronic links to GPs and the Prescription Pricing Authority;
- routinely considering telemedicine and telecare options in all Health Improvement Programs;
- offering NHS Direct services to the whole population establishing local Health Informatics Services and producing rational local implementation strategies;
- completing essential national infrastructure projects including the networking infrastructure, national applications etc.;
- opening a National Electronic Library for Health with accredited clinical reference material on NHS VPN accessible by all authorized NHS organizations;
- planning and delivering education and training in informatics for clinicians and managers.

2.2. International Requirements

Functional and technological regional and international interoperability of National Health Systems, focused to meet EU eHealth goals in order to serve any requirement for primary healthcare of non-resident during his/her stay in Croatia.

2.3. Functional Specifications

PHIS is logically divided into two parts: Central Information System to which all GP practices are connected and Client Information Systems at GPs.

2.3.1. Primary Healthcare Information System - High Level Functional Specifications – Central Information System

The Central Information System contains:

- ***Primary healthcare information system management****:* health insurance management, patient management, electronic health documentation management, extended communications management, health information system reporting management;
- ***Clinical Information System Management:*** service management, data access and protection management, clinical documentation management, health related registers management (state, local), HL/7 communication system, clinical data management, "virtual" electronic health and electronic medical record management;
- ***Administrative and business support****:* Global registration management, health insurance database management, personal ID-management, national MKB-10 classification system, drug, pills, orthopaedic supplement list management, list of services and procedures;
- ***Privacy and security management****:* Smart card technology driven privacy and security for patients and healthcare professionals, PKI infrastructure, role based data access control;
- ***Technical and technological integration with the:*** Hospital information systems and information systems of Croatian National Institute of Public Health, Croatian Institute for Health Insurance and Ministry of Health and Social Welfare;

2.3.2. Primary Healthcare Information System - High Level Functional Specifications – Client Information System.

The Client Information System contains:

- ***Health Professional****:* Role based Health Profession Identification, Authentication and administration services, Patient care service workflow, Diagnostics, Referrals, Prescriptions, Medical Services, patient health and medical document generation, Encounter Management, Laboratory services, Calendar and administrative Management, Comprehensive Reporting System;
- ***Health and Medical Supporting services****:* Health documentation management, Clinical documentation management, Decease Related Drugs Recommendations, Drug Retrieval;
- ***Patient oriented services****:* Encounter registration and waiting room management, Patient identification, Authentication and administration services, Patient related medical documentation (laboratory, images, other), task list, procedures and memos;
- ***Patient Management:*** General Demographic Patient Data, Health insurance related data, Patient Health Data (Anamnesis, Risk factors, Allergies, Medical treatments, Health Problems, Chronic deceases,), Patient Medical Data, Vaccinations, Administrative document issued, Illnesses;
- ***Interoperability with Central Information System:*** XML/HL7 Client Agent communications services.

3. General Architecture of Croatian Primary Healthcare Information System

General architecture of NHIS consists of central components - The NHIS infrastructure, and contextual portals:

- ***Components of Central Information System****:* Core Networked Healthcare Repositories[3] (Population, Health Insurance, Public Health, Health Financials) along with acting Application Service Providers - ASPs (Primary Healthcare, Public Health, Health Insurance, Health Professional Associations):
- ***Contextual Portals****:* Ministry of Health, Public Health, Health Insurance, Primary Healthcare, Hospital, Pharmacy, Health Professional Associations, Professional and Public education, General Health Communications[4], Other health related portals, as presented in Figure 1. Portal implementations provide autonomy of professional functionalities and contextually "glue" all stakeholders in their mutual interactions.

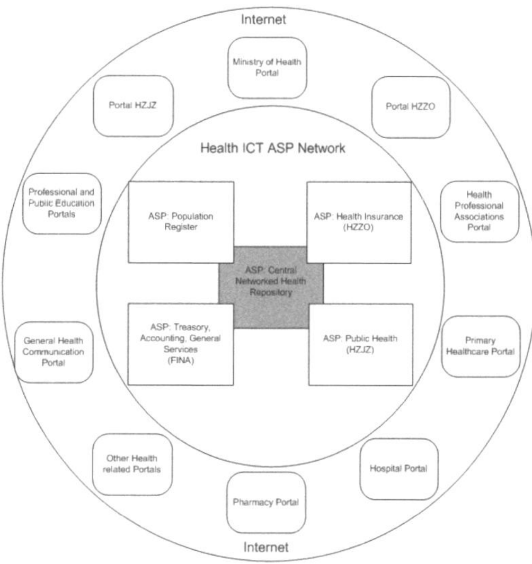

Figure 1: General Architecture of Healthcare Information System

4. Implemented Pilot projects

Based on the General Architecture and priorities given, the pilot projects was the necessary step in the procurement process and following results were obtained.

---

[3] With respective data, process and knowledge interdependencies

[4] General Health Oriented Communications and Professional Communications. Telemedicine is an example of event driven temporal multipoint professional health communications.

4.1. *Primary Healthcare Information System (PHIS)*

Primary Healthcare Information System is designed and implemented as: Central Information System, and Client Information System.

4.1.1. *G1 – PHIS Central Information System*

PHIS Central Information System implements functional requirements in the form of Integrated System. Integration is based on interoperability standards.

Central Component of PHIS integrates: Ministry of Health Information System, Health Insurance Information System, Hospital Information System, Information System of Public Health, National Certification Authority, Pharmacies, laboratories, Primary Healthcare Teams and Patients. Illustration of integration is presented in Figure 2.

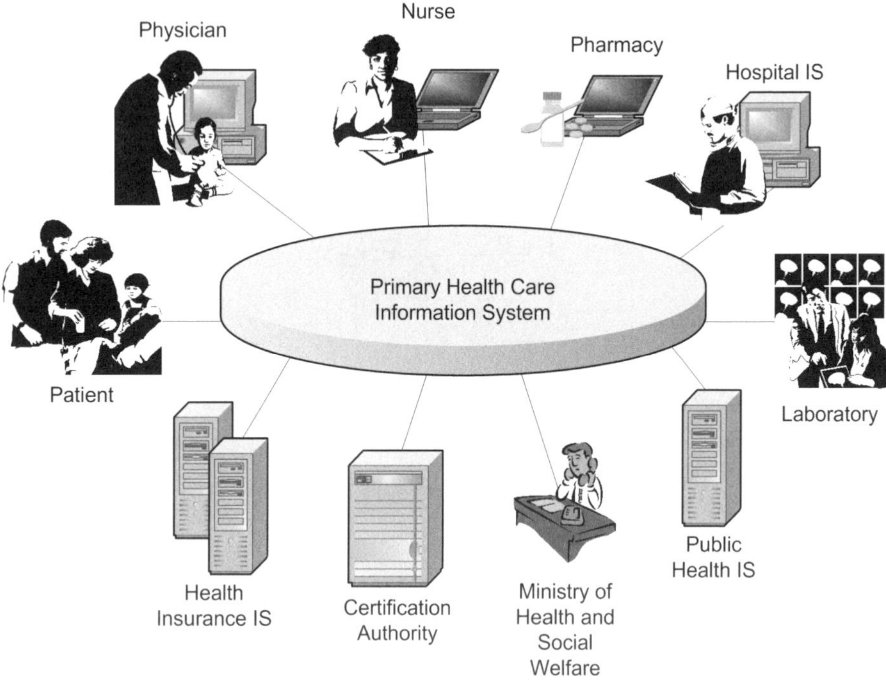

Figure 2: Basic entities in Primary Healthcare Information System

Program Architecture is implemented on three layers (Figure 3):

- **Open Application Layer:** Applications related to PHC Teams (doctors, nurses), Laboratories, Public Health, other;
- **Middle Layer:** Middle Layer implements **common health services** (Electronic Health Record Management, Patient Record Management,

Resource Management, Terminology Services, and Authorization) and common general services (coding schemes, directory management, transaction tracing, message interchange, and authentication);
- **Communication Layer:** open authenticated communications.

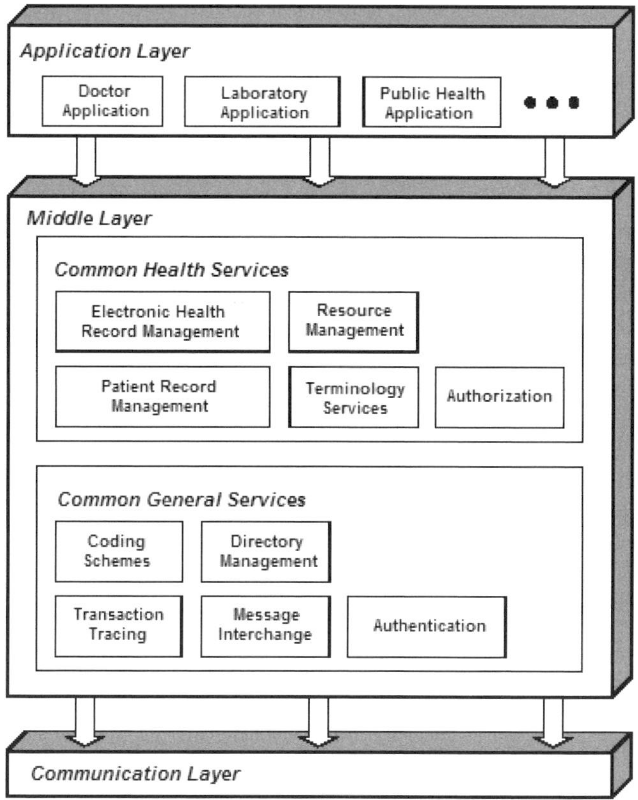

Figure 3: Referent PHIS Program Architecture

Portal technology implemented in Middle Layer integrates Data Layer (Intranet databases: health resource registers, population register; Internet databases: electronic libraries, knowledge bases, clinical recommendations) and Presentation Layer (Web server, e-mail server).

4.1.2. Croatian Model of Electronic Health Record

Croatian model of Electronic Health Record is developed as Integrated Care Electronic Health Record (ICEHR) and is based on the nationally adopted European norm ENV 13606. The further step was developing HRN ENV 13606 norm and adding elements which are required for meta-data analyses. Its structure and basic elements are listed in Figure 6.

- **Case** is defined by any occurrence which is reflected on health and can be described by a single entity (code and description) of ICD – 10 classifications. Typical case could be an occurrence of illness. In the case of chronic illness, Case once registered, stays with the patient for the rest of his life. Acute cases are registered always as a new Case;
- **Encounter** is a form of health care event and it is represented by any contact with the primary care system;
- **Medical episode** is defined by the processing of individual case during an encounter, while it actually structurally within itself integrates two concepts which are often separated in literature: episode of illness and episode of care. Medical episode is primarily defined by the processed case; while it contains the information on diagnostic processing and the plan of therapy concerning the relative case, which were collected during particular encounter;
- **Collection** was introduced in order to bypass the complicated organization imposed by HRN ENV 13606 and to simplify the presentation of structure. The Collection implies the architectural components specified by norm (Root Architectural Component, Folder, Composition, Headed Section etc.) and their specialization;
- **Archetypes** represent definitions of the structure of clinical concepts, in other words, the rules which disclose storages inside the electronic health record structure of the information related to particular concept.

4.1.3. Management potentials in central PHIS

Management and control in Health System: strategic and operational patient relationship management, drug prescription, referrals, therapeutic processes performance and drug efficiency assessments.

GP teams: Authorized access to distributed EPR and related medical document resources, emergency and crisis management, personal performance management, health and medical reporting system.

Public health: Healthcare Intelligence, evidence based management in public health, public health dynamics based on Population register.

Ministry of Health and Social Welfare: Healthcare Intelligence, Health Performance Management, Business Intelligence, Health resources management.

Health Insurance Institute: Direct HL/7 communication on healthcare activities, ICPC-2 activity based costing; Evidence based Planning, Budgeting and Monitoring, Pharmacy management, drug consumption management.

Patient: Direct control on Patient electronic record, Quality of service assessment and review, Patient Relationship Management, Privacy Audit and Reporting, Healthcare Service Ordering System, Public Related Health education, Discrete Selection/Change of GP.

Public: Health condition of the population, transparency and benchmarking of public health services.

4.1.4. G2 – PHIS, Client Information System

PHIS Client Information System implements client system functional requirements, customized for the dedicated application area.

Interoperability standards as the prerequisite for the integration in PHIS Central Information System allow for open competition in client application developments as well as implementations and maintenance.

Context sensitive navigation and correspondent workflow is applied for the patient, doctor, nurse. Illustrative example of patient context "chronic deceases" is presented IN Figure 4.

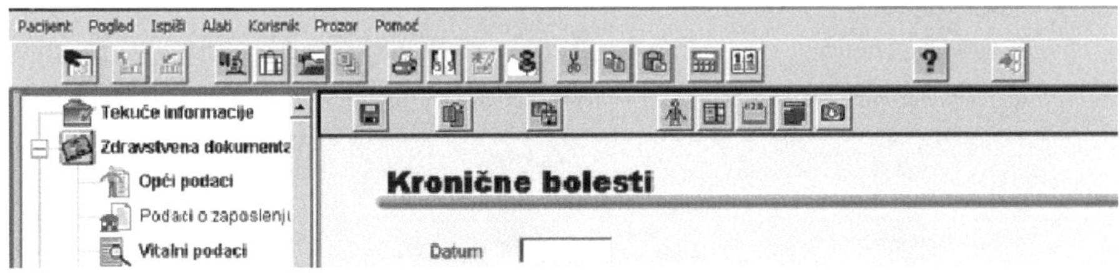

Figure 4: Example of context sensitive navigation

4.2. Communication System

Two components of communication system have been implemented for the pilot implementations.

Primary Healthcare Communication Architecture (Figure 5.) Agent based software technology and implemented XML/HL/7 standards are supporting networked asynchronous execution of all health related activities.

PHIS Virtual Private Network (PHIS VPN) (Figure 5.) PHIS implementation is based on Elaboration of Government Computer and Communication Network as one instance of it, thus enabling wide connectivity and interoperability of health as well as government and public services.

Computer resource has been formed by central and backup PHIS Computer Resources, Health Insurance Health Computer Resources, Public Health Computer Resources, GPs offices. PHIS VPN connects all above mentioned resources into primary healthcare computer and communication network.

4.3. National Health Card

Smart cards can add mechanisms to the Internet to implement security (data protection and anonymity-confidentiality) which are easy to use.

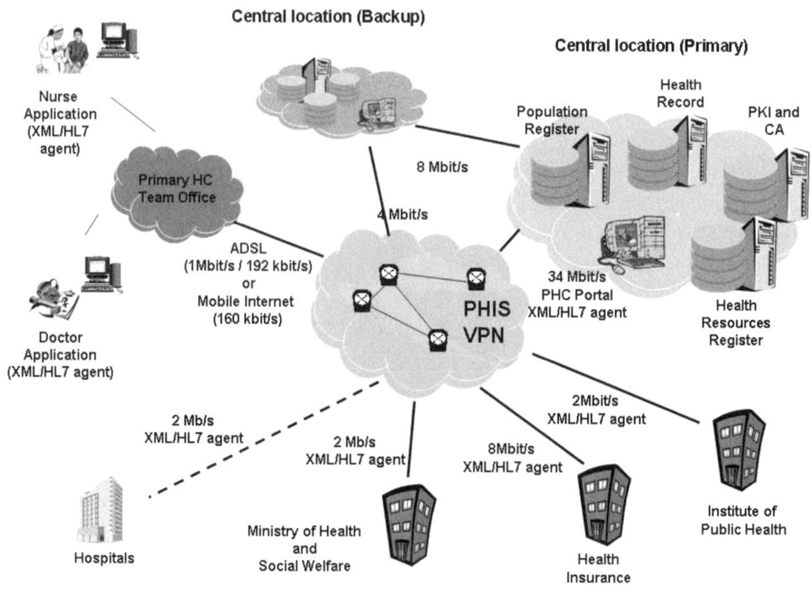

Figure 5: Primary Healthcare Communication Architecture and system PHIS VPN

National health card in pilot project, based on smart card functionality, implemented two basic functionalities:

- For professional usage - health practitioner card for secure access to patient data, with security components;
- For citizen's/patient's usage - Insured patient's card which includes: administrative data, medical data and security components.

4.4. Pilot implementation metrics

4.4.1. Primary healthcare teams

Sixty primary healthcare teams, consisting of the physician and the nurse, were selected and trained to implement G2 component of PHIS. In order to reduce pilot costs, pilot locations clustered on the cities of Zagreb, Čakovec, Požega, Split, Koprivnica. Standardized hardware and communication equipment has been installed at the PHC team's premises.

4.4.2. Health Insured Individuals

More than 100.000 health insured individuals were included in respective PHC team files.

4.4.3. National Health card

Number of issued cards: 120 professional cards. Implemented functionality: Electronic ID, Advanced electronic signature.

4.4.4. Implemented Security levels

Smart heath card: identity card, advanced electronic signature, assigned attributes (roles);

　　Application: role based access control (HL/RBAC), certification of applications;

　　Message and messaging agents: digital signature of message encryption;

　　Equipment: server security, desktop security, mobile desktop (authentication, integrity, encryption);

　　Network security: local area network access control (router/firewall), virtual private network implementation of Internet protocol security with IPv4IPv6 (IPSec – Internet engineering task force standard).

5. Project implementation

5.1. Primary Healthcare Information System (PHIS)

After the pilot phase, the procurement part of the process has successfully end with one signed contract for PHIS Central Information System and five contracts with five different vendors for PHIS Client Information Systems (all of them signed at the end of 2003.). During 2004 there has been little progress on the implementation of the Central Information System and Client Information System due to organizational problems on the government side. In early 2005 the new initiative to push project implementation further has come from the government side with the new PMU in place and implementation has started.

5.2. G1 – PHIS Central Information System

The focus of the implementation was according to the contract with supplier and specification from pilot phase on building Central Information System ready to accept connections from around 2300 different GPs locations. The Central Information System was build according to the specification from pilot project, as described above.

　　However, several changes to the original project have been implemented on the way, in order to enable project to succeed:

- Project was divided into two parts: first one was building of base ICT software infrastructure for Messaging system between Client Information Systems and Central Information System. Second part was modelling and implementing Electronic Healthcare Record System in order to enable existing health system to migrate from paper based documents exchange to electronic one;
- Scope of the Project was extended to existing information systems of Croatian National Institute of Public Health and Croatian Institute for Health Insurance. This was necessary in order to prepare those information systems for communication with Central Information System;

- Health PKI infrastructure was built as an integral part of the all health information systems. Two types of smart cards (healthcare professional usage and patient's usage) were merged into one physical smart card that can perform both functions.

Implemented systems communication architecture was the same as in pilot. However, in the first phase connections to the PHC Portal, GPs, and health insurance and public health institutions have been established. Connections to hospitals and laboratories will be established in the later phases of the project. By the late 2006 the Central Information System has been fully functional.

5.3. G2 – PHIS Client Information System

Implementation of the Client Information Systems has been according to the specification of the Client Information System in the pilot phase, described above.

Several changes to the original concept have been implemented and they are:

- Originally five vendors were selected for supplying application for client Information System throughout Croatia and they have exclusive rights to do so. The change have been that so that there don't have an exclusive rights to install their application in GPs, but other vendors can participate as well if they fulfil process of the certification of their application for GPs. This was done because the model where there are only five companies that can offer software to GPs is distortion of the free market forces and could potentially lead to formations of cartel and thus eventually increase the cost and deteriorate their efficiency in providing applications to GPs;
- There has been change in the organization of the first level support. Originally it was planned that first line of support would be done by government agency. This solution proved inefficient and costly since government agency would provide support for five different software solution and second the cost to do so would be substantially higher than if this task done by software providers for GPs themselves.

By the end of the 2006, according to official statements, there have been around 350 GPs connected to the PHIS Central Information System. Croatian Institute for Health Insurance is putting in their contracts with GPs saying that all GPs have to be connected to PHIS Central Information System in 2007.

6. Embedded Standards

International Interoperability requires implementation and maintenance of a large set of international standards. Two important subsets are presented as ICT related standards and health related standards.

6.1. ICT related standards

ICT related standards implemented are:

- **Interoperability:** Object Management Group OMG, W3C, XML, GIF (UK Government Interoperability Framework);

- **IT and Software Engineering:** Software Engineering Standards (IEEE SECS), Imitational Organization for Standardization / International Electro technical Commission (ISO/IEC JTC1/SC7), Data Interchange Standards Association, CENELEC - the European Committee for Electro technical Standardization, CEN/ISSS (European Committee for Standardization - (Information and Communications Technologies) activities., FIPS (Federal Information Processing Standard), National Institute of Standards and Technology (US NIST), American National Standards Institute (ANSI), The Foundation for Intelligent Physical Agents (FIPA);
- **Smart card:** identification cards – physical and electronic characteristics, dimension and location of the contacts, inter-industry commands for interchange, system and registration procedure for applications identifiers, inter-industry data elements, machine readable cards for healthcare applications, security categorization and protection for healthcare cards specification standards (ICO/IES 7816-1-10, 8824-8825; CEN/EN 726-1-7, CEN/ENV 1257/1-3, 1284, 1387, 1867, 12018, 12388, 12924, 13729; smart card interoperability specifications and "Open Smart Card Infrastructure for Europe) (OSCIE) common specifications (3).

6.2. Health related Standards

Health related standards were specified as a set of requirements, an consequently implemented as a prerequisite for [5] preventing health hazards (e.g. drug allergy, hypersensitivity), patients starting to demand that 'their' data should be available on-line, improved efficiency by enabling professional co-operation in new ways, Quality management requirements on aggregated data, Integration of modular systems from different suppliers, Lowered costs and facilitated procurement, and primarily the national, regional European and global interoperability and action.

6.2.1. Health standardization institutions referenced

- **CEN/TC 251** – (Committee European de Normalization) - European Standardization of Health Informatics Technical Committee 251 - Healthcare information interchange within Europe;
- CEN/TC 224 – Machine-readable cards, related device interfaces and operations;
- **ISO TC 215** – "Health Informatics" (Messaging standards for information exchange between healthcare information systems; WG 5 – Health Cards)
- **ASTM** – (American Society for Testing and Materials - Interchange of data between medical information systems)
- **ACR/NEMA** – (American College of Radiology / National Electronic Manufacturers' Association: Digital Imaging and Communication in Medicine – DICOM; Program of Assertive Community Treatment - PACT)

---

[5] Health On-line, eEurope, CEN/ISSS, 2002

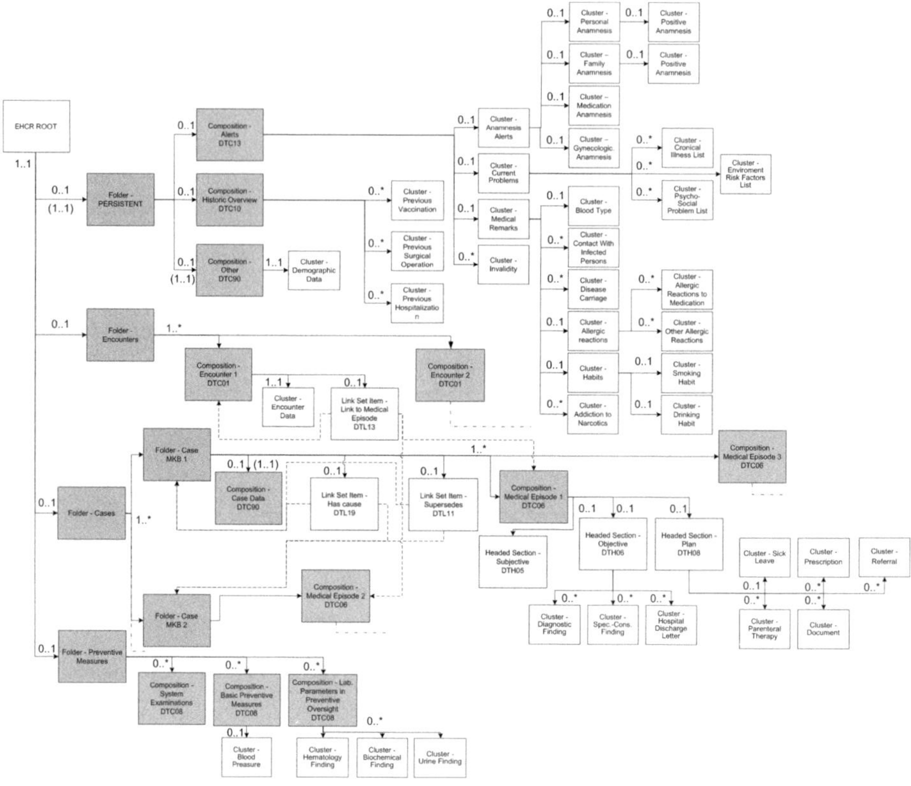

Figure 6: Croatian model of Electronic health record in accordance with ENV 13606

6.2.2. Implemented Standards and Classifications

- **ICD-10** – Classification of diseases for the collation of medical statistics
- **DRG** – *Diagnoses Related Groups*
- **ATC** – *Anatomic Therapeutic Chemical Code*
- **IEEE/P1157** – Standard for Healthcare Data Interchange (Standards for moving data from medical devices to computers and vice versa along standardized hardware buses and interfaces)
- **ANSI HL7** – Standard for electronic data exchange in healthcare environments
- **ENV 13606** – European standard which defines architecture, organization and communication of Electronic Health Records.

7. Conclusion

Design of the complex national primary healthcare information system is based on corresponding national and international strategic documents, precise definitions of functional requirements and the results of started pilot project implementation (trial run). The implementation phase brings reality checks of the accepted design and necessary fine tuning in order to achieve implementation goals. The most common cases of the fine-tuning in this case were: less than expected capability of other government bodies to support project and less than expected GPs level of sensibility to the importance of this project.

Hierarchical and functional project management showed good results since it enabled fast decisions supported by the sponsors of the projects. as well as to building capacities for accelerated implementations of the project extensions in the years to come.

Aligned with international standards and implementation policies for information societies, healthcare information system provides the drivers for national, regional and international interoperability.

References

[1]   A. Pavelin, I. Klapan, M. Kovač, M. Katić, R.Stevanović, M. Rakić, N. Klapan,   A Functional Telemedicine Environment in the Framework of the Croatian, Healthcare Information System // Remote Cardiology Consultations Using Advanced Medical Technology (Applications for NATO Operations) / I. Klapan,, R. Poropatich (ed.).Amsterdam, Netherlands, *IOS Press*, Inc., 2006.

[2]   Stevanovic, R. Pristas, I. et all. Development and deployment of a health information system in transitional countries (Croatian experience) // Medical and Care Compunetics 2 / Bos, Lodewijk ; Lexminarayan, Swami ; March, Andy (ed.).Amsterdam : *IOS Press*, 2005, 82-87

[3]   R, Stevanović, A. Stanić, G. Galijašević, M. Mauher, Development of Informatic's System and Telemedicine in Croatian Primary Healthcare // Med e-tel, The International trade event and Conference for Health, Telemedicine and Health ICT/Collignon Jean-Michel (ed.). Luxembourg : Med e-Tel, 2005. 58-59.

Medical and Care Compunetics 4
L. Bos and B. Blobel (Eds.)
IOS Press, 2007

CCR Exchange: Building a Patient-Driven Web-Based Healthcare Community Around an Emerging Personal Health Record Standard

Steve Chi-Hung Lu[a], Ph.D.
CCR Exchange, Inc.

Abstract. This document demonstrates how we use open source software in building an Internet healthcare community around an emerging Personal Health Record standard called Continuity of Care Record (CCR) format, and how members of the community can share healthcare information securely and efficiently while retaining total privacy.

Keywords. Continuity of Care Record, Web Community, Open Source Software, Public Key Infrastructure, Key Management, Key Recovery, Two-Factor Authentication, XMLSignature, XMLEncryption

Introduction

The Continuity of Care Record[1] (CCR) is an XML-based electronic health record format that is quickly gaining acceptance in the Healthcare industry as a vehicle for exchanging clinical information among providers, institutions, or other entities. Because of the platform-agnostic property of XML, CCR is an ideal format for a patient to keep either as a brief summary of recent care or as a life-long record of medical history. Furthermore, because of XML is a well-supported format by database vendors, importing into existing EMR systems involves only simple XML transformations (XSLT) for converting CCR into native schema.

CCR Exchange Network is a web-based infrastructure that provides patients, physicians, and clinicians a secure environment to share CCRs over public network. By taking advantage of the recent advent on information and security technologies and standards, CCR Exchange was built with special attention to security both in its design and implementation. A list of security services that CCR Exchange Network offers includes:

- Strong Two-Factor Authentication,
- Data Integrity and Confidentiality,
- Patient-Centric Discretionary Access Control,
- CCR Document Revision Control,
- Integrated Key Management,

---

[a] Corresponding Author: CCR Exchange Inc. E-Mail: steve.lu@ccrexchange.com

- Facility for Key Backup and Recovery,
- Security Audit and Data Access Monitoring,
- Secure Messaging and Conferencing.

In the remainder of this document, we will show how CCR Exchange implements these services using technologies freely available on the Internet. At the end of this document, we will demonstrate a scenario whereby a patient consults with his primary care provider and the provider in turn refers him to a specialist.

1. A Brief Introduction to CCR

Continuity of Care Record, or "CCR", was developed in response to the need to organize and make transportable a set of basic patient information consisting of the most relevant and timely facts about a patient's condition. These include patient and provider information, insurance information, patient's health status (e.g., allergies, medications, vital signs, diagnoses, and recent procedures), recent care provided, as well as recommendations for future care (care plan).

To ensure CCR documents are truly transportable, each document must abide by the latest CCR schema specification which dictates not only the set of valid CCR tag names but also the order by which tags and their child tags appear in the document.

The service of validating each CCR document is built into the CCR Exchange client and only documents that pass the schema validation is admitted into the Network.

2. Public Key Infrastructure

The basis of the security service provided by CCR Exchange is the underlying Public Key Infrastructure (PKI) built into both the CCR Exchange server and client.

- **CCR Exchange Server** plays the dual role of certificate issuing authority and the registration authority. During the registration process, a certificate request submitted by the Browser is automatically accepted and stored in the server's registration database. By eye-balling the submitted data from an administrative web page, an administrator can grant or deny the issuing of the certificate. This manual process ensures the integrity of the user data and also prevents denial of service attack on the registration process itself. Following the administrator's decision, a notification email is automatically sent to the applicant. For a qualified applicant, the email contains both links for downloading certificate and the CCR Exchange Client software. Apache, PHP, OpenSSL, and MySQL were used in implementing these server processes.

- **CCR Exchange Client** is a Firefox extension that, in addition to CCR viewing, editing, and validating capabilities, performs security tasks such as member authentication, authorization, and enforcing access control rules. The core of the CCR Exchange client is a compiled XPCOM component acting as the security monitor that marshals all client/server communications requiring read/write access to server data. The Graphical User Interface (GUI) and user interactivities are implemented by plaintext XHTML and XUL pages and embedded JavaScripts. Using Mozilla's XPConnect technology, embedded JavaScripts can call into XPCOM component to request web service from the CCR Exchange server. The clear code boundary that lies between the GUI components and the XPCOM engine helps preventing rogue script attack on the server while making CCR Exchange Client more temper-proof (see section 2.1 for a detailed exposition on this topic.) Mozilla's Network Security Service (NSS) is an important part of the core.

A typical setup of the CCR Exchange network is shown in Figure 1.

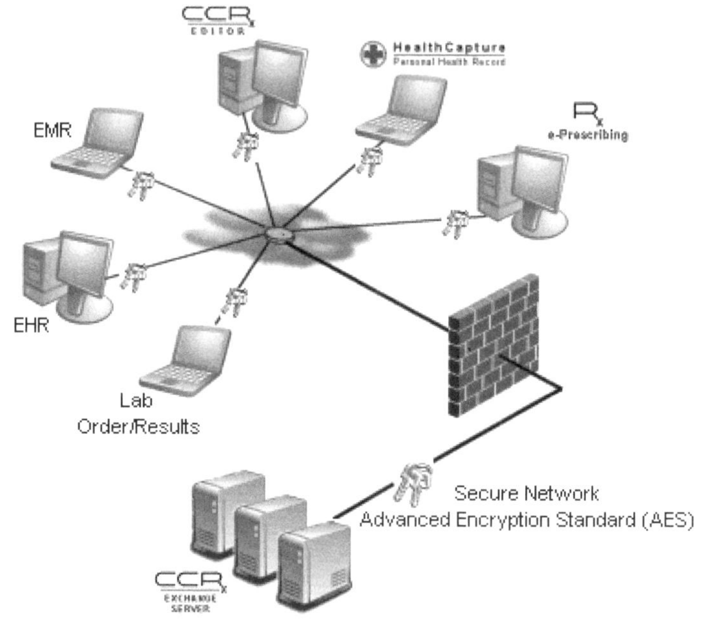

Figure 1. CCR Exchange Network.

2.1. JavaScript and XPCOM Security

The default security policy governing a JavaScript file's access to the interface exposed from an XPCOM component is the *same-origin* policy. That is, they must come from the same domain for a XPConnect call to be successful. In the case of CCR Exchange client, most of the XPCOM functionalities are not accessible from JavaScript files downloaded from the Internet, since the component resides on localhost and is considered to be a different domain.

However, in order to edit CCR records downloaded from CCR Exchange server, this policy is relaxed for a subset of the XPCOM interface – those that are editing related. This by no means compromises the overall security of the CCR Exchange client, since only local JavaScript files are allowed to create an Editor Object in XPCOM, and any remote JavaScript file trying to access the editing functions would fail since the required Editor Object has not been created within the same security context.

2.2. Two-Factor Authentication

After a successful enrollment, a CCR Exchange member would have in possession a CCR Exchange certificate and his/her signature key, both are stored in the Firefox's soft token – a database that holds both user certificates and signature keys. To subsequently sign on to the CCR Exchange Network, a member must provide both a valid password and a Proof of Possession (POP) showing he/she is the rightful owner of the key.

Using a challenge-and-response type of protocol, the POP is technically a digitally signed server challenge. A server challenge is a random binary string concatenated with a shared secret that is issued to the client by the CCR Exchange server upon each log-in request. The CCR Exchange client constructs the POP by encrypting the challenge blob with the current user's private key. And upon receiving the POP returned by the client, the server decrypts it using the corresponding public key. By comparing the unwrapped challenge and shared secret to the original copies, the server effectively verifies the authenticity of the client.

The benefit of using two-factor authentication is that, in an unlikely event of password being compromised, the perpetrator can not log into to the CCR Exchange network without the signature key. However, the enhanced security necessitates a user to transport his/her credential, both certificate and signature key, in order to log in from a different computer.

2.3. Data Integrity and Confidentiality

During each CCR Exchange session, all data uploaded to the server is encrypted using a session key generated by the client upon log-in and disposed of after log-off. Not using the same session key twice adds further data protection against a single compromised key.

Accompanying the encrypted data in each upload is the session key itself in a protected format. The session key is first encrypted with a transport key derived from a shared secret between the server and the client. The outcome is then digitally signed with the user's private key. On the server side, the key blob is first decrypted/verified with the user's public key and then re-encrypted with the server's master key before it is entered into the database along with the encrypted data.

For CCR documents, the encryption takes the form of XMLEncryption standard. Each document is also digitally signed with the user's private key, following the XMLSignature standard.

Each upload request from the client within a session, as mention earlier, is marshaled by the XPCOM component. To prevent replay attack, the XPCOM component adds to each outbound request a header containing the user id, a session id, a timestamp-based identifier and a hash. The hash is the SHA-1 hash of the user id, a password-based hash, and the timestamp identifier. This guarantees that no two request headers are alike and makes replay attacks impossible.

2.4. Patient-Centric Discretionary Access Control

In the CCR Exchange Network, each member has full control of who may or may not read or write to his/her CCR files or other data resources. This access control rule is enforced by the XPCOM component acting as the security monitor. The actual rules for all system wide data resources are stored on the server.

Mechanisms are provided in the CCR Exchanged client for a member to modify the access control rule associated with each of his/her owned data resource. The member can also create a public or private group and assign arbitrary members to it. Using groups, a member can allow many members access to his/her data at once.

2.5. CCR Document Revision Control

For each CCR document uploaded, the CCR Exchange server maintains a history of past revisions starting with revision 0 – the original document. Each subsequent revision is a standalone CCR document containing just the modification. This is called an Incremental Revision.

Each Incremental Revision contains 2 extra signatures. The first signature is produced from a snapshot of the latest revision signed with the current author's private key. The second signature is produced from the newly added modification using the same key. This way, the order of the revisions applied to the document is made non-repudiable as the modification itself.

All revisions are viewable as either HTML or raw XML from within the CCR Exchange client.

2.6. Integrated Key Management

To share CCR documents and other data resources (images, text, or PDF files) with members of the CCR Exchange network, the document owner's encryption key needs be securely delivered to the requesting member for decryption. Once the key arrives at the requesting client, it becomes short-lived and is securely deleted in memory after the decryption is complete. This process of secure key sharing is integrated into the CCR Exchange Network and is completely transparent to the user.

As pointed out earlier, all data resources in the CCR Exchange Network are stored in an encrypted form using the owner's session key - the session key that was generated when the data resource was first uploaded to the server. This session key is also stored on the server, however, it is encrypted with a transport key and then by the master key of the CCR Exchange server. When a member, with owner's permission, is requesting the data object, the server decrypts the session key blob with the master key and then encrypts the resulting blob with the requesting member's public key. The server sends down both the data object and the key blob. This guarantees that the only person that can recover the key and thus the data is the person with the private key matching to the encrypting public key.

2.7. Facility for Key Backup and Recovery

All data encrypting keys on the server are doubly encrypted by a Transport key and a Master key. In cases when the owner of the key can not be reached to authorize document accesses, such as a medical emergency when the patient is incapacitated, a procedure is in place to allow Key Recovery. Usually, one signature from the CCR Exchange security officers (or administrators) and one signature from the patient's primary care physician (or other physicians) are required to authorize the key recovery process. Once authorized, the requesting member will then gain access to the patient's data object as if the patient has granted the access himself.

2.8. Security Audit and Data Access Monitoring

All service requests from the CCR Exchange client are logged and entered into the server database with restricted access. A security officer can log into the administrative web page to query for a particular member's past activities for any time period and/or for any specific type of events (e.g. file upload, file download, log-in, log-off, file rename, access control list modification, admin login, etc.).

Each event is tagged with the user id, session id, time-stamp, and attributes. Attributes are information important for a particular type of event such as the new file name for a file rename event.

Time-stamps throughout the CCR Exchange Network are provided by one unique time source – the CCR Exchange server. These include time-stamps used in digital signature and messages submitted in discussion forums.

2.9. Secure Messaging and Conferencing

CCR Exchange provides separate discussion forum for each stored data object. These forums allow physicians and patients to convene and exchange information on documents of mutual interest. Similar to CCR documents, all messages are encrypted by the respective owner's session key, both in transit and in storage. The CCR Exchange server manages and supplies all the keys necessary for decrypting all past messages pertaining to the data object under discussion.

2.10. Application Level End-to-End Security

The security services provided by the CCR Exchange Network is built at the application level and does not rely on transport layer security protocols such as SSL and TLS, albeit they provide additional protection if enabled. The benefit of application level security is that it makes possible end-to-end data confidentiality from the CCR Exchange Client to the MySQL database where the data is stored and stays encrypted. The SSL/TLS data encryption, on the other hand, ends at the web server and therefore leaves open the opportunity for data hijacking by system or network administrators at the hosting company.

All data objects inside the CCR Exchange Network, whether in storage or in transit, are encrypted with the owners' session keys and only the owner or members with owner's specific permission are able to decrypt and view plaintext data inside the CCR Exchange Client.

3. Conclusion

Health care consumers expect their medical information to be appropriately safe-guarded. CCR Exchange Network provides the necessary infrastructure for protecting consumer privacy and information security that is also compliant with government's security and privacy law (HIPPA[2]). And because of its uses of open format and technologies, it can easily be adopted into existing IT systems and readily supports future extensions such as smartcards and directory services.

References

[1] Standard Specification for Continuity of Care Record (CCR). ASTM International E2369-05, http://www.astm.org, 2007.
[2] Health Insurance Portability and Accountability Act of 1996, http://aspe.hhs.gov/admnsimp/pl104191.htm.

Medical and Care Compunetics 4
L. Bos and B. Blobel (Eds.)
IOS Press, 2007

Access Control: how can it improve patients' healthcare?

Ana FERREIRA[abd], Ricardo CRUZ-CORREIA[cd], Luís ANTUNES[b], David CHADWICK[a]

[a]*Computer Laboratory, University of Kent*
[b]*LIACC- Faculty of Science of Porto*
[c]*Biostatistics and Medical Informatics Dept. of Porto Faculty of Medicine*
[d]*CINTESIS – Center for research in health information Systems and technologies*

Abstract. The Electronic Medical Record (EMR) is a very important support tool for patients and healthcare professionals but it has some barriers that prevent its successful integration within the healthcare practice. These barriers comprise not only security concerns but also costs, in terms of time and effort, as well as relational and educational issues that can hinder its proper use. Access control is an essential part of the EMR and provides for its confidentiality by checking if a user has the necessary rights to access the resources he/she requested. This paper comprehensively reviews the published material about access control in healthcare. The review reveals that most of the access control systems that are published in the literature are just studies or prototypes in which healthcare professionals and patients did not participate in the definition of the access control policies, models or mechanisms. Healthcare professionals usually needed to change their workflow patterns and adapt their tasks and processes in order to use the systems. If access control could be improved according to the users' needs and be properly adapted to their workflow patterns we hypothesise that some of the barriers to the effective use of EMR could be reduced. Then EMR could be more successfully integrated into the healthcare practice and provide for better patient treatment.

Keywords. Computer Security, access control, computerized patient record

Introduction

The widening use of healthcare information systems such as the Electronic Medical Record (EMR), which allows for the collection, extraction, management, sharing and searching of information, is increasing the need for information security (e.g. confidentiality, integrity and availability) [1], [2].

Although the EMR is a significant support tool for patients and healthcare professionals there are still some barriers that prevent its successful integration within the healthcare practice. These barriers comprise not only security concerns [3] but also costs, in terms of time and effort, as well as relational and educational issues that can hinder the proper use of the system [4], [5]. Relational issues may exist when, for example, the relationship between patient and physician is affected. Educational issues relate to the fact that healthcare professionals need to learn how to use and adapt the system to their own needs [6]. They are usually not consulted when the system is designed and implemented and therefore are most of the time forced to use the system and need to redesign their workflow patterns around it [5].

Access control is essential to provide for the confidentiality of the EMR because it is part of the authorisation process where the system checks if the user can access the resources he requested. The study of access control policies, models and mechanisms that are commonly used in healthcare and within the EMR can help us understand how access control can affect the success of EMR integration and how this can be used to minimize the barriers that are usually present.

The main objective of this paper is to review how access control has been studied, designed and implemented in general and compare this to similar research in the healthcare domain, more specifically within EMR systems. This review will help identify what are the main issues regarding healthcare professionals' needs in terms of access control, and identify the barriers that usually prevent the successful integration of access control systems into EMR. If the improvement of access control development and usage can reduce some of the EMR integration barriers then we hypothesize that patient treatment and support can be improved.

This paper is structured as follows. Section 1 briefly introduces the concept of access control and some of the complexities involved in its design and implementation. Section 2 presents some of the problems with EMR and how access control relates to them. Section 3 describes the methodology used for the review and section 4 presents the results obtained from the review. Section 5 analyses and discusses the results and suggests some ways to improve the design and use of access control and its integration with EMR in healthcare practices. Section 6 concludes the paper.

1. Access Control

Information security is usually defined by three main characteristics [2], [7]:
- confidentiality - the prevention of unauthorized disclosure of the information
- integrity - the prevention of unauthorized modification of the information
- availability - the prevention of unauthorized withholding of the information.

Confidentiality is often used interchangeably with privacy but they are not exactly the same. Privacy is the right of an individual to not have their private information exposed (and this is usually enforceable by law), whilst confidentiality is limiting access to information to authorised individuals only.

The complexity of building secure information systems relates mainly to three fundamental and competing factors: i) the complexity of the security technology itself, ii) the difficulty of classifying the information that is to be protected and iii) the use of the technology by humans. This last factor is normally the most problematic [8] because it deals with the interactions between humans and systems. Other important but secondary competing factors are: protecting information from unauthorised access whilst needing to be able to access it for audit or law enforcement purposes; and making it easy for an authorised user to gain access to the information but complex for an unauthorised user to do the same.

In order to securely access information within a system three steps are usually required: identification (where a user says who he is, e.g. with a login username); authentication (where a user proves his identification given in the first step, e.g. with a password or a PIN number); and authorisation (where access rights are given to the user). Whilst access control is conceptually part of the authorisation process that checks if a user can access the resources he requested, we are including all three steps within the scope of our review since the first two steps are necessary precursors to the third. Furthermore many implementations combine the three steps together into one access control decision, by having the implicit access control policy that everyone who is successfully authenticated can have access to the resource. This is the coarsest granularity of access control policy, in which everyone has the same access rights. Thus the authentication mechanism becomes a combined authentication and authorisation mechanism.

The design of access control systems is very complex and should start with the definition of structured and formal access control policies as well as access control models [9]. An access control policy must describe the rules that need to be enforced in order to provide the information security requirements of the organization. Afterwards, an appropriate access control model must be chosen in order to model the rules defined within the policy. Examples of common access control models are: Role-Based Access Control (RBAC) that associates rights to groups of users according to their roles within the organization; Identity Based Access Control (IBAC) that associates rights to specific users depending on their needs; and Mandatory Access Control (MAC) that defines mandatory rules for all the users of the system. A model can also be hybrid and include more than one model in order to tackle the more heterogeneous needs of an organization. Only after the access control model is chosen can the right technology and both authentication and access control mechanisms be selected and implemented. Authentication mechanisms provide for the identification and authentication of a user to the system - the first 2 steps above - (e.g. login/password; fingerprint) while access control mechanisms protect against unauthorized use of the requested resources (e.g. access control lists, security labels) [10]. Both mechanisms should perform in a correct and consistent way according to the access control policy and model defined.

The means of providing access control has become more challenging as policies become more complex. These need to be studied carefully within the healthcare environment so that access control can be correctly developed and applied without hindering the system's use.

2. The Electronic Medical Record

Access control is of vital importance in healthcare. Confidentiality is a main concern when it is related to patient clinical information that needs to be private. It is essential to protect this information from unauthorized access and, therefore, misuse or legal liability.

The introduction of the EMR within healthcare organizations has the main goal of integrating heterogeneous patient information that is usually scattered throughout different locations [11], [12]. This is why the EMR is becoming an essential source of information and an important support tool for the healthcare professional. There is also an increasing need to access healthcare information at remote locations [13]. This and the distributed nature of the information stress the need for access control requirements to be taken seriously [14].

Although the EMR is an essential tool for the healthcare professional, the reality is that it still does not integrate easily and effectively with healthcare professionals' daily workflow and processes [15]. Several obstacles are mentioned by healthcare professionals concerning the use of EMR. The obstacles are associated with a concern for patient privacy and other security vulnerabilities related to the easy distribution, sharing and wider online access of the information [16], [17].

Other barriers that prevent the successful integration and use of EMR are mostly related to human interactions with the system. These include the time taken by healthcare professionals to learn and to use the system, and the consequent extra time and costs the patients may incur if they have to wait longer to be seen and treated. In addition, relational and educational barriers also hinder the right use of the EMR. Relational barriers include the perceptions that the physician and the patient have about the use of the EMR and how their relationship can be affected by it. Educational barriers comprise the lack of proficiency and difficulties that healthcare professionals have whilst interacting with the EMR to perform their daily tasks [6].

Taking into account the problems mentioned above and considering that the main factor that is driving the integration of EMR systems is the need to improve clinical processes and workflow efficiency [13], a deeper understanding of how access control systems can affect this integration and how they are being developed within the EMR is required. This analysis is done in the following sections.

3. Methodology

In order to deepen the understanding of the design and implementation of access control systems, two reviews were performed. The first review comprised an analysis of the design and implementation of generic access control policies, models and authentication mechanisms, where the latter incorporated an implicit access control function, whilst the second review was similar but applied specifically to the healthcare environment.

3.1. Review for Generic Access Control

This review comprised full articles from the last 10 years (1996 until mid 2006) whose content covered generic access control policies, models and authentication mechanisms that incorporated an implicit access control function.

Searches were made in IEEE Xplore and ACM (Association for Computing Machinery) conference databases as well as SACMAT (Symposium on Access Control Models and Technologies) and ESORICS (European Symposium on Research in Computer Security). Specific queries were made in IEEE Xplore (access control<in>metadata) and ACM with "access control".

The review method was done in several stages. We started by reading the titles and the abstracts from the list of articles retrieved by the queries. We tried to summarise in a table the most important topics about access control that we wanted to study. We included articles that described at least one of the following topics:

- **Type of access control policy**: Institutional, Legislation, End-user, override and other.
- **Type of access control model**: RBAC, IBAC and DAC, MAC, Hybrid and other.
- **Study and/or implementation**: Access control policy, access control model and Authentication Mechanisms with an implicit access control function.

- **Authentication mechanisms**: Login/password, Single Sign on, smartcard, fingerprint, digital signature, certificates and other.
- **Results**: Just build the model; prototype or real set implementation.
- **Problems**: The limitations.
- **Successes**: The advantages and benefits.

Articles that applied specifically to the healthcare domain were excluded from this review but included in the next one.

From the articles selected we tried to search the full articles and read them. The table was filled with the necessary information whilst the full articles were being read.

3.2. Review for Access Control in Healthcare

This review comprised full articles from the last 10 years (1996 until mid 2006) whose content covered access control policies, models and authentication mechanisms (that incorporated an implicit access control function) when applied in the healthcare environment.

Searches were made in medical databases such as Medline (that included the BMJ-British Medical Journal) as well as IEEE Xplore and ACM.

As one query was not sensitive enough several queries were made in Medline - "computer security access", "access to information" and "security", "access to information" and "confidentiality"; IEEE Xplore - (access control and health<in>metadata), ("access control' and health"<in>metadata), (access control and health<in>metadata), (pki<in>metadata) and patient; and ACM - "access control" and "electronic patient record" and "security" and confidentiality".

The review method used was similar to the one presented in the previous section. We started by reading the titles and the abstracts from the list of articles retrieved by the queries. We tried to summarise in a table the most important topics about access control that we wanted to study. We included articles that described at least one of the following topics:

- **Type of access control policy**: Institutional, Legislation, End-user, override and other.
- **Type of access control model**: RBAC, IBAC and DAC, MAC, Hybrid and other.
- **Study and/or implementation**: Access control policy, access control model and Authentication Mechanisms with an implicit access control function.
- **Authentication mechanisms**: Login/password, single sign on, smartcard, fingerprint, digital signature, certificates and other.
- **Healthcare Institution**: Hospital, hospital department, primary care, private care and other.
- **Healthcare Information System**: EMR/EPR/CPR, prescription and consultation.
- **User Groups**: Medical doctors, nurses, patients and other healthcare professionals.
- **Portal/Internet access**: Healthcare professionals, patients and other.
- **Results**: Just build the model; prototype or real set implementation.
- **Problems**: The limitations.

- **Successes**: The advantages and benefits.

Next we tried to find the full version of the articles selected according to their titles and abstracts. The summary table was filled whilst the full articles were being read.

4. Results

The review results are presented below and analysed in section 5.

4.1. Review for Generic Access Control

351 articles were obtained within the search queries. After reading titles and abstracts 80 full articles were selected and read. Of these, 59 articles were deemed to be in scope and were included in the review.

As can be seen in Table 1, from the 17 articles that mentioned the definition and use of an access control policy only in 1 case was it implemented, and this was a prototype system. From the 59 articles that mentioned access control models, 52 concentrated on the study of an access control model and in only 8 cases were these studies implemented, mostly as prototypes with only 1 of these being implemented in a real scenario.

Table 1. No of papers reviewed covering access control policies, models and mechanisms between 1996 and 2006.

	1996-99	2000-03	2004-06	Total
Access Control Policy				
Study/Analysis		4	12	**16**
Implementation			1	**1**
Access Control Model				
Study/Analysis	4	11	37	**52**
Implementation		2	6	**8**
Authentication Mechanisms with an implicit access control function				
Study/Analysis		5	10	**15**
Implementation		1	2	**3**

The most commonly used access control model was RBAC, being covered in 38 articles out of 52. The most commonly studied and prototyped authentication mechanism was digital signatures with public key certificates (9 out of 15).

During the last ten years the 3 countries with more publications in this particular area are the USA with 40, UK with 8 and Germany with 7.

4.2. Review for Access control in Healthcare

1453 articles were obtained from the Medline search queries, 234 from the IEEE queries and 200 from the ACM queries. These articles relating to access control in healthcare were reviewed according to their titles and abstracts. From these, 77 full articles were selected and read. Of these, 59 articles were deemed to be appropriate and were included in the review.

From a total of 27 articles that refer to the system's implementation, 25 were built as prototypes whilst 2 were built in a real life scenario.

From the 34 published articles that mention access control policies, Table 2 shows that 22 refer to the study and analysis of those policies, whilst only 4 of them actually implemented policy based systems as prototypes. In 14 out of these 34 papers, the policies were institutionally or legislatively defined, whilst in only 4 of those 34 articles is it mentioned that end-user can set policies. But none of these 4 policies were actually implemented, not even as prototypes. Further, none of the 34 articles that mention access control policies included the end-users of the system as part of the group that designed and developed those policies.

Finally, 7 articles refer to the need for an override policy definition i.e. an access control system which allows the user to override the current policy in times of emergency, and gain access to patient confidential information that they would not otherwise be able to see.

As for access control models, from the 40 articles that refer the use of access control models, 24 of these mention its study and analysis whilst in 8 articles the models were implemented as prototypes only.

Table 2. No of papers reviewed covering access control policies, models and mechanisms in healthcare between 1996 and 2006.

	1996-99	2000-03	2004-06	Total
Access Control Policy				
Study/Analysis	2	8	12	**22**
Implementation		3	1	**4**
Access Control Model				
Study/Analysis	6	10	8	**24**
Implementation	1	6	1	**8**
Authentication Mechanisms with an implicit access control function				
Study/Analysis	6	10	8	**24**
Implementation	1	6	1	**8**

The most commonly used access control model was RBAC (22 from 40) whilst the most tested authentication mechanism was digital signatures with public key certificates (29 from 41).

Focusing now on the EMR and its users, Table 3 shows the type of information systems that were implemented and in which healthcare institutional setting they were implemented. It also presents the most common types of user groups for those systems.

Table 3. Healthcare institutions, information systems and user groups.

	1996-99	2000-03	2004-06	Total
Healthcare Institution				
Hospital	3	10	7	**20**
Hospital Department		2		**2**
Primary Care		1	1	**2**
Private Care		1	3	**4**
Other		2	5	**7**
Total	**3**	**16**	**16**	**35**
Healthcare Information System				
EPR/EMR/CPR	5	14	15	**34**
Prescription		2	1	**3**
Consultation			1	**1**
Total	**5**	**16**	**17**	**38**
Portal/Internet Access				
Healthcare professionals		1	1	**2**
Patients		1		**1**
Total		**2**	**1**	**3**
User groups				
Medical doctors		2	2	**4**
Nurses		3	2	**5**
Patients		1	4	**5**
Others (HPs,GPs,IT,Pharmacists)	2	13	9	**24**
Total	**2**	**19**	**17**	**38**

Most of the information systems are EMR (34 from 38 articles) and were implemented within hospitals (20 from 35 articles). The end users of the system are mostly healthcare professionals (HPs), general practitioners (GPs), IT and pharmacists. Only in 5 articles is it mentioned that patients might have access to their healthcare information but none of these systems were being used in a real environment.

Table 4 shows the usability problems that were encountered as described in the published articles.

Table 4. Usability problems that were encountered.

Problem type	No of occurrences
Educational Barriers	5
Disruption to workflow & performance	7
Relational Barriers	1
Increase in time for patient session	1
Security concerns	1
Cultural barriers	2
Management problems	4

During the last ten years the 3 countries with more publications in this particular area were the USA with 15, UK with 10 and Greece with 7.

5. Discussion

The main observation from the first two tables was that the results were very similar and access control in healthcare reflects what is happening generally concerning access control in information systems.

Both reviews showed that there is a great interest in defining and studying access control models. However, without a proper access control policy definition, a model cannot be properly implemented and configured, and will never accurately represent both the organization and users' needs in terms of access control. Still, this kind of academic modelling approach works because the vast majority of the models were not implemented in practice. They are analysed as models or, at most, implemented as prototypes. Proper system evaluation is needed before one can conclude that these models are either appropriate or effective.

The preference for using RBAC as the starting point to build an access control model can be explained by the fact that this model allows easier administration and more flexibility in order to be adapted to the workflow and hierarchical needs of a heterogeneous organization.

In terms of authentication mechanisms, the most studied was digital signatures with public key certificates in a Public Key Infrastructure (PKI). Similar results were obtained from both the healthcare domain and the general domain. The use of PKI is extremely complex and usually requires expensive resources, both in terms of manpower expertise and software. At the time the articles under review were written (mostly prior to 2004) PKI systems had not been widely implemented and used in real and complex healthcare scenarios such as public hospitals and other large organizations where resources are usually scarce. After 2004 we could find only one study where PKI was implemented in a real healthcare scenario, but not within an EMR [18]. This study describes a web-based system to access healthcare brain injury information in a regional area. They use digital certificates for authentication. Although this kind of approach deemed to be successful the researchers concluded also that certificates' management is time consuming and requires a strong technical infrastructure and human resources that require continuous monitoring.

Nevertheless, the situation today is changing, although these later developments are not usually reported in research articles. Several national PKI systems have been rolled out, for example, the US Federal PKI system [19], and the Italian identity card system [20], whilst several national healthcare PKI systems now exist e.g. in the UK [21] and Australia [22]. But there is little published research about them.

From this review we found that most healthcare information systems that need access control are EMR systems built within heterogeneous and complex organizations such as hospitals. EMR is becoming more available because its advantages are well acknowledged [13]. However, according to the review, access control policies and models in EMR are usually not implemented and used in real life environments. Some national health services have started to work on such services, e.g. the UK NHS [23], but they are not fully implemented yet.

From those which were implemented within a real setting the end users of the system did not participate in its development and, most of the time did not support its introduction and use [13]. It is also relevant to note that none of the access control systems used within the EMR and in a real environment were being accessed by patients. This situation does not appear to be any better in the national systems that are currently under development, since the patients are not even being informed that their records will be held electronically in these systems, let alone be invited to participate in the design [24]. According to the European legislation [25] patients should be able to access their medical information whenever they request and in an understandable format. Several studies refer to the importance of the benefits to be gained from patients accessing their medical records [26], [27], [28]. However, only one of the analyzed studies [29] provided patients with access to their information, this being via an Internet portal prototype. Again, both healthcare professionals and patients did not participate in the development of this access control system, even though the system focused on patients' access to medical information with the objective of providing for their needs and subsequent healthcare support.

Most access control policies and systems are implemented following legal and institutional requirements. Littlejohns' study [30] shows very clearly the practical problems of implementing information systems within hospitals. According to Littlejohns, the problems arise due to not ensuring that the end users of the system knew why and how the system was being implemented, and for not recognising that education is an extremely important factor to take into account prior to systems' implementation. Further, the complexity of healthcare tasks and processes was underestimated and therefore could not be modelled accordingly. Miller's study [5] analysed the most important barriers to the successful integration of EMR within healthcare practice and found that there were many difficulties with the technology as well as the need for complementary changes and support to be implemented in order to use EMR. These increased the time and costs of implementation while at the same time reduced physicians' use of EMR and consequently the improvement in quality that had been expected. The study also concluded that most physicians needed to spend a great deal of time customizing their electronic forms and had to redesign their workflow processes to use the EMR. Miller et al believe that some of these problems can be reduced with the definition of both public and private policies that can better adapt EMR functionalities, including security, to the needs of its users.

Hackos [31] conclude that the development and implementation of similar projects must start with a realization and understanding of the following: the precise purposes for creating a system; the people who will use the system; what tasks the system will be used for; and where and how the users will use the system. In this way, users' more specific needs such as workflow processes and activities as well as cultural issues will also be taken into account and modelled.

6. Conclusion

Despite the benefits of EMR, there are some barriers (that may include access control systems) that hinder users from fully taking advantage of them and improving their workflow patterns.

Although access control is a security service that has been widely studied and applied in healthcare systems such as EMR, the fact is that the most interested parties, the users (both healthcare professionals and patients), are not usually consulted when the access control policies are integrated into these systems, and when the system is integrated within their workflow environments. Healthcare professionals usually needed to change their workflow patterns and adapt their tasks and processes in order to use the systems.

We believe that if healthcare professionals and patients support and participate in the access control systems' development process and the access control policy definition then some of problems described above can be minimized ensuring that EMR can be more effectively used in order to provide for better healthcare.

Future work that we propose to undertake includes the development of an access control policy that can incorporate all the stakeholders' needs and views regarding access control (including healthcare professionals and patients) and a further definition of an access control model that can effectively represent these policy rules. We will then proceed with the implementation and evaluation of this access control model within a real healthcare scenario in order to assess whether the improvement in access control systems within EMR, according to the users' needs and workflow patterns, can reduce some of the barriers to the effective use of EMR and therefore provide better healthcare and patient treatment.

References

[1] CERT Coordination Center CMU. CERT/CC Overview Incident and Vulnerability Trends. Carnegie Mellon University; 2003.
[2] Gollman D. Computer Security. 1st ed: John Wiley & Sons; 1999.
[3] Knitz M. HIPPA compliance and electronic medical records: are both possible? . Graduate research report: Bowie State University. Maryland in Europe; 2005.
[4] Sprague L. Electronic health records: How close? How far to go? NHPF Issue Brief. 2004 Sep 29(800):1-17.
[5] Miller RH, Sim I. Physicians' use of electronic medical records: barriers and solutions. Health Aff (Millwood). 2004 Mar-Apr;23(2):116-26.
[6] Becker MY, Sewell P. Cassandra: flexible trust management, applied to electronic health records. 2004; 2004. p. 139-54.
[7] Harris S. CISSP All-in-One Exam Guide. 2nd ed: McGraw-Hill Osborne Media; 2003.
[8] Schneier B. Secrets and Lies: digital security in a networked world: Wiley; 2004.
[9] Blobel B. Authorisation and access control for electronic health record systems. Int J Med Inform. 2004 Mar 31;73(3):251-7.
[10] ISO – International Organization for Standardization. ISO 7498-2: Information processing systems - Open Systems Interconnection - Basic Reference Model - Part 2: Security Architecture. 1989.
[11] Waegemann C. EHR vs. CPR vs. EMR. Healthcare Informatics online. 2003 May 2003.

[12] Cruz-Correia R, Vieira-Marques P, Costa P, Ferreira A, Oliveira-Palhares E, Araújo F, et al. Integration of Hospital data using Agent Technologies – a case study. AICommunications special issue of ECAI. 2005;18(3):191-200.

[13] Institute MR. 7th annual survey of electronic health record trends and usage for 2005. Medical Records Institute. 2005. Medical Records Institute: Medical Records Institute; 2005.

[14] Bakker A. Access to EHR and access control at a moment in the past: a discussion of the need and an exploration of the consequences. Int J Med Inform. 2004 Mar 31;73(3):267-70.

[15] Lehoux P. The Problem of Health Technology: Policy Implications for Modern Health Care. 1st ed: Routledge; 2006.

[16] Knitz M. HIPPA compliance and electronic medical records: are both possible? . Graduate research report: Bowie State University. Maryland in Europe; 2005.

[17] Miller RH, Hillman JM, Given RS. Physician use of IT: results from the Deloitte Research Survey. J Healthc Inf Manag. 2004 Winter;18(1):72-80.

[18] Lemaire E, Deforge D, Marshall S, Curran D. A secure web-based approach for accessing transitional health information for people with traumatic brain injury. Computer Methods and Programmes in Biomedicine. 2006; 213-219.

[19] Alterman P. The US federal PKI and the federal bridge certification authority. Federal PKI steering committee.2005. Available at: http://www.cendi.gov/presentations/alterman_pki_05-13-01.ppt. Acessed on the 20th March 2007.

[20] The Italian electronic identity card. The Italian Ministry of interior. Cybertrust. 2005. Available at: http://www.cybertrust.com/media/case_studies/cybertrust_cs_ital_1.pdf. Accessed on the 20th March 2007.

[21] PKI advaice for Caldicott Guardians & Delegate Authorities. NHS – NSTS phase 2b briefing paper. 2005.   Available   at: http://www.connectingforhealth.nhs.uk/nsts/docs/pki_advice_caldicott.pdf. Accessed on the 20th March 2007.

[22] Public Key Infrastructure (PKI) Security - About PKI. Australian government – Medicare Australia. 2007 Available at :   http://www.medicareaustralia.gov.au/vendors/security_technology/pki_security/ about_pki.shtml. Accessed on the 20th March 2007.

[23] Security   and   access   –   staff   access.   NHS   –   Department   of   Health.   Available   at: http://www.nhscarerecords.nhs.uk/nhs/security-and-access/staff-access. Accessed on the 20th March 2007.

[24] The British Medical Association is urging doctors to begin telling their patients about the new electronic   health   recordKable's   Government   Computing.   2006   Available   at: http://www.kablenet.com/kd.nsf/Frontpage/7A8A73686DE734478025722700554CFC?OpenDocument. Accessed on the 20th March 2007.

[25] Recommandation n° R (97) 5 relative à la Protection des Données Médicales. Comité des Ministres aux États Membres. 1997.

[26] Ross SE, Lin CT. The effects of promoting patient access to medical records: a review. J Am Med Inform Assoc 2003 May-Jun; 10 (3):294.

[27] Honeyman A, Cox B, Fisher B. Potential impacts of patient access to their electronic care records. Inform Prim Care. 2005;13(1):55-60.

[28] Ferreira A, Correia A, Silva A, Corte A, Pinto A, Saavedra A, Pereira A, Pereira AF, Cruz-Correia R, Antunes L. Why facilitate patient access to medical records. Studies in Health Technology and Informatics. 2007. (To be published).

[29] Masys D, Baker D, Butros A, Cowles K. Giving patients access to their medical records via the Internet: The PCASSO experience.

[30] Littlejohns P, Wyatt J, Garvican L. Evaluating computerised health information systems: hard lessons still to be learnt. BMJ. 2003;326:860-3.

[31] Hackos J, Redish J. User and Task Analysis for Interface Design 1st ed: Wiley; 1998.

Medical and Care Compunetics 4
L. Bos and B. Blobel (Eds.)
IOS Press, 2007

Why Facilitate Patient Access to Medical Records

Ana FERREIRA[a,b,d], Ana CORREIA[c], Ana SILVA[c], Ana CORTE[c], Ana PINTO[c],
Ana SAAVEDRA[c], Ana Luís PEREIRA[c], Ana Filipa PEREIRA[c],
Ricardo CRUZ-CORREIA[b,c] and Luís Filipe ANTUNES[d]
[a] *Computer Laboratory at the University of Kent*
[b] *CINTESIS – Center for research in health information Systems and technologies*
[c] *Biostatistics and Medical Informatics Dept. at the Faculty of Medicine in Porto*
[d] *LIACC – Faculty of Science of Porto*

Abstract. The wider use of healthcare information systems and the easier integration and sharing of patient clinical information can facilitate a wider access to medical records. The main goal of this paper is to perform a systematic review to analyze published work that studied the impact of facilitating patients' access to their medical record. Moreover, this review includes the analysis of the potential benefits and drawbacks on patient attitudes, doctor-patient relationship and on medical practice. In order to fill a gap in terms of the electronic medical record (EMR) impact within this issue, this review will focus on the use of EMR for patients to access their medical records as well as the advantages and disadvantages that this can bring. The articles included in the study were identified using MEDLINE and Scopus databases and revised according to their title and abstract and, afterwards, their full text was read considering inclusion and exclusion criteria. From the 165 articles obtained in MEDLINE a total of 12 articles were selected. From Scopus, 2 articles were obtained, so a total of 14 articles were included in the review. The studies revealed that patients' access to medical records can be beneficial for both patients and doctors, since it enhances communication between them whilst helping patients to better understand their health condition. The drawbacks (for instance causing confusion and anxiety to patients) seem to be minimal. However, patients continue to show concerns about confidentiality and understanding what is written in their records. The studies showed that the use of EMR can bring several advantages in terms of security solutions as well as improving the correctness and completeness of the patient records.

Keywords. Computerized, Medical Records, Patient Access to Records

Introduction

The wider use of healthcare Information Systems and the easier integration and sharing of patient clinical information can facilitate patients to access their own medical records. With the paper version only, there was the need to gather all the information into a single copy of the scattered medical record and patients had to obtain a formal authorization to access it [1].

According to the European legislation patients should be able to access their clinical information whenever they request and have means to control who can see and change that information [2]. However, this is still not common practice mostly because of logistic and also cultural issues. The general idea is that healthcare professionals think this may negatively affect their relationship with the patients whilst patients themselves do not know if they want to see their medical record and if they do, will it be helpful and will they understand it anyway.

Nevertheless, nowadays, patient access to paper records can be fairly common in some places. Countries like United Kingdom, New Zealand, Canada and USA have enacted legislation to ensure patient access to health records [3]. In 1996, it was stipulated by the HIPAA Act (Health Insurance Portability and Accountability Act) in the USA that patients must be able to access and get a copy of their medical records and correct them as needed [4].

Apart from some disadvantages already mentioned, Ross et al. [1] describes that patient access to medical records can facilitate doctor-patient relationship by enhancing doctor-patient communication, which allows the flow of information among them and helps reducing errors and improve quality. However, it can, at the same time, undermine the trust and so harm doctor-patient relationship.

If, on one hand this access can potentially bring some effects on the patients like improving satisfaction, autonomy or self-efficacy it can, on the other hand, cause confusion and anxiety [1,5]. Outside the health care sector, personal health records can influence many aspects of life, such as obtaining employment, life insurance or consumer credit [3].

The example of a scenario done within the UK NHS (National Health Service) introduced the opportunity of patients to get copies of their referral letters [6]. Although White et al. [6] claims that there has been little empirical research done in this area, with this case they expect patients to better understand their situation as well as improve doctor-patient relationship and the quality of medical information.

A review done in 2003 of published material that analysed the effects of promoting patient access to medical records concluded that the revised material consistently showed that it enhances doctor-patient communication [1]. Further, the patient satisfaction is high compared with very few records that found that patients were upset with what they saw.

This same review also indicated that the future is likely to involve EMR and future research will show if this technology will influence positively or negatively patient satisfaction, understanding or any other factor that would affect healthcare. Although EMR may be able to facilitate the access to clinical information by the patients the fact that it is sometimes fragmented across multiple treatment sites can pose an obstacle to clinical care, research and public health efforts [7] as well as security [8].

The objective of this paper is to perform a systematic review to analyze published work that studied the impact of facilitating patients' access to their medical record. Moreover, this review includes the analysis of the potential benefits and drawbacks on patient attitudes, doctor-patient relationship and on medical practice. In order to fill a gap in terms of the EMR impact within this issue, this review will focus on the use of EMR as well as the advantages and disadvantages that it can bring.

The next section presents the methods used for the review while Section 2 presents the most relevant results. Section 3 discusses those results and the last section gives some hints on what should be the trend to follow when facilitating or not patients' access to their medical records.

1. Participants and Methods

A systematic review based on articles written between 1990 and 2005 was performed. The dependent variable was *the effects on medical practice* and the independent variable was *patients having access to records*. The target population was adult patients and studies that gave parents access to paediatric records were excluded.

The articles were identified using MEDLINE and Scopus. The resulting query used in MEDLINE was ("Medical Records Systems, Computerized"[MeSH] OR "Medical Records"[MeSH]) AND "Patient Access to Records"[MeSH] NOT (pediatric[All Fields] AND ("records"[MeSH Terms] OR records[Text Word])) AND ("1990"[PDAT]: "2005"[PDAT]). As more medical records are being computerized the mesh term *Medical records systems, computerized* was added to analyse the access to records through computers. The publishing type *Review* was excluded as well as the parents' access to paediatric records, in order to focus the study in the impact of a patient reading their own records. In Scopus search, 3 queries were applied: ALL ("Medical Records Systems") AND ALL(Computerized) AND ALL("Patient Access to Records") AND PUBYEAR AFT 1990; ALL("Medical Records Systems") AND ALL(computerized) AND ALL("Patient Access") AND PUBYEAR AFT 1990; and ALL("Medical Records Systems") AND ALL(electronic medical record) AND ALL("Patient Access") AND PUBYEAR AFT 1990.

To increase the sensibility of the selection new rules were established. We included articles that analysed the effect of patients' accessing their medical records and also studied the consequences on patients, health care providers, medical practice and doctor patient relationship. The articles referring to the access of medical records through electronic files were also included. The languages selected were English, Portuguese, French and Spanish.

Excluded from this review were articles referring to specific cases that analysed the property of medical records, the patients' rights, judging cases, identification of gametes donators and legal documentation.

The articles were distributed by two groups of three people and each group read the titles and abstracts considering the established criteria.

Figure 1 shows the method used to select the articles for the review.

In a second step, the methodological quality of the articles was evaluated. In order to extract data from the articles we fragmented our main theme in 14 topics. Only 10 of these were explored: *Patient Interest and Acceptance, Confusion and Misunderstandings, Patient Education, Creating Anxiety, Providing Reassurance, Promoting Adherence, Concerns about Confidentiality, Improving Doctor-Patient Relationship, Correcting Errors, The Use of Electronic Medical records.*

Each article had a grade between 0 and 22 based on 6 criterions. The criterions taken into consideration were: (1) *Objective of the study* – if it fully coincides with ours it should be given 14 points; 0 points if it has nothing to do with it; and 1 point for each topic it referred; (2) *The kind of study* – if it was a letter or an editorial it should be given 3 points; (3) *Type of sampling* – 2 points were given for a randomized sample and 1 point for a non-randomized; (4) *Size of the sample* – if the article studied a sample of [0–50] people it should receive 0 points and if it studied a sample with more than 50 people it would get 1 point; (5) *Method used to collect data* – if it was considered appropriated for the conclusions we wanted to achieve it was given 1 point otherwise it should receive 0 points; (6) *Concordance between the results and the initial objective*

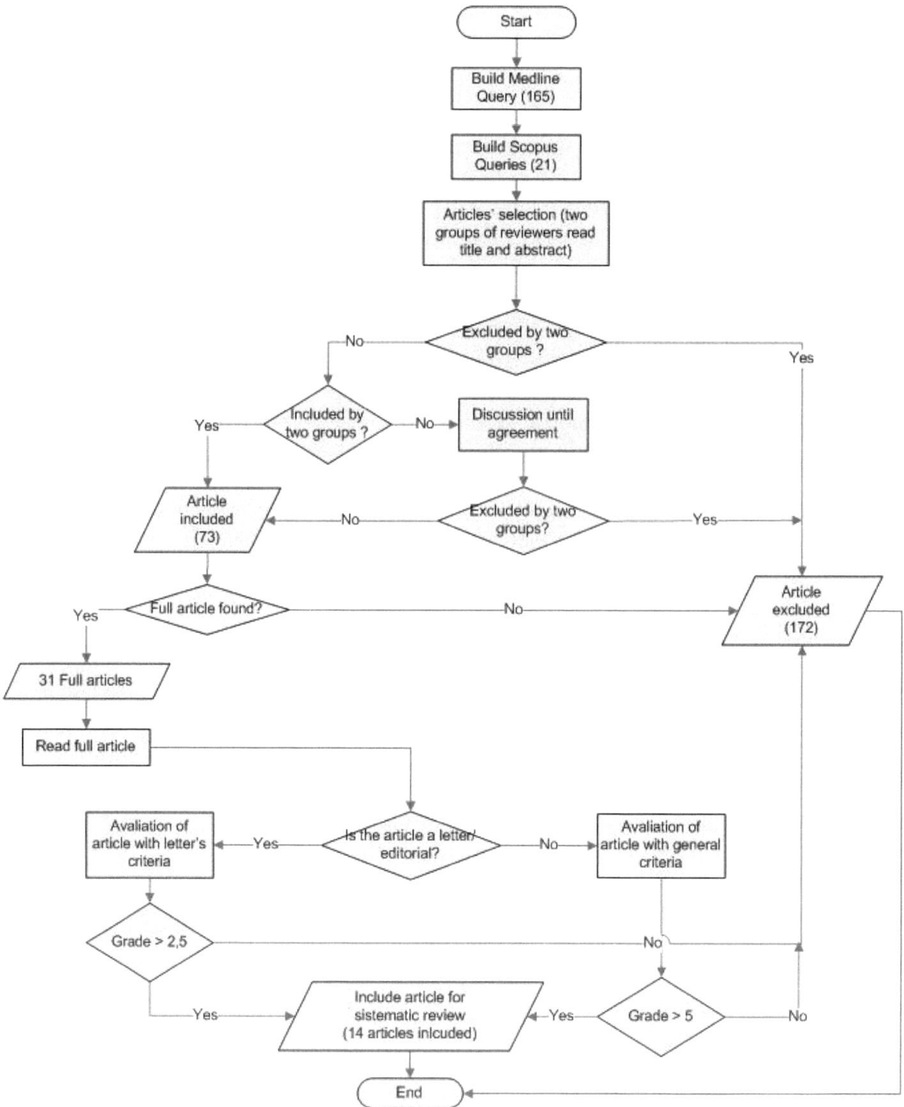

Figure 1. Method used for the systematic review.

of the study (objectivity of the study) – if there was concordance it should be given 1 point and if there was not any concordance it should be given 0 points.

After analysing all the articles and considering these criterions, we excluded the ones that received a grade inferior to 11.

As there were not many scientific studies available for the studied theme we decided to include letters and editorials in the review. For these, the last four criterions

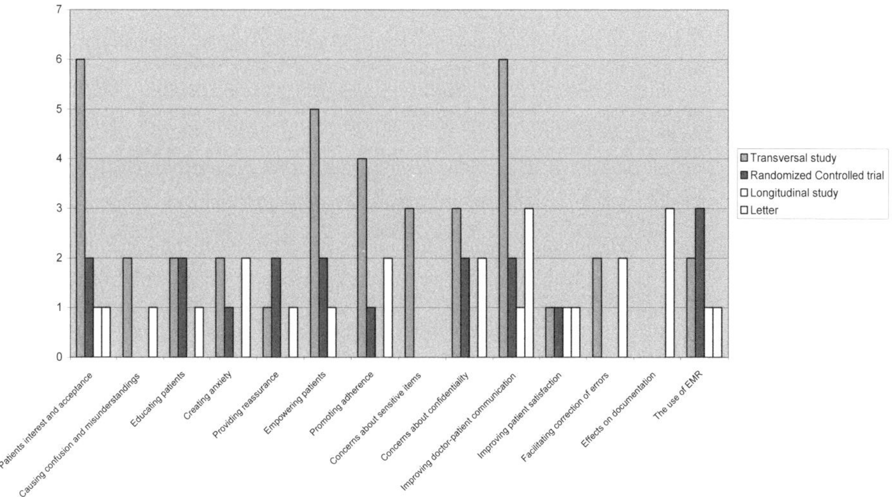

Figure 2. Number and type of articles referring each topic.

did not apply, so they were given a grade between 0 and 17. If they had a grade superior or equal to 6 they were included. This means that a letter or editorial to be included had to mention at least 4 topics (Table 1 – Appendix).

2. Results

2.1. Search and Selection of the Articles

From 165 articles obtained in MEDLINE search queries, 52 were selected after titles and abstracts were read. Then 22 full articles were found and analyzed considering the quality criterions explained in the previous section. From these 10 were excluded. A total of 12 articles were included from the MEDLINE search.

On Scopus a total of 21 articles were obtained. From these only 9 were included and we managed to get 3 full articles. The quality criteria selected only 2.

A total of 14 articles have been reviewed to write this paper.

2.2. Data Extraction

As described before, in order to extract data our main theme was subdivided in 14 topics. Figure 2 shows the number and type of article that mention each topic.

The results presented in this section refer to only 10 of those 14 topics. *The Effects on documentation, empowering patients, concerns about sensitive items* and *improving patient satisfaction* were not analyzed. Table 1 presents the articles that mention each one of the topics.

Table 1. Number of articles that referred each one of the 10 studied topics

Topics	No of Articles	
	YES	NO
Patient interest and acceptance	5 [5] [10] [12] [20] [21]	1 [14]
Confusion and misunderstandings	3 [15] [16] [21]	
Patient education	2 [4] [17]	
Creating anxiety	1 [15]	4 [4] [5] [10] [16]
Providing reassurance	2 [10] [17]	
Promoting adherence	1 [7]	1 [11]
Concerns about confidentiality	3 [4] [5] [17]	
Improving doctor-patient relationship	2 [4] [17]	
Correcting errors	1 [19]	
The use of Electronic Medical Records	8 [4] [5] [7] [9] [11] [12] [17] [21]	1 [10]

The following section describes in more detail the results obtained for each topic.

2.3. Patient Experience with Access to Medical Records

2.3.1. Patient Interest and Acceptance

In a study with cancer patients, 91% of the patients declined the offer to see their medical records and the reasons given were: they trust totally on what the doctor had told them, they think that they knew enough or they would not understand it anyway [14]. The ones that inspected their medical records affirmed they did not obtain any new information and believed that any questions they might have could be answered by the clinical nurse or doctor.

Although the situation referred above presents us a very strong percentage of people who refused the access to their medical records, the interest of patients in seeing their records is generally high [5,10]. This is revealed by the answers of the patients that were asked about shared records in general, and about shared records online, in particular [20]. 95% of the patients agreed with the statement: "Overall, I think it is a good idea for patients to be able to routinely review their outpatient medical records". It is also confirmed by this study that the interest was age dependent reducing steadily from 95% for those aged 21–30, down to 68% for those aged 71 and over. Most patients knew that they had the right to access their records and control those accesses although only 5% had actually accessed them.

Some studies have demonstrated that patients' interest in accessing their medical records was related with factors such as: general concern about health, independency of health status, interest in health information, concerns about patient safety, having a less trusting relationship with their primary physician and also the desire to be more involved in their own care [10,21]. Ross et al. [11] showed that interest was not, however, health status or health care use related nor was it education or income related. This same study concludes that a vast majority of patients endorse the concept of patient-accessible medical records and about half support online access. This survey further demonstrates that these attitudes are shared even by patients in ethnically diverse and socio-economically disadvantaged populations. Focusing the access to the medical records via Internet, this study also revealed through a multivariate analysis that demographic features such as age, gender, race and education did not influence the interest in online patient-accessible records. The primary predictor was previous experience with the Internet, followed by expectations of the benefits and drawbacks of reading the medical record.

Other studies have concluded that patients who have looked at their medical record in the past remain interested in reading it [10,11]. Patients who did not know that they had the legal right to inspect their records were more than twice as likely to be very interested in reading their record [9]. Another aspect revealed was that women are more interested in accessing their medical records than men.

Other findings were that patients were more interested in seeing their laboratory results followed by the physician's notes [10,12]. Patients were least interested in seeing past medication [10]. Most of the patients were interested in reading their medical record at regular intervals but not very frequently.

2.3.2. Confusion and Misunderstandings

Some studies have revealed that incomprehensible jargon or pejorative comments will understandably confuse or distress the patients [15,16]. This was an argument used many times in order to keep the medical records secret.

Another study refers that patients of community health centers were more likely to be confused by various parts of the medical record and also embarrassed or offended bydoctors' notes, in comparison with academic primary care clinical patients [21].

2.3.3. Patient Education

The articles collected refer that in the majority of the cases an advantage to access the medical records is patients' education. The access to the records helps patients to understand their health condition as well as what the doctor thinks [4,17].

Patients who had access to their electronic medical records improved their own knowledge about their disease and increased the sense of ownership of their health care. This fact helped them to be more involved in their treatment and increased their ability to coordinate their care. It also allowed them to confirm the doses of medications and to provide laboratory results or medical information to other doctors. This has promoted patients' sense of personalized support and capacity to look up their results [10,12].

A disadvantage referred by some patients is the difficulty to understand medical records because of the use of technical language.

2.3.4. Creating Anxiety

Although seeing their medical records can cause patients some anxiety or upsetting at times [15], recent studies and letters demonstrated that this is, in a vast majority of the cases, not true [4,5,10].

Recent experiences with patients who had access to their own records showed that doctors and patients considered the experience positive and did not cause any kind of anxiety or upset [16].

Psychiatric patients may respond less favourably than other patients. In spite of causing distress in a short term, in a longer term the access to records may be therapeutic. In a transversal study using adult psychiatric patients who had access to a written clinical summary about themselves, only 28% of the patients were upset with what they had read and 51% rated the written assessment as having provided helpful information [15].

2.3.5. Providing Reassurance

After reading and understanding what their doctor wrote about their health treatment the patients felt more reassured about their disease or health condition [10].

Patients felt reassured and more relaxed because their records gave them clear ideas about their health condition [17].

2.3.6. Promoting Adherence

In agreement with an American study based in the analysis of the American legislation about this theme, the simple fact of opening access to medical records can improve patients' adherence to treatment, the efficiency of the service and strengthen the role of the profession [7]. A descriptive article about adherence shows that patients' interest in viewing records increases after one interview which explains the objectives or the consequences of that access. In these cases, patients change their life style. They try to be more careful in order to follow medical recommendations.

However, a randomized controlled trial study revealed that the access to an informatics' program that provides patients' access to their clinical notes did not result in any significant differences in their health status, clinic visits or hospitalizations but increased in 31% the messages sent to the system. The patients can have more interest in accessing their medical records but that does not mean that they will, most of the times, change their way of life [11].

2.3.7. Concerns About Confidentiality

When patients were questioned about electronic access to their medical records they were worried about the security of some sensitive items. Although they find the inclusion of these items appropriate, they also think that they could be identified by a code [5].

In a randomized controlled trial several individuals voiced theoretical concerns about the security of their online records and were particularly concerned that their records could become available to employers or government agencies without their permission, although many did not mind sharing the records with close family members [17].

In another study, 24% of the patients expressed concerns about the confidentiality of their medical records which included the ability of others to get into the system where the health records were available. They did not trust the staff people and did not know how the system worked, which caused insecurity [4].

2.4. Effects on Doctor-Patient Relationship

2.4.1. Improving Doctor-Patient Relationship

In a transversal study, over 75% of the respondents stated that having access to their notes would break down the barriers between them and the doctor and give information which one was not sure about. Over 70% felt it would give them more confidence in the doctor and over 65% felt it would help them to understand their condition and feel that their doctor understood them. 67% of the patients disagreed that it would give them less confidence in their doctor [4].

In another study the majority of patients and doctors were unanimous in their belief that the impact of the access to electronic health records was positive for both and improved the level of communication between them [17].

2.5. Effects on Medical Practice

2.5.1. Correcting Errors

Although patient accessible medical records offer them the opportunity to correct errors within the record, patients may also introduce errors if they make unauthorized additions or deletions to the medical record.

The utility of auditing and of patients being able to correct their computer held records has been shown in several studies, including studies of administrative records in hospitals, outpatients clinics and general practice.

In general practice, 24% of the patients said that there were mistakes, 30% found omissions within their medical record including allergies, dates of birth, addresses, current drug treatments, items on the problem list, smoking details, height, weight, alcohol history and family history [19].

2.6. The Use of Electronic Medical Records

In eight of the fourteen selected articles the patients were given access to their electronic medical records [4,5,7,9,11,12,17,21].

In some randomized clinical trials patients and doctors were given access to health records through the internet and electronic systems [11,12,17]. In the end, the majority of patients and doctors found this kind of systems easy to use, useful and considered that it can improve their communication with health care providers and their health care quality.

In another randomized clinical trial the patients were given access to their electronic records in the waiting room through a secure access system that used fingerprint recognition technology [4]. When these patients were asked how interested they were in seeing their electronic records, a mean of 8.05 was obtained (in a scale of 0 to 10). Some of the patients said why they were interested on accessing electronic records: "not taking up anyone's time", "no bother for anyone" and "can just come in and sit down (at the computer)". 41 patients were asked if they were interested in looking at their electronic records over the internet: 18 said they were very interested and 14 not interested at all. Some of them even added the comment: "do not think it should happen at all".

56% of the patients agreed with the statement "Overall, I think it's a good idea for patients to be able to review their outpatient medical records using the Internet", meaning that about half of the patients support online access [21]. This study also concluded that previous experience with Internet, expectations of the benefits and drawbacks of accessing their medical records were the primary predictors of an interest in online patient-accessible records.

In another study, patients were divided in terms of the preferred mode of access to medical records: through a paper copy of their medical record (49.3%) or through an electronic version at a secure, private web site (43.8%) [10].

In an editorial was said that by allowing patients interaction with the EMR physicians have much more accurate and up-to-date information for managing therapy [20]. However, there are still certain problems with access that must be overcome, such as ensuring privacy of personal medical data and determining the ways in which patients should be able to influence their charts.

3. Limitations

Our review presents some limitations such as: not all the studies included in the review were randomized trials and, in general, their sample size was small. Most studies did not use standardized methods and the number of full articles found to include in the review was not very high. As the number of scientific articles found was quite reduced, we decided to include letters and editorials, which usually do not comprise the quality of a scientific study.

4. Discussion

Overall, the studies revealed that patients' access to medical records is beneficial both for patients and doctors, since it enhances communication between them whilst helping patients to better understand their health condition.

Accessing medical records has also shown improvements on patients' education, a better knowledge of the disease and more participation in their health treatment. Improvements on adherence made patients more careful in following medical recommendations and provided for self-empowerment. It allowed them more autonomy and self-efficacy by increasing a sense of ownership to their medical records.

However, patients find some parts of the medical records difficult to understand because some notes are unintelligible or illegible to them. The access to medical records helps correcting errors and omissions but patients can also make unauthorized additions or deletions. The use of EMR can facilitate this process, so patients' actions on their medical record must be ruled, monitored and controlled.

The EMR raises several concerns about the security of sensitive items and confidentiality of the records. Some suggest the use of codes to identify sensitive items. As for confidentiality the possibility that technology gives for using security or any other security device reassures patients. The use of EMR also implies previous technological knowledge, which can be a problem, especially for older people.

Nevertheless, the EMR makes it possible to solve some of the problems concerning the access to medical records, such as understanding doctor calligraphy. It can also reduce data errors by increasing the opportunities of patients to access their medical records as well as providing mechanisms to control the access, validate and correct information.

5. Conclusion

Most patients and healthcare professionals seem to be unanimous in their belief that the impact of patients' access to their medical record is positive for both.

Not only are there some real benefits in the patient accessing his/her medical record but also new technologies can help improving and supporting this access.

We agree that the EMR can bring some security solutions as well as the possibility of improving both the quality and completeness of the record allowing, therefore, for better treatment and trust in healthcare by the patients.

This review stresses the importance and need for this kind of study to be further pursued and done in a regular basis. It can also be used as a future platform for research in this area.

Acknowledgements

We would like to thank class 2 of the 1st year medical students from the 2005/2006 academic year at the Biostatistics and Medical Informatics Department of the Faculty of Medicine of Porto for their work and enthusiasm in the development of this project.

References

[1] Ross SE, Lin CT. The effects of promoting patient access to medical records: a review. J Am Med Inform Assoc 2003 May–Jun; 10(3):294.

[2] Recommendation No. R (97) 5 of the Committee of Ministers to Member States on the Protection of Medical Data. Council of Europe – Committee of Ministers. 1997.

[3] Carter M. Should patients have access to their medical records? Med J Aust 1998; 169:596–597.

[4] Honeyman A, Cox B, Fisher B. Potential impacts of patient access to their electronic care records. Inform Prim Care. 2005; 13(1):55–60.

[5] Pyper C, Amery J, Watson M, Crook C. Access to electronic health records in primary care – a survey of patients' view. Med Sci Monit, 2004; 10(11):SR17–22.

[6] White P. Copying referral letters to patients: prepare for change. Patient Educ Couns. 2004 Aug; 54(2):159–61.

[7] Mandl KD, Szolovitz P, Kohan IS. Public standards and patients' control: keep electronic medical records accessible but private. BJM 2001 Jun 2; 322 (7298):1368–9.

[8] Bakker A. Access to EHR and access control at a moment in the past: a discussion of the need and an exploration of the consequences. Int J Med Inform. 2004 Mar 31; 73(3):267–70.

[9] Winkelman WJ, Leonard KJ, Rossos PG. Patient-perceived usefulness of online electronic medical records: employing grounded theory in the development of information and communication technologies for use by patients living with chronic illness. J Am Med Inform Assoc. 2005 May–Jun; 12(3):306–14. Epub 2005 Jan 31.

[10] Fowles JB, Kind AC, Craft C, Kind EA, Mandel JL, Adlis S. Patients' interest in reading their medical record: relation with clinical and sociodemographic characteristics and patients' approach to health care. Arch Intern Med. 2004 Apr 12; 164(7):793–800.

[11] Ross S, Lin CT. A randomized controlled trial of a patient-accessible electronic medical record. AMIA Annu Symp Proc. 2003; 990.

[12] Cimino JJ, Patel VL, Kushniruk AW. The patient clinical information system (PatCIS): technical solutions for and experience with giving patients access to their electronic medical records. Int J Med Inform. 2002 Dec 18; 68(1–3):113–27.

[13] Warden J. Patients to see medical records. BMJ. 1991 Sep 7; 303(6802):538. e.

[14] Rostom AY, Gershuny AR. Access to patient records. Lancet. 1991 Nov 23; 338(8778):1337–8.

[15] Bernadt M, Gunning L, Quenstedt M. Patients' access to their own psychiatric records. BMJ. 1991 Oct 19; 303(6808):967.

[16] McLaren P. The right to know.BMJ. 1991 Oct 19; 303(6808):937–8.

[17] Earnest MA, Ross SE, Wittevrongel L, Moore LA, Lin CT. Use of a patient-accessible electronic medical record in a practice for congestive heart failure: patient and physician experiences. J Am Med Inform Assoc. 2004 Sep–Oct; 11(5):410–7. E pub 2004 Jun 7.

[18] Jones R, Cawsey A, Bental D, Pearson J. How should we evaluate patient access to their own records? An example with cancer patients in Scotland. Stud Health Technol Inform. 2003; 95:152–7.

[19] Jones R. Patient access to records must be acceptable to both parties. BMJ. 2001 Jun 2; 322(7298): 1368–9.

[20] Ross, S.E., Todd, J., Moore, L.A., Beaty, B.L., Wittevrongel, L., Lin, C.-T. Expectations of patients and physicians regarding patient-accessible medical records (2005) Journal of Medical Internet Research.

[21] Tsai, C.C., Starren, J.Patient participation in electronic medical records (2001) Journal of the American Medical Association 285 (13), p. 1765.

Appendix Table 1. Articles included with the Relevance/Quality criteria

Articles	Objective (14)	Kind of study (3)	Type of sample (2)	Size of sample (1)	Methods of data extraction (1)	Objectivity (1)	Total	Exclusion/ inclusion
AHIMA e-HIM Personal Health Record Work Group. Practice brief. The role of the personal health record in the EHR. J AHIMA.	0	–	–	–	–	–	0	E
[4] **Honeyman A, Cox B, Fisher B.** Potential impacts of patient access to their electronic care records. Inform Prim Care.	5	3	2	1	0	1	12	I
Waegemann CP. Closer to reality. Personal health records represent a step in the right direction for interoperability of healthcare IT systems and accessibility of patient data. Health Manag Technol.	0	–	–	–	–	–	0	E
[9] **Winkelman WJ, Leonard KJ, Rossos PG.** Patient-perceived usefulness of online electronic medical records: employing grounded theory in the development of information and communication technologies for use by patients living with chronic illness. J Am Med Inform Assoc.	4	3	1	1	1	1	11	I
[5] **Pyper C, Amery J, Watson M, Crook C.** Access to electronic health records in primary care-a survey of patients' views. Med Sci Monit.	9	3	2	1	1	1	17	I
Hassol A, Walker JM, Kidder D, Rokita K, Young D, Pierdon S, Deitz D, Kuck S, Ortiz E. Patient experiences and attitudes about access to a patient electronic health care record and linked web messaging. J Am Med Inform Assoc.	0	–	–	–	–	–	0	E
[10] **Fowles JB, Kind AC, Craft C, Kind EA, Mandel JL, Adlis S.** Patients' interest in reading their medical record: relation with clinical and sociodemographic characteristics and patients' approach to health care.	5	3	2	1	1	1	13	I

Appendix Table 1. (Continued.)

Articles	Objective (14)	Kind of study (3)	Type of sample (2)	Size of sample (1)	Methods of data extraction (1)	Objectivity (1)	Total	Exclusion/ inclusion
[11] **Ross S, Lin CT.** A randomized controlled trial of a patient-accessible electronic medical record.AMIA Annu Symp Proc.	8	3	2	1	1	1	16	I
Jones TM. Patient participation in EHR benefits. Health Manag Technol.	0						0	E
[12] **Cimino JJ, Patel VL, Kushniruk AW.** The patient clinical information system (PatCIS): technical solutions for and experience with giving patients access to their electronic medical records. Int J Med Inform.	5	3	1	0	1	1	11	I
Hughes G; American Health Information Management Association. Practice brief. Patient access and amendment to health records. J AHIMA.	0	–	–	–	–	–	0	E
Dyer C. Patient denied right to see medical records. BMJ.	0	–	–	–	–	–	0	E
[No authors listed] What's in my record? Lancet.	1	2	–	–	–	–	3	E
[13] **Warden J.** Patients to see medical records. BMJ.	4	2	–	–	–	–	6	I
British Medical Association. Patients' rights to see records. BMJ.	0	–	–	–	–	–	0	E
Jones R. Patient access to records must be acceptable to both parties. BMJ.	2	2	–	–	–	–	4	E
[14] **Rostom AY, Gershuny AR.** Access to patient records. Lancet.	4	3	1	1	1	1	11	I
[15] **Bernadt M, Gunning L, Quenstedt M.** Patients' access to their own psychiatric records.BMJ.	5	3	1	1	0	1	11	I

Appendix Table 1. (Continued.)

Articles	Objective (14)	Kind of study (3)	Type of sample (2)	Size of sample (1)	Methods of data extraction (1)	Objectivity (1)	Total	Exclusion/ inclusion
[16] **McLaren P.** The right to know. BMJ.	7	2	–	–	–	–	9	I
Reuler JB, Balazs JR. Portable medical record for the homeless mentally ill. BMJ.	0	–	–	–	–	–	0	E
[17] **Earnest MA, Ross SE, Wittevrongel L, Moore LA, Lin CT.** Use of a patient-accessible electronic medical record in a practice for congestive heart failure: patient and physician experiences. J Am Med Inform Assoc.	8	3	1	1	1	1	15	I
[18] **Jones R, Cawsey A, Bental D, Pearson J.** How should we evaluate patient access to their own records? An example with cancer patients in Scotland. Stud Health Technol Inform.	5	3	1	1	1	0	11	I
Ross, S.E., Todd, J., Moore, L.A., Beaty, B.L., Wittevrongel, L., Lin, C.-T. Expectations of patients and physicians regarding patient-accessible medical records (2005) Journal of Medical Internet Research	9	3	1	1	1	1	16	I
[20] **Tsai, C.C., Starren, J.** Patient participation in electronic medical records (2001) Journal of the American Medical Association 285 (13), p. 1765.	7	2	0	0	0	1	10	I
[21] **Kim, M.I., Johnson, K.B.** Personal health records: Evaluation of functionality and utility (2002) Journal of the American Medical Informatics Association	3	3	1	0	0	1	8	E

Medical and Care Compunetics 4
L. Bos and B. Blobel (Eds.)
IOS Press, 2007

91

The Value of Information for Decision-Making in the Healthcare Environment

Itamar SHABTAI[a] Ph.D., Moshe LESHNO[b] M.D., Ph.D.,
Orna BLONDHEIM[c] M.D. and Jonathan KORNBLUTH[d] Ph.D.
[a]*College of Management Academic Studies*
[b]*Tel Aviv University*
[c]*Clalit Healthcare Services – HMO*
[d]*Hebrew University of Jerusalem*

Abstract. With their ever-growing importance and usability, the healthcare sector has been investing heavily in medical information systems in recent years, as part of the effort to improve medical decision-making and increase its efficiency through improved medical processes, reduced costs, integration of patients' data, etc. In light of these developments, this research aims to evaluate the contribution of information technology (IT) to improving the medical decision-making processes at the point of care of internal medicine and surgical departments and to evaluate the degree to which IT investments are worthwhile.

This has been done by assessing the value of information to decision-makers (physicians) at the point of care by investigating whether the information systems improved the medical outcomes. The research included three steps (after a pilot study) – the assessment of the subjective value of information, the assessment of the realistic value of information, and the assessment of the normative value of information, the results of each step being used as the starting assumptions for the following steps. Following a discussion and integration of the results from the various steps, the results of the three assessment stages were summarized in a cost-effectiveness analysis and an overall return on investment (ROI) analysis. In addition, we tried to suggest IT strategies for decision-makers in the healthcare sector on the advisability of implementing such systems as well as the implications for managing them.

This research is uniquely pioneering in the manner in which it combines an assessment of the three kinds of measures of value of information in the healthcare environment. Our aim in performing it was to contribute to researchers (by providing additional insight into the fields of decision theory, value of information and medical informatics, amongst others), practitioners (by promoting efficiency in the design of new medical IS and improving existing IS), physicians (by enhancing the efficient use of information resources), patients (by improving healthcare services) and policy decision-makers in the healthcare sector (regarding the advisability of investments in such systems and suggestions for managing them).

Keywords. Medical Informatics, Patient Record Access, Medical Decision-Making, Value of Information

Introduction

The information revolution of the last few decades has brought about a massive adoption of information technology by organizations of all types and in all sectors of the economy, with the aim of reducing the uncertainty of decision-makers and improving the decision-making process. In fulfilling their function of supporting decision-making, information systems perform tasks such as collecting, organizing, processing and analyzing data reflecting the organization's activities. The information they provide is a critical resource that has significant impact on the outcomes of managerial decision-making [1].

However, information in itself is not the panacea of all ills. Indeed, one of today's main problems is information overload, and one of the most important issues in the area of research dealing with organizational information systems is assessing the value of information [2,3]. Understanding the importance of assessing the value of information and developing methods which provide the ability to assess the value of information can improve the processes of planning, designing, developing, building and managing of decision support systems (DSS).

Information technologies today are considered critical to the operational, managerial and strategic levels of the organization. They play a significant role in managing healthcare systems. Hospitals and health service providers aim to provide their customers with qualitative healthcare services and at the same time to be efficient and to optimally cope with complicated and varying environments and activities [4]. In order to provide the proper level of service, as well as to survive and compete, they need to use information efficiently.

Today, with the huge amounts of medical data and information and the growing number of medical information systems, there is an increasing need for medical information that is complete, homogeneous, precise, updated, reliable and accessible at the point of care. Information based on the historical medical data of the patient collected in real time from all relevant internal and external sources can be the basis for an optimal decision-making process [5]. This information is essential to insure the quality of the medical care process and healthcare service and it needs to be provided effectively and efficiently utilizing all the sophisticated techniques for collecting, browsing and presenting data that today's information technology has to offer.

This study deals with point of care information systems (POC IS) intended to improve physicians' decision-making.

Objectives

This study aimed to assess the contribution of information technology (IT) in improving the decision-making process in the medical environment and to examine the benefits of IT investments in the healthcare environment. In so doing, it assessed the value of information provided to the decision makers (physicians) at the point of care and checked whether the information systems improved the outcomes of the decision-makers.

Method

The assessment of the value of information was carried out in three steps using the methods common in the information systems research area – assessing subjective value of information, realistic value, and normative value.

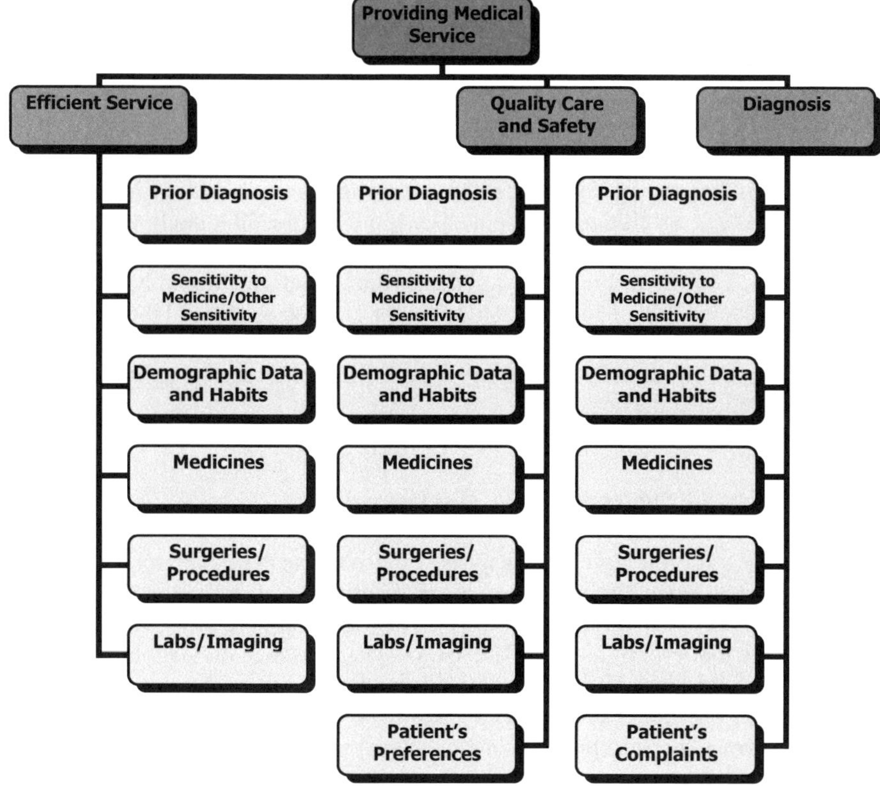

Figure 1. The Hierarchical Model.

The study was conducted on a sample group of physicians representing two different areas of specialization – surgeons and specialists in internal medicine, and two different levels of seniority and experience – experts and juniors. All of the subjects use the dbMotion system installed at hospitals belonging to the largest HMO in Israel, which covers all historical information about the patient from all points at which treatment has been received and documented in the HMO's information systems. The system was first adopted in the hospital sector and then in the community sector. This research focused on the hospital sector because it was the first to install the system and is now beyond the run-in period.

This research included three steps (after a pilot study):

1. Assessing the subjective value of information.
2. Assessing the realistic value of information.
3. Assessing the normative value of information.

The results of each step were used as the starting assumptions for the following steps. The pilot study carried out in the pre-test stage aimed at making an initial examination of the system in order to understand and estimate the extent and frequency of its use and the information it supplied. The pilot study also helped develop the hierarchical model (Fig. 1) which was used to determine the main mission, objectives and criteria of the physicians' actions at the point of care, and to identify which pieces of information were essential for them. This hierarchical model was the basis for the first step of the research – assessing the subjective value of information. The pilot study's method was based on semi-structured interviews with a sample of three interest groups associated with the system: (i) key users of the system, such as physicians and department managers; (ii) employees of the HMO who were involved in the planning, designing and developing of the system and who were responsible for its implementation (such as the CIO, the head of the steering committee, the project manager, etc.); and (iii) representatives of the software developing company. The results of the pilot study indicated that the adoption of the information system by the hospital sector had led to improvements in the physician's ability to browse and gather historical information in a way that improved outcomes. In addition, the pilot study results enabled us to build the hierarchical tree which described the main task, the targets and the information components required at the point of care. This structure was the basis for assessing the subjective value of information at the next step.

Step 1: Assessing the Subjective Value of Information

As the framework for our structural analysis, we use the analytic hierarchy processing (AHP) method developed by Saaty [6] to place the principal objectives and goals in the medical care process in a hierarchical tree [7]. The main objective of providing medical care is set on the top level of the tree. The main objective is then divided into three sub-goals on the second level of the tree: (a) diagnostic precision, (b) providing quality care including safety and (c) providing an efficient service. The next level in the hierarchical tree analyzes the information components (prior diagnostics, prior procedures, etc) needed in order to achieve each goal.

The physicians participating in the survey were asked to assess the absolute importance of each information component and then, in the next step, to compare between each pair of components in order to determine their relative importance.

Thus, analyzing the hierarchical tree enables us to find the value of the different information components and to rank them.

Results indicate that the importance and value of information is affected by several factors:

1. The goal which the physician has to achieve (i.e., the decision he has to make). Results show that when diagnosis is the major concern, the physicians seek information components different from those used in situations of treatment or medical service.
2. The subject's specialization – physicians who are specialists in internal medicine and surgeons differ in the information components they use from the patient's medical record.
3. The level of seniority and experience.

One of the main contributions of the research is that it enables us to specify the information components required by physicians to improve their decision-making. In addition, it enables us to identify the factors influencing the importance and value of information.

Step 2: Assessing the Realistic Value of Information

After understanding the subjective value and the way in which the physicians perceived the value of the information that they received, this second step aimed at finding out whether they really used the information system and how they did so. Another target was to find out whether the use of historical information improved their performance and the outcomes. The methods included a tracklog file analysis and an analysis of data regarding hospitalizations, which was collected during the second half of the year 2004 for the internal medicine and surgery departments of the Meir Hospital, Kfar Saba, Israel. The sample was the same as in Step 1. The data regarding the activities was used to assess the realistic value of the information and to find out whether the use and consumption of historical data did in fact reduce the amount and duration of hospitalizations and the consumption of other medical services.

The main results indicated significant differences between the internal medicine and surgical departments in the amount and frequency of use of historical information about patients. We found that while the surgeons mostly used the summary of the data screen, the internal medicine physicians preferred to browse the system for the lab results screens. There were no differences in the use of the rest of the information components. In the internal medicine departments we did not find any significant difference in the mix of patients from various HMOs, while in the surgical departments there was a significant difference between patients from Clalit and patients from other HMOs in their use of medical services. It is well known that in the internal medicine departments, patients arrive randomly and spontaneously while surgery is generally on an elective basis. Therefore, historical information is more important in the internal medicine departments. Sometimes the internal medicine department itself is the only source of historical information. In the surgical departments, the activity is more organized in advance and the historical information is collected and organized beforehand.

Results from the assessment of the realistic value of information show that in the internal medicine departments, the use of historical information affects the number of one-day hospitalizations. Using a stepwise linear regression procedure we found that the HMO, as an independent variable, significantly explained ($p<0.05$) the number of hospitalization days as a dependent variable. The rate of one-day hospitalized patients from Clalit was 22.2%, and from other HMOs it was 27.4%. That is, Clalit had 20% less one-day hospitalizations. Because historical information exists in the information system for Clalit patients only, and because of the fact that the main reason for one-day hospitalization is to collect and gather more information, we can conclude that historical information reduces the amount of redundant one-day hospitalizations.

Next, we examined whether we could explain the use and consumption of medical services – such as CT, MRI, X-Ray, etc, by the use of historical information. Results show that the use and consumption of medical services depend on the patients' specific problem. From a stepwise linear regression we found ($p<0.05$) that when physicians browse for historical information on prior examination results relating to specific problems, they again access the same medical services, probably because they need updated information.

Step 3: Assessing the Normative Value of Information

The aim of this part of the research was to estimate the added utility per patient (in QALY units [8]) derived from using historical information and to conduct a cost-benefit analysis in order to find the threshold [9] value per unit of QALY [10]. Results show that the utility of using historical information provided by the information system is 0.0687 QALY. The cost-benefit analysis showed that under the assumption that there were 10,000 patients per year in the internal medicine departments and that the cost for the first year of adopting the system was $1,000,000, the added cost per 1 QALY was $1,455.60 per patient. A Monte Carlo simulation of 10,000 trials resulted in a normal distribution in which the average was 0.067162 QALY and the standard deviation was 0.02357 QALY.

Contribution

The main contribution of this research is the assessment of the value of information by the rarely employed method of integrating three examinations in one study: subjective, realistic and normative. The study is also unique in that the three examinations were carried out sequentially and not in parallel. This method enabled the use of results from one step as the input assumptions for the following one, all by adjusting each step and the whole structure to the environment of healthcare information systems. This methodology is a "black box" model which can be implemented in the various situations of the heterogeneous medical environment.

Another contribution relates to the productivity paradox [11]. The study was conducted in the service sector and specifically in the healthcare services, where IT investments have been growing rapidly in recent years but little research has been conducted [12].

Following Wyatt and Spiegelhalter [13], the implementation of the three methods for assessing the value of information in the decision process in the healthcare environment can contribute in many ways, such as:

- Promotion of the use of information systems – in order to promote the use of information resources by physicians it is necessary to prove that they are both beneficial and reliable. The use of information systems can really improve the physicians' decision-making and help in providing better treatment and service to patients.
- Supporting and promoting the medical informatics discipline.
- Supplying feedback and control that can provide designers and developers of the systems with successful methods and techniques.

This study also has practical implications which can contribute to improving and promoting the activities surrounding medical informatics. In addition, it contributes to policy decision-making in the healthcare sector by enabling policy makers to estimate the value of investing in point of care information systems and determine the added utility in QALY units.

Summary

Assessing the impact of information technology on organizations is an important area of inquiry, from both the scientific and the practical points of view. Over the last few decades, organizations in all sectors of the economy have invested large amounts in information technology and the question of the return on investment (ROI) is critical. The processes for assessing the return are complicated, and there is no general agreement between researchers and practitioners about the best method of arriving at it. As the healthcare sector continues to adopt ever more IT, policy makers pay ever more attention to the issue.

One of the major roles of IT is to supply information to support the decision-making process. In the healthcare sector, physicians need information to help them accomplish the task of providing medical services, making the correct diagnosis, prescribing the best treatment, and ensuring safety and quality of service.

Assessing the value of information – subjective, realistic and normative, is one of the approaches to determining the contribution of such information systems, and this study aimed at adding more insight on the subject and the area of medical informatics.

References

[1] Ahituv, N., Neumann, S., (with Riley, N.), (1994), "Principles of Information Systems for Management", WM. C. Brown, 4th ED.

[2] Ahituv, N., (1989), "Assessing the Value of Information: Problems and Approaches", Proceeding of ICIS – 89, Boston, MA., pp. 312–325.

[3] Ahituv, N., (1980), "A Systematic Approach Toward Assessing The Value of an Information System", MIS Quarterly, pp. 61–75.

[4] Shortliffe, E.H., Perreault, L.E., Wiederhold, G., Fagan, L., M., (2001), "Medical Informatics – Computer Applications in Health Care and Biomedicine", Springer, 2nd Edition, New-York.

[5] Brailer, D.J., Terasawa, E.L., (2003), "Use and Adoption of Computer-Based Patient Records", Oakland, CA., HealthCare Foundations.

[6] Saaty, L.T., (1981), "The Analytic Hierarchy Process", McGraw-Hill, New-York.

[7] Saaty, L.T., (1987), "Concepts, Theory, and Techniques, Rank Generation in the A.H.P. Decision Process", Decision Sciences, Vol. 18, No. 2.

[8] Phillips, C, Thompson, G., (2001), "What is a QALY?", http://www.evidence-based-medicine.co.uk.

[9] Pauker, S.G., Kassirer, J.P., (1980), "The Threshold Approach to Clinical Decision Making", The New England Journal of Medicine, Vol. 302, No. 20, pp. 1109–1117.

[10] Williams, A., (1994), "Economics, QALYs and Medical Ethics: A Health Economist's Perspective", Center for Health Economics, University of York, No. 121.

[11] Brynjolfsson, E., (1993), "The Productivity Paradox of Information Technology", Communications of the ACM, 36(12), pp. 67–77.

[12] Goldschmidt, P.G., (2005), "HIT and MIS: Implications of Health Information Technology and Medical Information Systems", Communications of the ACM, Vol. 48, No. 10, pp. 69–74.

[13] Wyatt, J.C., Spiegelhalter D., (1990), "Evaluating Medical Expert Systems: What to Test and How?" Medical Informatics, 15(3):205–217.

Medical and Care Compunetics 4
L. Bos and B. Blobel (Eds.)
IOS Press, 2007

Management of the Electronic Patient Records in the Web Based Platform for Diagnosis and Medical Decision for Optimization in Healthcare-PROMED

Roxana ANTOHI [a], Cristina OGESCU [a], Livia STEFAN [b], Mircea RAUREANU [c], Mircea ONOFRIESCU [d], Marius TOMA[d]

[a] *The Company for Research, Development, Engineering and Manufacturing for Automation Equipment an Systems -IPA SA, Bucharest Romania*
[b] *Institute for Computers- ITC SA, Bucharest Romania*
[c] *National Institute for R&D in Informatics –ICI, Bucharest Romania*
[d] *University of Medicine of Iassy Romania*

Abstract. The paper describes a research–development which had the objective to implement and manage the Electronic Patient Record in a multifunctional pilot platform named PROMED. The Electronic Patient Record implemented by PROMED platform is mainly aimed to facilitate both patient and health providers access to the health records and to provide an optimization of diagnostic and decision in healthcare services based on patients' medical history and medical statistics. The project promotes modern information and communication technologies for increasing quality and efficiency of healthcare services in an information based society. The PROMED platform is expected to contribute specifically to the improvement of the healthcare services in Romania by offering a solution for the integration of the main stakeholders involved in national healthcare system: patients, health service providers and public health authorities. The pilot system is first implemented in the "Cuza Voda" Obstetrics and Gynecology Hospital in Iassy, an important universitary and cultural city in the North East of Romania.

Keywords: healthcare, patient, electronic patientl record, medical diagnosis, medical statistics, health information , Internet application , web portal, distributed applications, databases

Introduction

The PROMED - Multifunctional Platform proposes to integrate the entities involved in the care process of patients for a profitable influence to the health system.

The main part of the project is the design of a module which assigns and creates an electronic patient record for each patient who is introduced in the PROMED information system. The electronic patient records are saved in a central database and accessed through a web portal application. In this way the patient is offered the possibility to access its own ELECTRONIC PATIENT RECORD, to print it, from any location, at any time.

From the healthcare providers' point of view, the electronic patient record can be visualized and updates with new records when the patient requires for a new consultation, for an ambulatory or hospital treatment.

The PROMED platform defines different levels of data access and in the same time does not limit the access to the relevant patient's health history.

1. General description of the PROMED informational platform

The PROMED multifunctional platform is implemented as a web portal application, supporting:
- creation and management of the electronic patient records by hospitals and ambulatory healthcare providers;
- visualization of the electronic patient records by the patient;
- health statistics and medical research;
- healthcare providers directory lists;
- medical discussion forum for exchanging healthcare information among healthcare professionals;
- assistance for system users.

For emergency situations the system is able to provide and transmit the vital patient information through a wireless communication service respectively the blood group, the rhesus factor, allergies, chronic diseases, health risks.

The web portal application contains the following functional modules/services:
- The "Authentication" module;
- The "Electronic Patient Record Management" module with three sub modules;
  - o   The "Patient" module;
  - o   The "Physicians" module with 2submodules "Hospital Electronic Patient Record "module and "Primary Care Electronic Patient" module;
  - o   "Hospital Emergency Room"module.
- The "Health resources" module;
- The "Medical statistics and research "module;
- The "Emergency " module;
- The "Forum " module;
- The "Help" module.

1.1. The "Authentication" module

This module gives the authorized user access to specific functionalities of the PROMED platform.

1.2. The "Electronic Patient Record Management" module

This module represents the central part of the platform and provides functions for creating, editing, manipulating, and printing patient administrative and healthcare data.

The information is organized in keeping with data model of the record of the patient which is in use in the Romanian healthcare system.

The electronic patient record is structured in two main subsets: administrative data and medical data. The administrative data contains the following information: name, surname, national personal identification number, residency and home address, phone, education level, occupation, healthcare insurance level.

1.2.1. The "Patients" module

This module allows the patients to visualize their electronic patient record. It is accessed through a user authentication and a "patient "user role.

1.2.2. The "Hospital Emergency Room" module

The "Hospital Emergency room" module is the hospital reception module and manages the patient's administrative data.

After the patient's examination in the emergency room, the physician takes the decision either to hospitalize or to send home the patient with treatment recommendation. In this module the following information is registered:

- the patient administrative data if he is a new patient;
- the data about the medical examination of the patient in the emergency room.

1.2.3. The "Hospital Electronic Patient Record" module

This module allows the hospital physicians to update and manage the electronic patient record. It is accessed through a user authentication and a "hospital physicians" user role.

In this module the patient data is organized in two sections:

- a section which contains emergency information: the blood group, the rhesus factor, chronic diseases, allergies;
- a section which contains information about the consultations at the hospital reception (emergency room) and the hospitalizations.

This module contains more functional submodules: "Patients", "Hospital presentations" and "Hospitalizations".

The "Patients" submodule reports data about all the patients introduced in the PROMED system. In this submodule are available the patient's administrative data and a "Patient Anamnesis" section which manages the medical history data as it is declared by the patient. It has the subsections:

       o   The major illnesses, allergies, a.s.o.;

       o   The specific pathology (e.g. obstetrical anamnesis for women).

The "Hospital presentations" submodule reports the patients who were registered in the Hospital Emergency Room, waiting either for an ambulatory care or for a hospitalization.

The "Hospitalizations" submodule manages all the data referring to the hospitalized patients and has the following specific subsections:

- "Progress Note" – manages data about patient health status during the hospitalization;
- "Surgical interventions" – manages patient data about surgical interventions during the hospitalization;
- "Treatments" – manages data about treatments during the hospitalization;
- "Functional explorations" – manages patient data about the functional explorations during the hospitalization;
- "Laboratory Analysis" – manages data about laboratory analysis during the hospitalization;
- "Prescriptions" – manages data about medication prescription during the hospitalization;
- "Discharge" – manages patient data about heath status when leaving the hospital (diagnosis, health status, medication prescription, physician recommendation).

The access in "Hospitalizations" module is based on an authorization process and security mechanism for providing confidentiality and security of all patient data and data modification traceability.

1.2.4. The "Primary Care Electronic Patient Record"

This module is intended to be used by primary care providers (family doctors, ambulatory healthcare centers). If the patient is not yet registered in the system, his administrative data will be introduced in this module. The electronic patient record can be visualized and updated with the physician's recommendations.

1.3. The "Healthcare resources" module

This module manages information about resources related to the national healthcare system:

- Healthcare providers (hospitals, ambulatory centers, public health institutions);
- Physicians.

This module data are recorded by the system administrator for all participants interested in joining the PROMED platform and being publicly available.

That is why this module is freely accessible for the entire portal's users; it does not require any authentication.

1.4. The "Medical statistics and research" module

This module is intended to present synthetic information regarding the health status of the comply population. Various reports are designed to be used for medical research and statistics and for healthcare providers reporting needs. The reports comply with the privacy and confidentiality rules for medical data, revealing no information about individual patients. This module is also freely accessible for all the portal's users, except for the specific reports for hospitals and primary care centers.

1.5. The discussion forum for healthcare professional

The discussion forum is designed to facilitate the exchange of medical information among healthcare professionals in order to help solving various medical issues. The forum is allowed only for physicians registered in PROMED portal, that is why it is accessed through a user authentication and a "healthcare professional" user role.

The main features of this section are:

- The forum is organized into topics;
- For each topic, each user can send unlimited number of messages;
- Each user can read all the messages from all the other users;
- Anyone can propose a new topic;

The messages are edited online.

1.6. The "Emergency" module

In case of an emergency (life risk situation), this module will allow access to vital information regarding the health status of the patient, namely the blood group, the Rhesus factor, chronic diseases, allergies to drugs or other substances.

This module can be accessed only by authorized medical personnel without the patient's consent if he/she is unconscious or it is not able to give his/her consent. This module is designed to be accessed through mobile devices (smart phone, PDA).

1.7. The "Help" module

This module will assist the users in platform exploitation.

2. Technical description of the PROMED platform

The PROMED plartform is developed under the form of a WEB PORTAL which is able to record groups of various information (administrative and medical) and to allow the access of a large number of users by means of their specific role: patients, hospital physicians, nurses, ambulatory physicians, public health authorities, anonymus user.

The hardware architecture of the multifunctional platform provides the support for all the web portal modules and ensures   the stability of the main components:

- The database server;
- The web application server.

The hardware specifications of the system refers to high memory capacity, high processing capabilities for the database server and the web server.

The database server is Oracle 10 g which provides all functional and security features necessary for managament of data recorded in the system.

For the application development we took the decision to use PHP5 platform which integrates with Oracle libraries (php_oci8.dll).

The operating system installed on the central server is Window 2003 Server, including IIS 6.0 web server.

The hardware infrastructure of the Multifunctional Platform is shown in figure 1:

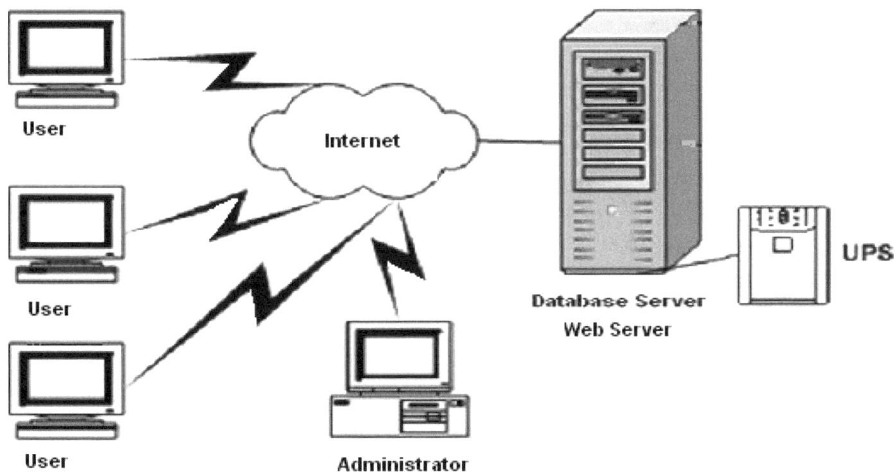

Figure 1 The hardware structure of the Multifunctional Platform

2.1 Technical specifications of the application program

The technical specifications of the application were established by means of diagrams to point the main action for :
–   Authentication;
–   Security;
–   Data Saving and Retrieving.

The diagnosis registered in the electronic patient medical record is compliant with ICD-10-AM (CIM – the 10 th OMS revision 2/2001VOL1 . The procedures for interventions in health field are from ICD-10-AM (CIM 10 –AM) revision 3/2002 edited by National Centre from Classification in Health Sydney, translated into Romanian.

The PROMED web portal contains functional sections comprising a number of web pages for data viewing, recording or modifying. The main sections of the portal are accessible through the following menu items:
-    Patients;
-    Physicians;
-    Hospital Emergency Room;
-    Resources;
-    Statistics;
-    News;
-    Help.

The "Emergency" module pages are designed for mobile devices and therefore is best viewed on such devices.

The PROMED web portal URL is www.rommed.ro/promed. A few screenshots are shown below:

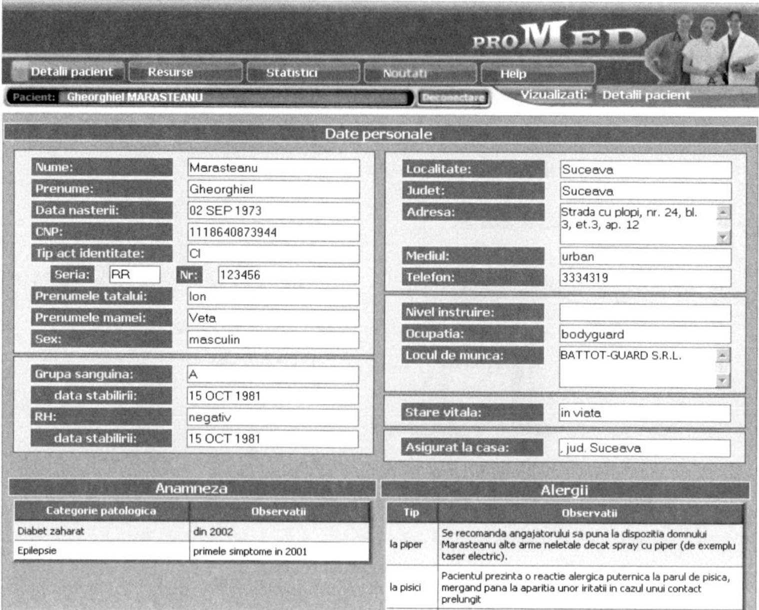

Figure 2 Patient Page (a)

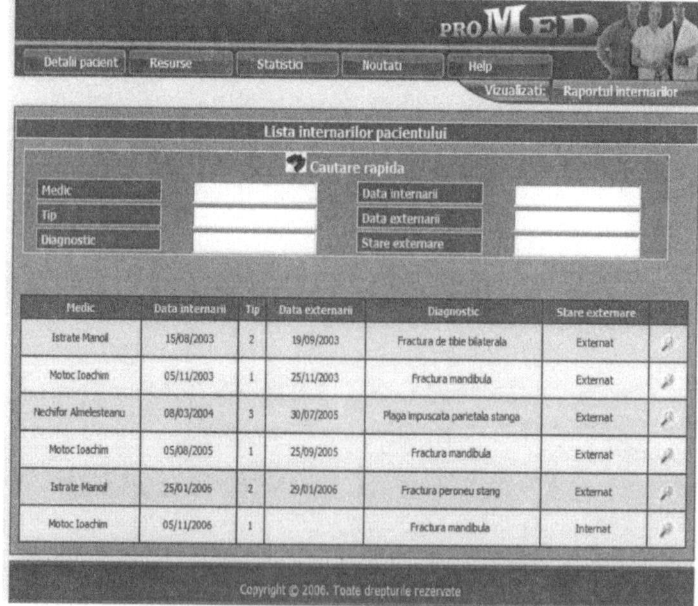

Figure 2 Patient Page (b)

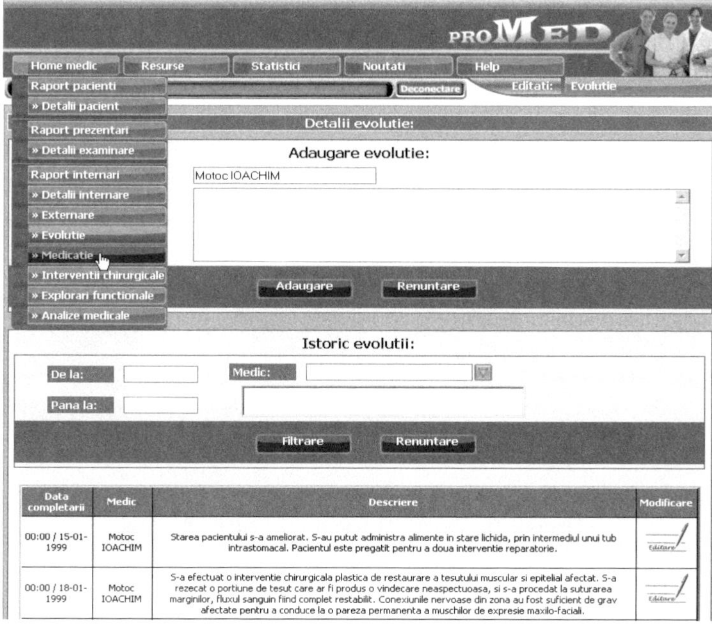

Figure 3 The "Physicians" page

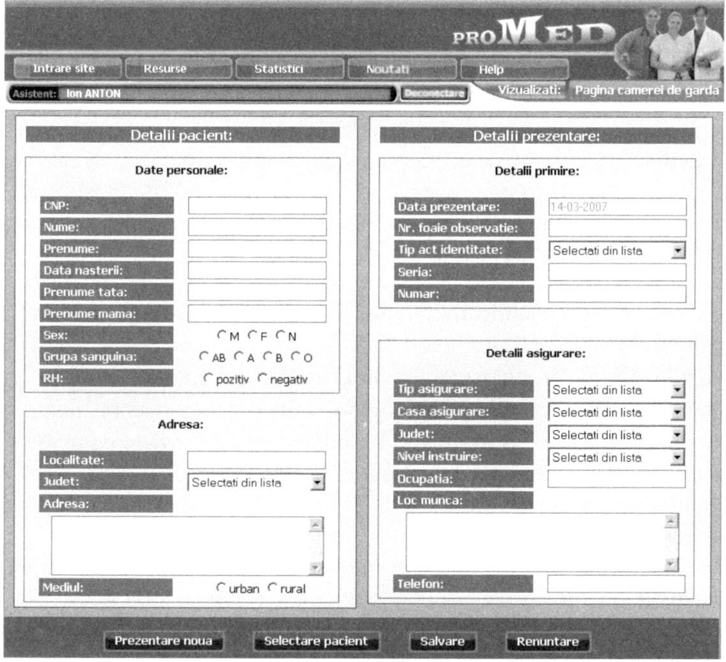

Figure 3 The "Emergency Room" page

The site map structure of the PROMED portal is presented in the figure 4:

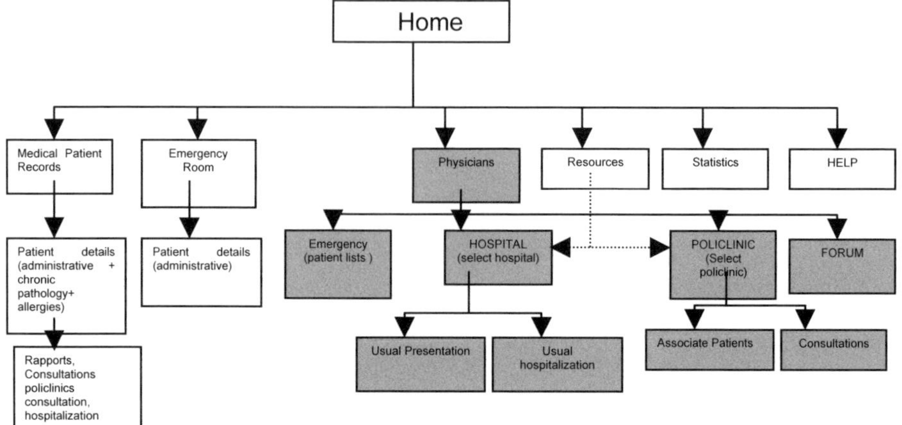

Figure 4 The site map structure of the PROMED portal

The portal will be accessed by four user categories:
- Patients;
- Medical personnel;
- Health authorities;
- Anonymous users.

Each user from these categories will have distinct rights to access ,view and modify various information from the database of the system .

 The medical resources and the official reports from the "Health statistics and research" module are unlimited accessible by any portal's user.

After a successful authentication in the "Patient" web page, the patients have the right to view the electronic patient record.

After a successful authentication in the "Physicians" web page, the physicians have the following rights:
- to view the electronic patient record for their patients;
- to update the electronic patient record only for the current patient;
- to view emergency information for all the patients registered in the system;

After a successful authentication in the "Emergency Room" web page, the nurses have the following rights:
- to register new patients;
- to amend the patient administrative information for patients reported to the hospital emergency room.

After a successful authentication in the "Health statistics and research" web page, health authorities have the right to view specific reports.

Conclusions

The PROMED platform represents an Internet access point and a web healthcare information system which provides various services for users (authentication, authorization, data and information management, reporting).

The platform will be used to support the healthcare services involved in the diagnosis and decision process and to manage the electronic patient records. It will allow the interaction between the three main actors in a health system:

- the patients, who will actively track their own healthcare status and have a electronic patient record updated and available anytime and anywhere;
- healthcare providers, who can find a patient and access its electronic patient record based on user access rights;
- public health authorities, who will be able to view various reports about the population health status and can elaborate prevention and warning plans against diseases.

On the platform there are also publicly available information regarding healthcare providers and official indicators.

The Promed platform supprt all the medical specialties except stomatology.

We consider that the PROMED healthcare information platform will eliminate many current problems occuring in the national health system, ranging from paper format healthcare records managing problems to cooperation between healthcare providers. Begining we will make experiments with PROMED platform in a pilot system with a 4G database. The PROMED Platform will be tested by physicians from two hospitals in Iassy and by physicians from Bucharest, Romania.

References

[1] ****   Health Informatics: Interoperability of Healthcare Multimedia Report Systems, CEN TC251 WG IV, and Version 1, 1999-05-28.
[2] **** European Committee for Standardization / Technical Committee 251 - Medical Informatics, Investigation of Syntaxes for Existing Interchange
[3] Kahn CE Jr. Design and implementation of an Internet-based health information resource. Compute Methods programs Biomed 2000 Oct
[4] Charles E. Kahn jr., - Bringing Computer-Based Decision Support and Education to the Point of Care, Medical College of Wisconsin, 2004
[5] *** HL7 Clinical Document Architecture, Release Two, January, 2003, San Antonio, Texas;
[6] www.oracle.com

Medical and Care Compunetics 4
L. Bos and B. Blobel (Eds.)
IOS Press, 2007

Towards a Partnership of Trust

Dr Amir Hannan, B.Sc., M.B. Ch.B, M.R.C.G.P. [a] & Fred Webber, B.Sc., Ph.D. [b]
[a]General Practitioner, "Information Management & Technology lead", "Clinical Governance lead", "Access, Booking & Choice lead", "Professional Executive Committee member", Tameside & Glossop Primary Care Trust. Member of the Records Access Collaborative. Member of the Clinical Leaders Network.
[b]Patient

Abstract: The relationship between doctors and patients is changing as patients live longer but with a greater incidence of chronic disease. An increase in the availability of information about health coupled with the Choice agenda and a patient-led NHS has encouraged patients to learn more about their own health. Patient access to their own GP-held records has led to the development of a Partnership of Trust whereby patients and their clinicians develop a shared understanding of their health and what each do for each other. This could potentially lead to significant patient and clinician benefits ultimately leading to better outcomes for individuals and societies.

Keywords: Records Access, Patient Empowerment, Trust, Doctor-Patient relationship

The traditional concept of the relationship between a doctor and patient is something that has remained relatively unchanged for generations. Generally speaking, this has taken the form of an adult/child, or teacher/pupil relationship. In such relationships the doctor has been the dominant component and the patient the usually passive recipient of the doctor's advice and guidance. Often the doctor was held in awe by the patient and typically there was little or no discussion during the consultation. When feeling ill the patient would visit the doctor and the main concern was to ask the doctor to "make it better" or to be given some medicine to ease the condition. This may partly explain why up to 40% of general practice consultations are for relatively minor conditions that could be managed without the need for a clinician or managed without a specific treatment [1].

However the nature of the relationship between doctor and patient is changing. Modern medicine is enabling patients to live longer but with a greater burden of chronic disease. The incidence of obesity and with it the risk of developing hypertension, diabetes, ischaemic heart disease and cerebrovascular accident [2] continues to rise in the main due to a poor lifestyle, poor diet, lack of exercise and genetic factors [3]. But it is also widely perceived to be readily controllable by the individual [4]. Patients and the medical profession have responded by trying to find pills for every ill [5] with little gain. At the same time, patients are increasingly being managed by teams of people from different disciplines and in different care settings. This may result in patients getting different messages depending on what information the clinician has before him [6].

Searching for a New Relationship

Patients and the general public are now looking for alternative ways to improve their health and reduce the burden of disease [7]. This is partly fuelled by an explosion in the quantity and quality of information that is now available via the internet [8]. However the resulting benefit is tempered partly because "further collaboration, training and evaluation of the information is required". But where can this come from and how can it be stimulated?

Self help groups such as the Alzheimers Society [9] and Diabetes UK [10] have responded by developing up-to-date web-sites providing information on their respective medical areas. They also try to link patients and their families with research data as well as specific lifestyle measures and other treatments that may help them improve their health and well being. Other groups have turned to alternative medicine [11] to find solace but this still sits uncomfortably next to traditional medicine for most clinicians.

The "Choice Agenda" [12] which enables patients to choose who provides hospital based treatment for them has encouraged the development of a multitude of web-sites [13], [14] to help patients to decide which organisation will best fulfil their needs. At the same time, a generation of people has grown up watching medical dramas depicting fictional medical problems and showing how stressed clinicians and patients or their families cope (eg Casualty, E.R.). This has helped to demystify medicine and enable the public to get a greater understanding of some of the complex problems clinicians and patients sometimes have to deal with. High profile cases in the news, e.g. issues relating to fertility treatment or end of life decisions especially around euthanasia, have further stimulated discussion and debate.

A patient-led NHS [15] encourages patients to take a more active role in the way the NHS delivers services. At the same time, clinicians are beginning to also appreciate the important role patients have in self-managing their conditions. The development of the Expert Patient Programme [16] alongside the introduction of NHS Direct, enables patients to get "instant" advice on medical matters via a telephone service manned by nurses 24 hours a day as well as the NHS Direct web-site and via digital television. [17] More recently the acceptance by the *National Institute for Health and Clinical Excellence* of the value of "pulmonary rehabilitation" [18] has further endorsed the view that patients can, when given the opportunity and some training, enhance their health and well-being over and above traditional medical treatments. Patients whose first language is not English have been given digital recording devices to take away from the consultation to review advice given by clinicians which has been particularly liked by elderly patients and those with memory problems. [19]. Patients have also been given patient-held guidelines to help encourage improved delivery of care. Whilst this has helped to reduce their anxiety, it has not necessarily led to an improvement in outcome [20]. At the same time, the sudden withdrawal of Vioxx from the market as a result of an increased risk of ischaemic heart disease has served to highlight the significant risk some modern medicines can pose despite the regulatory authorities and the best of intentions [21]

What is the Purpose of IT in Healthcare Delivery?

"A modern and dependable National Health Service needs accurate and instantly accessible information. It is vital for improving care for patients, for improving the performance of the NHS, and the health of the nation." [22]. The National Programme for IT was developed to help bring modern computing systems to the NHS. As the take-up of broadband increases, more people are using the internet seeking information eg the news [23], buying goods [24], [25] or cheap flights [26]. At the same time there has been a plethora of web-sites offering a wide variety of medical information within the NHS [27] and outside it too [28]. But to date the web-sites have offered generic information for a generic audience.

What if patients could be given patient-specific information to help link themselves to their health record and to the clinicians looking after them?

www.renalpatientview.org has been developed as a joint venture between renal patients, their clinicians and the laboratories. It enables patients to see their diagnoses, treatments and test results and share these with anybody anywhere in the world. More recently EMIS [29], a clinical supplier for general practices in the UK and PAERS [30] have developed a system that enables patients to access their full GP-held record over the internet without prior filtering. This includes seeing full notes of consultations, all results of tests as well as any letters or other documentation that has been attached to their medical record.

NHS CfH is about to start the early adopter implementation of the NHS Summary Record [31] via the Spine and enable this information to be seen via Health Space [32]. This will enable patients to record their personal demographic details and some medical values e.g. blood pressure and smoking status. It will also allow them to see a summary of their medical information e.g. current medication and list of allergies once these are available on the Spine. It will also allow patients to book appointments for hospital care or diagnostics e.g. CT scans or MRI scans at a time of their choice that providers can offer. These developments will further encourage patients to use the internet as a means of finding out more about their own health, what choices there are available and even to register their choices. The user experience is much more centred on the needs of the patient and not that of the system as has traditionally been the case

How does enabling patients to see their medical records over the internet lead to a Partnership of Trust?

Simply enabling patients to access medical records over the internet will not lead to better health outcomes. Patients need to feel there is some value in the record that could then benefit them. This "value" comes directly from the doctor-patient relationship or perhaps more correctly the clinician-patient relationship which recognises the important role nurses and other allied health professionals play in delivering health-care. If this is a strong relationship, where each party feels an equal partner, then they are more likely to share their ideas, concerns and expectations. "Shared decision making" may be regarded as an aspect of "patient centeredness" and can enhance patient autonomy as well as being associated with more positive consultations without increased anxiety [33]. The clinician can bring to the consultation his or her experience and knowledge of the medical world whilst the patients can bring their experience of the symptoms of the disease and how it is affecting them. Together they can build a "partnership". But for this partnership to be beneficial, it needs to provide something for each party. Trust is that basic commodity. The clinician needs to trust the patient who is telling them all they can about their illness whilst recognising that patients have their own agendas and may only tell them what they feel comfortable with. Similarly the patient needs to trust the clinician hoping that they will be given all the relevant information about their illness in a form they can understand. By accessing the medical records, the clinician is in effect telling the patient what their understanding of their illness is and what the plan of action may be. The patient is able to access this information, agree with it or refute it or identify any mistakes that may co-exist and then respond by determining what course of action to take. The more information there is, the greater the trust this breeds between the two parties. Trust can be broken and partnerships can split but when a Partnership of Trust is formed, it can create a synergy that enables the clinician and the patient to feel more in control and more at ease with their disease and enables patients to feel less ill (personal communication with patients of AH). A Partnership of Trust can exist without access to health records but this could be a false partnership that could result in great distrust if abused. Harold Shipman, the mass murderer is thought to have killed more than 200 patients during his career. He did this by amassing large quantities of diamorphine deceptively from patients to use against his victims and demonstrated how dangerous this can be if such a trust is misappropriated and a patient is unable to let others see what is happening. Record access for the patient enables a very open relationship and helps to prevent such a calamity from ever occurring again.

How can a Partnership of Trust help patients to achieve better health outcomes?

The underlying assumption is that patients wish to get better and feel less ill (although this is not always the case especially in a country with a well-developed welfare system). But to gain better health outcomes, patients need to understand their health better. That means gaining a better understanding of their health parameters eg blood pressure, body mass index, cholesterol, mental health status and knowing what these health parameters mean and what is normal for them.

Identifying what is normal for people can be problematic. [34]. Often the context is more important than the value itself. For instance, understanding the significance of a lipid profile depends on whether or not the blood test was taken fasting, the sex of the patient, their diabetes status, whether or not they suffer with ischaemic heart disease and what their blood pressure and smoking status is. It is also affected by their ethnic status and whether or not there is a family history of heart disease. As time goes on, we are likely to identify other risk factors which will further help to stratify risk. Clinicians may be able to identify these factors and use "risk calculators" or other tools to help patients to categorise their level of risk. Trying to explain this risk to patients and perhaps more importantly identifying what factors can be altered (e.g. smoking status or weight) to reduce that risk may help patients to modify their health risk and improve their health outcome. The Partnership of Trust is critical in enabling this because patients will need to change the way they live their lives in order to reap the rewards.

Simply telling people to do something will not work – they need to feel how important the change is and to feel that it is something achievable and worthwhile. This does not happen spontaneously: both parties have to work hard to learn to trust each other and in so doing respect each others' views whilst trying to move towards a common goal. Once this is reached, a Partnership of Trust is engendered which can then help the patient and the clinician to develop a bond that helps each to move forwards productively. – the patient gets a better understanding of their health and may feel more empowered; the clinician feels more valued by bringing his knowledge and experience forwards and enabling the patient to feel more happy and less ill.

What are the benefits of the Partnership of Trust?

By developing a Partnership of Trust, a more open relationship is formed where there is less hidden between the clinician and the patient. Giving patients access to the medical records further cements that relationship and helps to ensure that the expectations of the patient are matched by what the clinician can deliver. As new encounters happen and more information becomes available the records will continue to further develop the plan which can continue to be agreed by both parties. This empowers both clinician and patient by informing, enabling and ultimately sanctioning a course of action that can be adhered to and recorded for review at a later date. This leads to an improvement in the knowledge of both parties of each others' situation, helps to improve the skills to understand each other and may even change the attitude each has. Over time, both will learn to communicate better as further trust is gained, become more responsive to each others' needs and hence enable more timely interventions. But more importantly for both parties, the contact becomes more productive and more efficient with greater ability to develop the relationship in a way suitable for both parties. The Partnership of Trust enables both parties to decide when and where and even how to meet – in person face-to-face, over the telephone, electronically via e-mail or other secure web-messaging service or by paper. At present only the clinician can write to the medical record but for this to be an equal partnership, the record may become either a two-way communication channel or a separate channel may be used for clinicians to be "allowed" to view the patient held record, something that does not exist in the UK but does exist in the US (Personal Health Record).

While knowledge is one of the keys to forming a Partnership of Trust, another is the possession of the skills necessary to apply that knowledge for the benefit of the partnership. Many of the required skills may already be possessed and practiced by the partners - honesty, candour, tact, discretion, courtesy and mutual respect. Others may need to be developed. Patients, for example, may need to gain the confidence to ask questions of the doctor if he or she does not understand what is being explained about the condition, its cause, effects or treatment. When patients feel trusted by the doctor, patients are more ready to express their worries without being concerned about being disbelieved or dismissed as being silly. In addition to this, an informed patient, after some discussion of the condition with the doctor, may feel it necessary to question the conclusions reached by the doctor. In this circumstance, courtesy and tact will be particularly important on the part of the patient when raising the issue and the doctor who responds to it. Both need to recognise that it is possible and legitimate to disagree without the intrusion of any tension or offence between them.

The medical record consists of a wide variety of descriptions of symptoms, signs, diagnoses and treatment plans. Over time these may join up to provide a "clinical pathway" highlighting the journey a patient makes as they move from one stage of management to another. Tools are beginning to be developed to help clinicians to manage patients along clinical pathways derived from standards previously agreed. An example is the Map of Medicine [35] which NHS CfH has adopted. It is not clear how such a tool may be deployed. But in theory patients might be able to see such a pathway and assess their progress along it. As time passes, further tools may be developed for patients to help them at points where there may be choices for different courses of action. These are points in the clinical pathway that the patient and clinician may want to discuss things to help decide the optimal treatment plan.

The clinical pathway may stimulate discussions on when a patient or clinician may choose not to follow the ideal care pathway. There may be times when the ideal care pathway cannot be followed because the service is not available or not accessible to the patient close to home or simply has not been considered. This could stimulate the patient and clinician to take an active role within the local health community to help bring forward such services or at least ask why they are not available. This will help the health service to be more responsive to the needs of the patient and clinician whilst recognising that all services cannot always be made available to all people all the time in a constrained service. It does however encourage patients to get involved in such things as Patient Participation Groups [36] or on health committees to ensure their voice is heard and that decisions are made taking into account patient's views. This is even recognised in the World Health Organisation report "Preventing Chronic Disease – a vital investment" [37].

Denmark already leads the world by enabling all its citizens to see medications and results of blood tests on-line [38]. This helps to stimulate a healthy Partnership of Trust. It encourages patients to see their clinician when they really need to rather than as a routine visit just to find out what is happening. This also means that the clinician can spend more time discussing the implications of the condition or treatment rather than just re-iterating the contents of a letter or informing the patient of a test result. The patient and clinician can then discuss the implications of the results rather than just the tests themselves.

As a Partnership of Trust is established, what can we go on to hope to achieve?

Health records contain information which hitherto has been mainly for fellow clinicians to see. The "copying letters to patient" initiative [39] has encouraged clinicians to change the style of writing to ensure patients can also understand what they have written. Otherwise patients may come back to them for further clarification. As patients begin to realise they have the right to access their medical records and the technology becomes more widely available, more patients will request access to their full medical records. Clinicians will need to respond by enabling patients to see records that they understand. This style will gradually develop as the Partnership of Trust shapes the skills and attitudes of the clinician as well as the patient. The clinician may have to adjust by being more prepared to enter into meaningful discussions with patients; to allow patients to participate in decisions about choice of treatment; to present information to the patient which may be unpleasant or potentially upsetting, honestly, and with full candour; to recognise that some patients are competent to make and record some of the more straightforward indicators, such as blood pressure, blood sugar, and to regard these as useful additional information, if appropriate; to recognise and accept that in some cases a patient may actually know as much, or even more than the doctor about a medical condition. Long term chronic conditions may stimulate patients to research their complaint in considerable depth. In other cases an obscure or rare condition might also stimulate extensive studies on the part of the patient. This situation may be difficult to concede by some doctors but its recognition does help to enhance the Partnership of Trust. Patients, too, may need to modify their approach to the clinician. For some there may be the need to overcome the natural or traditional reticence to engage in genuine two-way discussions with the doctor; to become better informed about their medical conditions, together with the initiative to find ways of doing so; to ensure their medical record is correct and free of error [40]; to cooperate with the doctor by taking more responsibility for their own health and welfare; to keep a close eye on dates and be proactive in making appointments for regular tests, etc., without having to be reminded; to become more involved in the activities of the practice. Patients can gain a better understanding of the workings of the health services in general and of the practice in particular. Patients have already started to help stimulate such discussion and debate [41], [42]. As this develops further, other interested groups e.g. Diabetes UK or the Alzheimers Society may produce specific advice for patients and clinicians to help further support the relationship between patients and clinicians. Groups such as the Patient Information Forum [43] are also likely to become more influential in supporting the transition of the patient from a passive recipient of care to an active partner.

Health Space [32] enables patients to store basic medical information such as current medication, allergies, blood pressures and peak flows. This facility will need further development so that complete medical information is available to help patients and clinicians to be aware of all information that is stored about their health in all care settings. This will help to stimulate many different Partnerships of Trust between many different clinicians, acknowledging the multi-disciplinary nature of modern healthcare.

The internet, like illness and disease, does not have national boundaries. People are now travelling further afield for business and / or pleasure. As the prevalence of chronic diseases continues to rise, many of them may have conditions that need to be managed whilst they are away from their home. They will therefore need access to high quality information about their own health and about the healthcare services specific to the country they are visiting. UK based web-sites may not be appropriate when in Africa or the Far East. But how can an individual know that the information they are receiving abroad is appropriate? How can the clinician whom they trust give appropriate advice about where the patient can get appropriate information whilst abroad? The World Health Organisation may have a role in developing standards for stimulating discussion and debate amongst member countries and relevant organisations to help produce a quality marker so that patients and clinicians can easily identify and use the information.

Clinical software to date has been largely focused on the needs of the clinician. This is not necessarily conducive to encouraging a Partnership of Trust. The next generation software needs to be developed for both patients and clinicians together in partnership so that it will encourage patients and clinicians to further develop and improve the clinician-patient relationship. This will support clinicians and patients to learn from each other and develop further mutual respect whilst recognising the critical role patients have in attaining better outcomes for themselves. This will be even more important as healthcare organisations move away from simply treating disease to promoting health and well-being and ultimately happiness. Already evidence is accruing that electronic health records contain sufficient information to help patients to identify the level of their personal cardiovascular risk [44]. Seeing this personalised information will encourage patients to consider their personal risk and plan life-style changes for reducing that risk.

Clinicians are concerned about the conflict of helping patients to self manage whilst enabling professional responsibility, accountability and contextual factors that drive behaviour such as consultation length [45]. Anecdotal evidence suggests that the time taken is typically much less because all information is to hand for the patient to see prior to the consultation. The frequency of consultations decreases but the quality of the consultation improves as the discussion focuses mainly on the implications for the patient as opposed to merely informing the patient of the results of tests or other communications that have been received. This however needs to be further researched and formally evaluated.

Ultimately it is hoped that a Partnership of Trust will support an open policy for patients and clinicians to feel comfortable with sharing all information that is available. Information unjustifiably locked in patient-sealed envelopes (preventing the clinician from seeing) or clinician-sealed envelopes (preventing the patient from seeing) [46] could build distrust and harm to both patient and clinician. It is however recognised that sealing may be necessary in some circumstances for a healthy relationship to exist e.g. the minutes from a child protection meeting. There needs to be a balance between enabling an open relationship whilst recognising the need for withholding some information so long as this is to the advantage of the clinician-patient relationship. A local Health Care Record Board made up of local clinical leads, managerial leads, information governance leads and patients could be an important group to manage and perhaps police the utilisation and development of patient access and clinician access to health records.

We hope that enabling patients to readily access their medical records will lead to an improvement in the health outcomes of individuals. In societies where patients have this facility they can enjoy living and celebrate the benefits of having information about their health linked with high quality information. This in turn will help them to continually improve their health as well as their relationship with their clinician: a true Partnership of Trust.

The authors would like to thank David Lerner, a patient of Dr Hannan, who originally coined the phrase "A Partnership of Trust"

References

[1]   Porteous T, Ryan M, Bond CM & Hannaford P. Preferences for self-care or professional advice for minor illness – a discrete choice experiment. *British Journal of General Practice* 2007; 57:911-917

[2]   www.gpnotebook.co.uk/simplepage.cfm?ID=705036330

[3]   Moore H, Summerbell C D, Greenwood D C, Tovey P, Griffiths J, Henderson M, Hesketh K, Woolgar S, Adamson A J. Improving management of obesity in primary care:cluster randomised trial. *BMJ* 2003; 327:1085-1089

[4]   Brown I, Thompson J, Tod A & Jones G. Primary care support for tackling obesity – a qualitative study of the perceptions of obese patients. British Journal of General Practice 2006; 56: 666-672

[5]   Kamerow D. Diet change vs pills for better health. *BMJ* 2005; 331:362

[6]   Alazri MH, Neal RD, Heywood P & Leese B. Patients' experiences pf continuity in the care of type 2 diabetes – a focus group study in primary care. *British Journal of General Practice* 2006; 56: 488-495

[7]   Meryn S. Improving doctor-patient communication. *BMJ* 1998;316:1922-1930

[8]   Reviewed by Birte Twisselmann. Health Information on the Internet: A Study of Providers, Quality, and Users. *BMJ* 2006; 333:607

[9]   www.alzheimers.org.uk

[10]   www.diabetes.org.uk

[11] Owen DK, Lewith G, Stephens CR. Can doctors respond to patients' increasing interest in complementary and alternative medicine? BMJ *2001; 322:54-158*

[12]   www.dh.gov.uk/PolicyAndGuidance/PatientChoice/fs/en

[13]   www.nhs.uk/England/Choice/

[14]   www.patientopinion.org.uk

[15]www.dh.gov.uk/PublicationsAndStatistics/Publications/PublicationsPolicyAndGuidance/PublicationsPolicyAndGuidanceArticle/fs/en?CONTENT_ID=4106506&chk=ftV6vA

[16]   www.expertpatients.nhs.uk/public/default.aspx

[17]   Ryan A, Greenfield S, McManus R & Wilson S. Self-care – has DIY gone too far? *British Journal of General Practice* 2006; 33:07-908

[18]   www.nice.org.uk/page.aspx?o=375979

[19]   Jackson M & Skinner J. Improving consultations in general practice for non-English speaking patients. *British Journal of General Practice* 2006; 29:27-628

[20]   McKinstry B, Hanley D, McCloughan L, Elton R & Webb DJ. Impact on hypertension control of a patient-held guideline – a randomised controlled trial. *British Journal of General Practice* 2006; 56: 842–847.

[21]   Krumholz H M, Ross J S, Presler A H, Egilman D S.What have we learned from Vioxx? *BMJ* 2007; 334:20-123

[22]   Information for health 1998. www.dh.gov.uk/PublicationsAndStatistics/Publications/PublicationsPolicyAndGuidance/PublicationsPolicyAndGuidanceArticle/fs/en?CONTENT_ID=4002944&chk=kwk%2BJz

[23]   www.bbc.co.uk

[24]   www.ebay.co.uk

[25]   www.tesco.com

[26]   www.easyjet.com

[27]   www.nhsdirect.nhs.uk

[28]   www.patient.co.uk

[29]   www.emis-online.com

[30]   www.paers.net

[31]   www.connectingforhealth.nhs.uk/delivery/programmes/nhscrs/adopterprogramme

[32]   www.healthspace.nhs.uk

[33]   Siriwardena AN, Edwards AGK, Campion P, Freeman A & Elwyn G. Involve the patient and pass the MRCGP – investigating shared decision making in a consulting skills examination using a validated instrument. *British Journal of General Practice* 2006; 56:857-862.

[34]   www.bbc.co.uk/radio4/science/am_i_normal.shtml

[35]   www.mapofmedicine.com

[36]   www.napp.org.uk

[37]   www.who.int/chp/chronic_disease_report/part4_ch1/en/index18.html

[38]   Protti D, Wright G & Treweek S. Primary care computing in England and Scotland: a comparison with Denmark. *Informatics in Primary Care* 2006; 14:93-99

[39]www.dh.gov.uk/PolicyAndGuidance/OrganisationPolicy/PatientAndPublicInvolvement/CopyingLettersToPatients/fs/en

[40]   Powell J, Fitton R & Fitton C. Sharing electronic health records: the patient view. *Informatics in Primary Care* 2006; 14:55-57

[41]   www.usercare.info

[42]   www.foldercare.com

[43]   www.pifonline.org.uk

[44]   Marshall T. The use of cardiovascular risk factor information in practice databases: making the best of patient data. *British Journal of General Practice* 2006; 56:600-605

[45]   Blakeman T, Macdonald W, Bower P, Gately C & Chew-Graham C. A qualitative study of GPs' attitudes to self-management of chronic disease. *British Journal of General Practice* 2006; 56:407-414

[46]   www.connectingforhealth.nhs.uk/crdb

Medical and Care Compunetics 4
L. Bos and B. Blobel (Eds.)
IOS Press, 2007

Introducing Guideline Management in the Healthcare Information System Architecture

I. Román[a], L.M. Roa[b], G. Madinabeitia[a] and A. Millán[c]
[a]*Group of Telematic Engineering, University of Seville, Spain*
[b]*Biomedical Engineering Group, University of Seville, Spain*
[c]*Dept. of Internal Medicine, Virgen Macarena Hospital of Seville, Spain*
Escuela Superior de Ingenieros. C. de los Descubrimientos, s/n 41092 Sevilla (Spain)
isabel@trajano.us.es

Abstract. This paper analyses different benefits of the full integration of components for clinical guideline management in the information system architecture of a healthcare organization. Subsequently, we propose a methodology for the development of these components based on the European prEN12967 standard, in order to facilitate this integration. Benefits are studied from several viewpoints. First, from the healthcare professional user viewpoint, as a powerful decision support tool, by which the Electronic Health Record of a specific patient could suggest the appropriate guidelines to apply and a particular assistance plan for him or her. We are centered in co-morbidity patients because these tasks are especially difficult to accomplish in this kind of patients. Second, from the guideline creation viewpoint, we analyze how the tacit knowledge implicit in the healthcare information system could be the base for the explicit representation of knowledge in a guideline and the posterior validation of these guidelines. Our approach is in agreement with today's new paradigm for evidence-based medicine demanded by healthcare professionals. The proposed method for guideline management components development is compliant with CEN's prEN12967 European standard, and consequently follows ITU-T's ODP methodology.

Keywords. Guideline, standardization, prEN12967, ODP, integration, comorbidity patient.

Introduction

Knowledge Management (KM) research is considered the key to success for healthcare in the 21st century by many authors. Professionals from this domain have attempted to bring together different aspects on how healthcare related information can best be disseminated to support the acquisition, generation, codification, transfer and recycling of knowledge in the context of specific organizational processes, leading to the emergence of the knowledge age in health care [1].

Knowledge is traditionally categorized into explicit and implicit, or tacit [2]. Explicit knowledge is the abstract, symbolic type of knowledge present explicitly and formalized or codified in some way, such as textbooks, guidelines or papers in a bibliographic database. It is applicable to both specific and generic problems and relies on explicit reasoning mechanisms. It requires the knowledge to be represented in a manageable, reproducible and clear way, facilitating knowledge processor to construe the meaning of concepts and to make automatic reasoning. Tacit or implicit knowledge is the rich, experimental, sensorial kind of knowledge that a knowledge processor acquires when immersed into an environment, or presented with detailed representations of that environment. It is very well applicable to specific instances of problems and relies on processing mechanisms such as feature selection, pattern recognition and associative memory [3].

The current understanding of Evidence Based Medicine (EBM) is the management of available explicit medical knowledge. EBM aims to provide doctors with conscientious, explicit, and judicious use of current best evidence in making decisions about the care of individual patients [1]. It is also essential for decision makers in healthcare systems in order to improve healthcare quality, facilitating clinical and health policy choices that provide the most efficient use of limited resources to promote personal and public health.

But some core problems have been identified in the current paradigm of EBM. The search of the best evidence for practitioners is not always an easy task; time constraints, out-of-date textbooks, difficult access to specific journals and the use of disorganized or non-systematic approaches have been identified as barriers to reaching the required information. Another problem in the use of available evidences is that patients are often selected to give the trial treatment maximum scope to show an effect, but these highly selective results are going to be applied to real-life patients. To alleviate these problems some intermediate 'information to knowledge' strategies have been developed, such as meta-analyses and major systematic reviews, that provide guidelines, clinical decision rules and treatment recommendations, published in libraries as Cochrane [4] and proposed to facilitate evidence-based decisions for a particular clinical problem in order to assess the evidence at an individual level for a particular patient.

On the other hand, publication bias and intermediates for knowledge generation introduce potential for even greater degradation of information quality due to the subjective inclusion/interpretation of data, inappropriate data gathering techniques, or rejection of contradictory data. Meta-analysis and systematic review methods not always provide an unbiased assessment of the evidence. Research sponsors, but also investigators, journal editors and peer reviewers all play a part here, and publication tends to favors studies with positive or striking results [5].

More complex issues have to be considered for the development of useful and reliable tools to assist clinicians in the management of the tacit knowledge. The extraction of this knowledge directly from the healthcare information systems, without 'information to knowledge' intermediates, is the new EBM paradigm that healthcare professionals are demanding lately.

This new paradigm is being fostered by the development and application of intelligent tools that help to accumulate and process data and make use of them. It bridges several areas, including databases, statistics, modeling, machine learning, and human-computer interaction. Nowadays, different researches are obtaining promising results focused on the direct use or integration into specific solutions in the healthcare domain, but these are only first steps.

Any KM research that provides really innovative and relevant conclusions must consider a great amount of information, referred to several issues inside the healthcare organization such as clinical, demographic, resources, staff… The full management of this information implies global access to knowledge and networking capacities by solving difficult integration issues.

Knowledge and business logic common to different sectors of the healthcare organization shall therefore be integrated in a specific architectural layer of the underlying information system and shall be accessible through services based on public and stable interfaces. The ultimate objective of such a structure is to build an open federation of complementary heterogeneous systems, spread over the territory, individually autonomous but also capable of interworking to meet effectively different needs in the healthcare environment as care, social, research or administrative, increasing the overall effectiveness of the activities carried out.

The goal can be achieved through a unified, open architecture based on a middleware independent from specific applications and capable of integrating knowledge and business logic and of making them available to diverse, multi-vendor applications. The architecture is intended as a basis both for working with existing systems, allowing specific models to be integrated, as well as for the planning and construction of new systems [6-8].

The focus of this work is centered on guideline management research from the perspective of the exposed EBM paradigm, exploiting the full tacit knowledge of the healthcare organization for the development, validation and the personal application of the guideline.

We are designing methods and techniques for the components developed for guideline management that could be easily integrated in the information system architecture of a healthcare organization.

1. Material and methods

1.1. Integration issues

Integration is the technique that permits a variety of components to work together in a seamless way, as if they were a single system. The use of fully interoperable components greatly facilitates the integration process.

As far as integration is concerned, standardization is a cornerstone. Standards already exist and will continue being defined for supporting specific requirements, both in terms of in-situ user operations and with respect to communication procedures. Some healthcare middleware approaches are developed by standardization organizations, like CEN [9] or OMG [10].

Our approach is based on the three-part draft European standard prEN 12967-1,2,3 [6-8] for a healthcare service architecture. The purpose is to allow describing the architecture of any generic healthcare information system as a federation of components interacting and co-operating to offer a set of information management services.

An important basis for the production of this service architecture standard is the ODP methodology [11-13] (Open Distributed Processing). ODP provides a five-layered approach to the definition of information services. However, only the three upper levels, Enterprise viewpoint, Information viewpoint and Computational viewpoint are used to produce prEN 12967. The two lower levels are certainly useful but should be considered in a specific implementation context.

- The enterprise viewpoint shall provide a guideline for the definition of the requirements for information exchange within a healthcare enterprise, with a focus on the purpose, scope and policies of the system.

- The information viewpoint is concerned with the kinds of information handled by the system and constraints on the use and interpretation of that information. It provides a methodology for detailing the semantics of the information to be processed as an information model and considering those provided by other standards for health informatics. This viewpoint supports the solution of semantics conflicts in the integration of systems.

- The computational viewpoint shall give guidance on the distribution through functional decomposition of the system objects that interact at defined interfaces. This is the basis for the solution of functional integration of systems inside the healthcare organization.

1.2. Clinical context

A significant amount of patients who are assisted either in the hospital scope (at a specialized level), and in the extra-hospital scope (at a level of general practice), suffer more than only one disease. In addition, many of the most frequent diseases affect several organs or systems.

In the hospital scope, within an Internal Medicine Service, the prevalence of patients with numerous disorders (comorbidity patients), is in the range between 21% and 75%. This group also includes patients showing special susceptibility and clinical fragility due to a progressive functional deterioration together with a gradual reduction of autonomy (frail elderly people), having professional and social implications.

In the extra-hospital scope, comorbidity patients represent about 5% of the population assisted in Primary Healthcare Centers. This group requires over four times the average of patient resource allocation, due to their higher number of consultations, complementary necessity of home visits, tests, multiple admissions at the hospital, and higher drug prescriptions [14].

Although this problem is not new, the increment of life expectancy in our society, and the consequent population ageing, anticipate that the health sector must respond to the challenges of the new scenario.

The clinical context in this paper is the assistance to comorbidity patients. The high degree of the clinical complexity of comorbidity patients entails that in these cases healthcare is delivered by numerous specialists, while the concurrence of several diseases implies that different guidelines could be applied. Consequently the elaboration of the appropriate plan for the personal assistance of a particular patient is complex and must be designed from his/her EHR, different clinical guidelines and the correct coordination of diverse professionals maintaining the integral view of the patient.

We are analyzing how the effective management of the implicit knowledge inside a healthcare information system architecture could provide several benefits related to guideline management and practical use [2], like:

- Suggestion of the best applicable clinical guidelines based on the particular EHR of a patient.

- Suggestion of a specific plan for a patient, considering his/her particular EHR and different applicable guidelines.

- Support to the conversion of tacit knowledge inside the healthcare organization information systems into explicit knowledge in the form of clinical guidelines.

- Help to the validation of clinical guideline's effectiveness.

1.3. Objectives

The main objective of our work is the design of methods to integrate clinical guidelines management from a KM viewpoint in the healthcare organization systems architecture. Our work is in the framework of the prEN12976 and follows ODP methodology.

Our approach considers the assistance to comorbidity patient and consequently the use of several guidelines, related to different health issues, for the development of the personalized plan for a patient.

2. Results

2.1. Contributions to the enterprise viewpoint

The clinical guideline management inside a healthcare organization has to be considered from a KM perspective, and this implies two different consequences:

First, knowledge about a particular patient, in conjunction with any other relevant knowledge inside the healthcare organization, may suggest the clinical guidelines that better fit the patient profile.

The combination of the suggested clinical guidelines, together with the knowledge about the patient, in special that stored in his/her EHR, suggests the better assistance plan for this patient. This is a powerful decision support tool, especially when several guidelines are relevant for the assistance of a comorbidity patient.

Second, the implicit knowledge stored in the organization information systems can be used for the validation of the guideline's effectiveness and can be processed and formalized into explicit knowledge in the form of clinical guidelines.

2.2. Contributions to the information viewpoint

In the context of the HISA standard the concept of clinical guideline refers to a set of systematically developed statements to assist the decision of health care providers about activities to be provided with regard to a specific health issue.

A plan is a bundle of activities addressing the treatment and care of a particular health issue of a specific Subject of Care, as defined by a healthcare provider as a standard planning element encompassing all activities to be performed to achieve the specified clinical objective for the given health issue.

A protocol is a set of systematically developed statements specifying the roles and dependencies between planned activities as part of a plan.

Figure 1 shows the relation among these concepts, and between them and the clinical information inside the organization. We have included some relations, shown in dotted lines in the figure, for the improvement of the model in order to support the management of clinical guidelines from a knowledge management viewpoint. Only relevant cardinalities are shown. We have changed the cardinality of the relation *"suggest"*, from clinical guideline to plan. With this change the model is better adapted to the assistance to a comorbidity patient, where several clinical guidelines, each related to a different health issue, have to be considered.

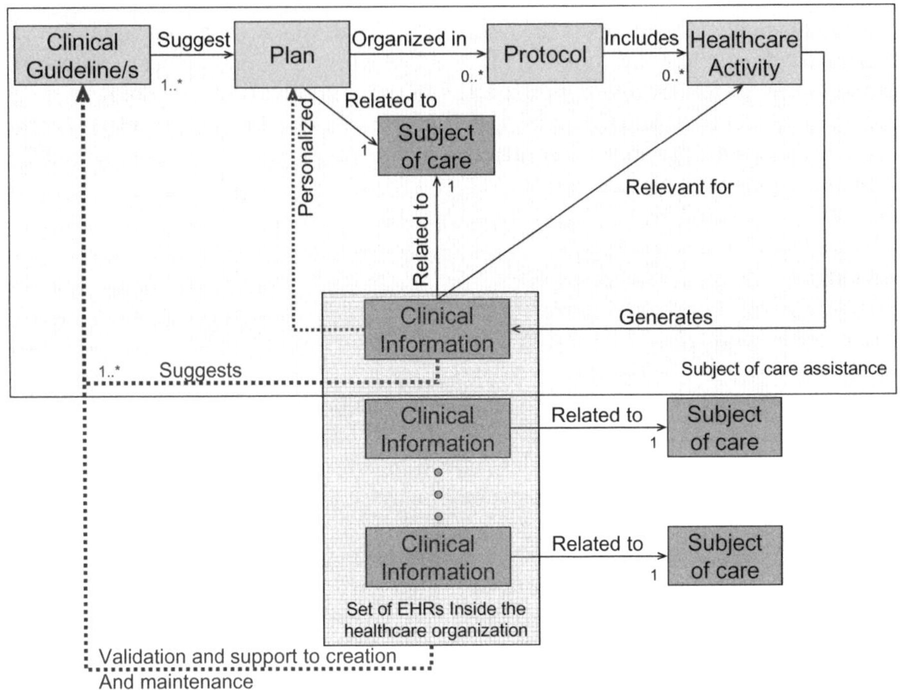

Figure 1. Adaptation of complex Clinical Guidelines management in the prENV12967 context

2.3. Contributions to the computational viewpoint

We have made a brief classification of services related to clinical guideline management.

Services for guidelines suggestion: applying KM techniques to the patient's EHR, the most suitable clinical guidelines are shown. Search criteria are based on organizational and personal parameters. The use of standard terminologies (CIE, SNOMED, UMLS, LOINC…) in the EHR is a valuable help to improve this search. We have been working with some public available services and databases [15] to develop some of these services.

Services for the creation of the assistance plan: these services help the physician to the definition of the best assistance plan for a particular patient. For comorbidity patient, incompatibilities between different guidelines applicable to a patient must be discovered, and the best choice should be suggested based on his/her personal clinical information. The plan could be organized in one or several protocols that include different healthcare activities, and must be planned and executed following the organization's processes and procedures. Of course, guidelines have to be written in a formal language for their effective management [16;17].

Services for the validation of guidelines: based on the analysis of the knowledge stored in the system about patients whose assistance plan were based in particular guidelines, these services help to the quality assessment of the guideline and could suggest changes for an improvement in this guideline.

Services for the creation of guidelines: these services are based on KM techniques. Exploiting the knowledge stored inside the organization systems could assist in the creation of guidelines considering not only the analysis of explicit knowledge compiled in publications but also combining the implicit facts inside the organization information systems [18].

3. Discussion

New EBM paradigms must be supported by the correct management of the implicit knowledge inside the information systems of healthcare organizations. The design of clinical guidelines will be based not only on published evidences and studies but in the information stored in the organization systems. Moreover the validation of clinical guidelines effectiveness and the measurement of quality parameters in guidelines could be improved with the management of tacit knowledge about patients that have been assisted following specific guidelines.

Furthermore clinical guidelines in combination with the knowledge about a patient can be automatically processed to assist the clinician in the design of the best personal plan for his/her assistance. A more personalized assistance, combining the best current evidence, available as explicit knowledge in clinical guidelines, in combination with the tacit knowledge about the patient, implicit in the organization systems, will assure the best diagnosis, treatment and prevention interventions, improving patient's assistance, health and quality of life.

The design of clinical guideline management components conform to prEN12967 standard and using ODP methodology and KM techniques is the key to success in this new challenge. The standard will need extensions and revisions for the inclusion of these components and of course organization's requirements and special conditions will impose design decisions in every scenario.

This is not an easy task and needs the cooperation of several professionals in an interdisciplinary team, considering issues as integration, normalization, distributed computing, KM advances, including those in ontologies, formal terminologies and structured representation languages, and obviously clinical domain expertise and experience.

Acknowledgements

This work has been partially financed by the Spanish Science and Education Ministry (TIN2006-15460-C04-03)

References

[1]   Bali RK, Feng DD, Burstein F, and Dwivedi AN, "Introduction to the special issue on advances in clinical and health-care knowledge management," IEEE Transactions on information technology in biomedicine, vol. Vol. 9, no. 2, pp. 157-161, June 2005.

[2]   P. Ciccarese, E. Caffi, S. Quaglini, and M. Stefanelli, "Architectures and tools for innovative Health Information Systems: The Guide Project," International Journal of Medical Informatics, vol. 74, no. 7-8, pp. 553-562, Aug. 2005.

[3]   S. Pantazi, J. Arocha, and J. Moehr, "Case-based medical informatics," BMC Medical Informatics and Decision Making, vol. 4, no. 1, p. 19, 2004.

[4]   "Cochrane collaboration web site: http://www.cochrane.org/," 2006. Notes: Last visited July 2006

[5]   A. H. Morice and M. Parry-Billings, "Evidence based guidelines--a step too far?," Pulmonary Pharmacology & Therapeutics, vol. 19, no. 3, pp. 230-232, June 2006.

[6]   CEN /TC 251.Secretariat: SIS, "Health Informatics - Service Architecture (HISA). prEN 12967-1 Part 1: Enterprise viewpoint," 2005.

[7]   CEN /TC 251.Secretariat: SIS, "Health Informatics - Service Architecture (HISA).prEN 12967-2 Part 2: Information viewpoint," 2005.

[8]   CEN /TC 251.Secretariat: SIS, "Health Informatics - Service Architecture (HISA). prEN 12967-3 Part 3: Computational viewpoint," 2005.

[9]   "CEN's web site: www.centc251.org,". Notes: Last visited February 2007

[10]   "CORBAmed web site: http://healthcare.omg.org/Roadmap/corbamed_roadmap.htm," 2006. Notes: Last visited July 2006

[11]   ITU-T, "Rec. X901-Information technology – Open distributed processing – Reference Model: Overview," 1997.

[12]   ITU-T, "Rec. X.902-Information Technology-Open distributed processing-Reference model:foundations," 1995.

[13]   ITU-T, "Rec. X903-Information technology – Open distributed processing – Reference Model: Architecture," 1995.

[14]   Zhan JX, Rathouz PJ, and Chin MH, "Comorbidity and the concentration of healthcare expeditures in older patients with heart failure," J Am Geriatr Soc, vol. 51, pp. 476-482, 2003.

[15]   "Entrez Web site: http://www.ncbi.nlm.nih.gov/Database/index.html,". Notes: Last visited February 2007

[16]   P. A. de Clercq, J. A. Blom, H. H. M. Korsten, and A. Hasman, "Approaches for creating computer-interpretable guidelines that facilitate decision support," Artificial Intelligence in Medicine, vol. 31, no. 1, pp. 1-27, May 2004.

[17]   K. Kaiser, C. Akkaya, and S. Miksch, "How can information extraction ease formalizing treatment processes in clinical practice guidelines?: A method and its evaluation," Artificial Intelligence in Medicine, vol. 39, no. 2, pp. 151-163, Feb. 2007.

[18]   R. Serban, A. ten Teije, F. van Harmelen, M. Marcos, and C. Polo-Conde, "Extraction and use of linguistic patterns for modelling medical guidelines," Artificial Intelligence in Medicine, vol. 39, no. 2, pp. 137-149, Feb. 2007.

Digital Homecare

Medical and Care Compunetics 4
L. Bos and B. Blobel (Eds.)
IOS Press, 2007

An RFID-Based System for Assisted Living: Challenges and Solutions

Judith SYMONDS [a], David PARRY [a,b] and Jim BRIGGS [b]
[a] *School of Computing and Mathematics, Auckland University of Technology, New Zealand*
[b] *School of Computing, University of Portsmouth, United Kingdom*

Abstract. Radio-frequency Identification (RFID) offers a potentially flexible and low cost method of locating objects and tracking people within buildings. RFID systems generally require less infrastructure to be installed than other solutions but have their own limitations. As part of an assisted living system, RFID tools may be useful to locate lost objects, support blind and partially sighted people with daily living activities and assist in the rehabilitation of adults with acquired brain injury. This paper outlines the requirements and the role of RFID in assisting people in these three areas. The development of a prototype RFID home support tool is described and some of the issues and challenges raised are discussed. The system is designed to support assisted living for elderly and infirm people in a simple, usable and extensible way in particular for supporting the finding and identification of commonly used and lost objects such as spectacles. This approach can also be used to extend the tagged domain to commonly visited areas, and provide support for the analysis of common activities, and rehabilitation.

Keywords. RFID, Assisted Living, Object Location, Rehabilitation

Introduction

Assistive technology has been recognised as a vital component of care for the increasing numbers of elderly and chronically sick people in western countries who will require help to stay in their homes and carry out the activities of daily living [1]. Therefore, there is a need for homes and the objects within them to become intelligent – that is to be able to actively assist their inhabitants. The concept of the "intelligent home" is not particularly new; [2] describes a "Smart House", including a network for home automation. More recently work has been done on the use of instrumented houses as technology test beds [3], and there has been increasing recognition that networking and computer control of electronic devices in the home is only one element of a solution for a supportive environment. A recent paper [4], gives an overview of some of these requirements. Appropriate interface design, context-awareness, standards for interoperability and, most importantly, usefulness are necessary for success.

1. Scenarios for Assisted Living

1.1. Object Location

Finding objects in the home is a task that everyone performs. Given the size of houses, location to around +/– 1 metre or even higher resolution is required. Houses also have structures – such as walls and furniture – that are a barrier to humans, but not radio waves. Lost objects or landmarks may not be in line of sight to the users. Memory failure is a common problem in the elderly with 25–50% of people reporting it [5]. A system to assist with finding objects in the home may therefore be useful for supporting elderly people in tasks of daily living.

Essentially the object location problem either requires a direct triangulation of the object, by the object having some sort of beacon attached, or the recording of the object's location in relation to some sort of map, which can be stored in a computer. An example of the first sort of system is the object finder [6], or the common sound-activated key rings. In this approach, the device emits a sound when the search function is activated. The user then follows the sound. Obvious disadvantages to such a system include the fact that many elderly people are deaf, and that precise object location by sound is difficult. In addition, the active beacons require batteries, and the beacons can themselves be quite large and interfere with the use of the object.

1.2. Object Identification and Characterization

In the object identification scenario, characteristics of the object being examined are important. This becomes important when there is some mismatch between the user's ability to perceive the attribute, and the requirement to know it in order to undertake certain tasks. Examples include identifying use-by dates, correct washing or cooking methods, instructions relating to the taking of prescribed drugs, the presence of gas or water leaks and interaction with mechanical and electronic devices.

Traditionally these requirements are met using visual indicators, whether symbolic or textual, in the form of instructions. Other sensory clues are also given – such as smell or sound. Even when the object incorporates specific affordances such as a handle or knob, vision assists in orientation. People with very poor eyesight may not be able to identify the colours of clothes, which can restrict their ability to dress themselves effectively.

Issues therefore arise for those with loss of vision, people who have difficulty reading, or those who are not speakers of the language in use. Loss or restriction of other senses can often raise problems when sound or smell is used as for attention focusing (such as a doorbell) or as a warning as in the odorant mixed with natural gas. In addition, the complexity of instructions and the number of possible interactions can give rise to difficulties if concentration or memory is impaired.

1.3. Activity Measurement and Person Tracking

One of the major concerns facing elderly people living alone is suffering a fall or other incapacitating event and being unable to summon help. Falls remain a common cause of morbidity and are difficult to prevent [7]. Changes in levels of activity can indicate exacerbations of chronic disease – e.g. Chronic Obstructive Airways Disease (COAD). Some people with dementia may require warnings when they venture outside the home or begin wandering. Brain injured patients and others with some types of memory loss may have difficulty completing tasks that need to be undertaken in a sequence, and will require reminders and training to allow them to finish them.

Gross activity measurement has been performed by many groups. A recent paper [8] has used information fusion from a number of sensors to monitor activity, and wrist-based sensors have also been used for this purpose. Fall alarm systems have become popular and more sophisticated [9]. However, such systems do have their drawbacks. In particular the activity-monitoring systems tend to measure gross activity, rather than whether the activity is directed and purposeful. Systems to notify carers of people straying are effective, but are single-use and tend to only perform this task [10].

2. A Review of the Technology of Object Identification and Location

GPS systems are difficult to use within buildings, because of reflection and attenuation with walls and other factors. Although this problem has been addressed [11], the solution involves triangulation of several different types of data. Any such system also requires that the plan of the building and furniture be translated into appropriate coordinates, so that the location of an object with respect to walls etc. is known. Triangulation techniques using either WiFi or mobile phone networks require available availability of wireless network infrastructure and are generally imprecise on the scale necessary, although there are techniques to reduce this error.

RFID has been proposed for object detection by several studies and the limitations of such development are well documented. Some systems, such as the one developed by Intel [12], use short range technology and can trace when objects are used in the environment by recording when the glove or bracelet is in close proximity to a tagged object in the environment. It should be pointed out that the main aim of this project is in activity tracking rather than object detection. Another such system by GaTech called the memory mirror [13] tracks removal and return of items from a specific storage area. The limitation of these systems is that they can only detect the location of objects when they are within range of the bracelet/glove/sandal and, due to technical limitations, the range is very short. This problem has led to augmentation with other types of data such as video analysis [14], motion detection sensors [12] and sonic data [15]. A recent summary from the University of Essex [16] has covered a number of projects that use object recognition by visual means – for example, mobile phone based work on object recognition in museums, active tagging or triangulation. Object recognition has the disadvantage that the system is computationally expensive and relies on the user pointing the device in the right direction. The use of additional hardware and sensors also adds to the cost of the overall system. However, the main disadvantage of such systems is that they are really only useful for self location or object identification. Lost objects will not be findable with this approach.

Long range RFID hardware uses either high frequency with high power supplies or ultra high frequency technology. The read range achieved starts from around 30cm and extends out to 10 metres. The exact location of an object is derived by triangulating the time difference in communication between the tag and reader to calculate an exact location. An example of this is the Paric system [17]. This system is extremely precise but requires a network of active tags which may be expensive.

This difference in user requirements can be illustrated by the type and differences in the kind of information provided by topographical and topological maps [18].

Topographic maps show a scaled representation of the area in question and significant objects within it. A topological map does not attempt to accurately represent distances between objects or landmarks, but rather distorts the layout so that routes between significant locations can be clearly seen, although the actual distance and absolute bearings are not correct. In an environment where the exact route taken between landmarks is not important, or routes are constrained for some reason, topological maps

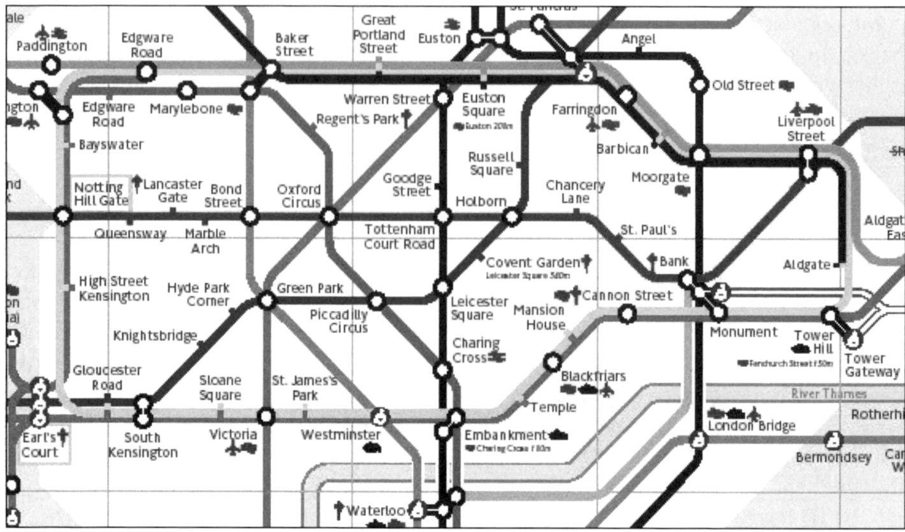

Figure 1. The Beck Map (copyright Transport for London).

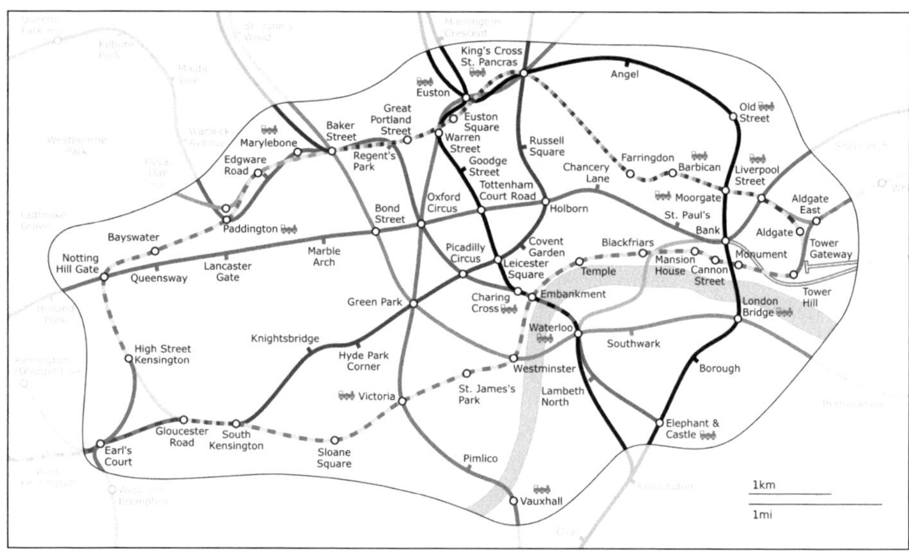

Figure 2. Topographic map of the Zone 1 area.

can be a great deal clearer than topographic ones. Topological maps are easily represented as a series of points and do not show exact coordinates.

A famous example of a topological map is the London underground map produced by Harry Beck in 1932 (Fig. 1). Compared to the topographic map in Fig. 2, the map is inaccurate in terms of location of stations, but it is extremely useful for route planning and progress monitoring.

In a system of object location using RFID, the Paric system referred to in the previous section would be very useful in preparing a topographic map of a room where the landmarks of the room were represented accurately to scale. However, such a system would be expensive overkill for preparing a topological map of the room in terms of providing the user with useful information.

3. Proposed System

3.1. General Characteristics of a Solution

According to our previous work [19] a system designed for the location of lost objects within the home as an assistive technology would have the following characteristics:

1. It should be relatively cheap
2. Objects should not have to be modified greatly
3. It should support multiple ways of searching
4. The interface and interaction should be intuitive
5. It must survive a reasonable degree of home rearrangement
6. It should not interfere with other occupants' lifestyle
7. A single system, rather than data fusion, is preferable for simplicity's sake

Fortunately, adding activity tracking and object identification is relatively straightforward. Object characterisation can be achieved by including more data – either embedded in the object or as data retrieved from a database using an object identifier such as a barcode. Activity tracking can occur as a by-product of object location – as the objects are picked up and landmarks passed.

Initially, losable objects (LO) and landmarks are labelled with RFID tags. A database in the interrogator system allows association between the tag ID (TID) and the description. For each TID a description that can be spoken and understood by the user is recorded. In choosing locations for landmarks, the user should have a higher density of landmarks near likely locations of loss as well as a regular pattern identifying navigation landmarks such as doorways, stairs etc. See Figs 3, 4 and for a potential scheme.

It may be useful to give such higher-level navigation tags high visibility colours so that they can be identified. Generally, higher-level navigation landmarks will require longer range detection, so tags with larger aerials may be used. The approach is similar to that of [20], where the "aura" component represents the final location of the object.

When the user is holding the losable object, the interrogator registers the presence of the object and records the high-level navigation tags that the user passes. The TID and timestamp are recorded in the database. Interrogation happens at around 10 millisecond intervals, depending on the number of tags within range. In order to reduce storage requirements, only the time of first detection and the time of last detection of a tag are stored for each tag detection episode. This avoids large amounts of data being stored when the user is stationary or holding an object. When the user drops the LO, then the system detects this by noting the absence of the LO's TID in the input stream. Any other navigation tags being detected at this point are noted.

When the user wishes to recover the LO, he or she names the object verbally and the speech conversion system finds the nearest LO name. When the required LO is identified, the topological map is searched via the timestamps, radiating outwards from the time that the LO was last detected. The navigation locations that were detected at

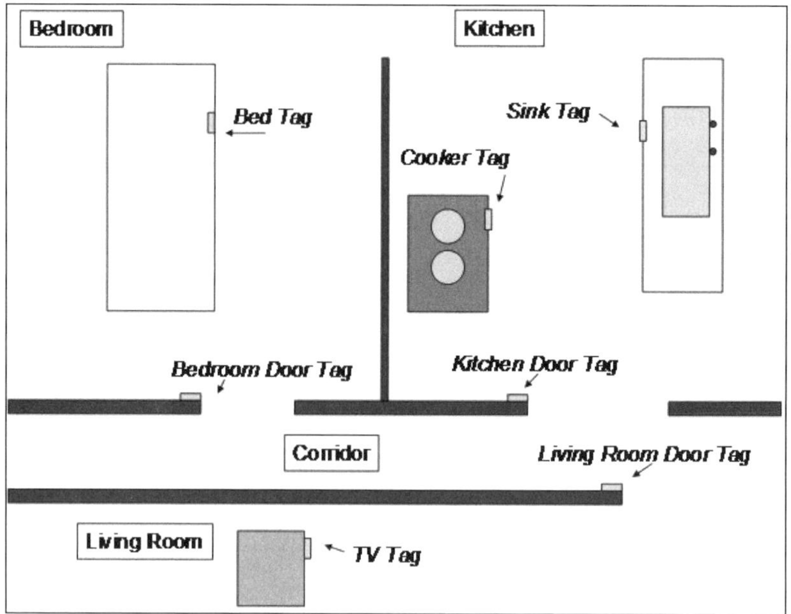

Figure 3. Topographic plan of the landmarks.

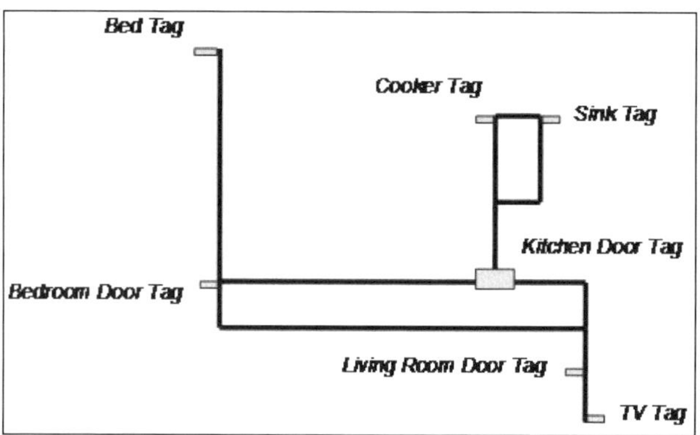

Figure 4. Topographic map of the landmarks.

the closest point to the dropping of the LO are declared. Should this not be clear, a dialogue could continue, with other nearby navigation points being declared until the user is satisfied that he or she knows the location of the object.

When the user gets to the nearest navigation point they can begin a detailed search for the LO. Patterns such as those used in avalanche search may be useful [21]. Another alternative is to retrace steps, where the system declares the sequence of navigation points around the time before and after the LO is dropped.

For object characterisation, the tags can either be used as the data storage medium, or as a pointer in a database stored in the interrogator or any central database. In some cases in the future many consumer items may have RFID tags already attached, which may provide some data or at least a unique identifier. Libraries may encode the name of the book although privacy issues may mitigate against this [22]. It may be more attractive to use this system to store user-generated data – for example whether the item of clothing is for warm or cold weather, along with any data that may be placed there automatically by the manufacturer. Short-range tags are most suitable for this application as the user will wish to distinguish between items that are stored close together.

Activity monitoring could use a number of approaches. The simplest is to measure movement of the user in relation to landmarks or tagged items. If the movement is below a certain amount, an alarm could be sent to a monitoring system. Adding the next level of complexity and invasiveness would identify landmarks that are the gateway to "no-go" zones (such as out of the front door). This would assume that the user is confused enough to wish to leave when they are at risk, but not determined enough to remove the interrogator device. A warning to the user that they were at risk from the device may be helpful. There is no reason why different zones may not be set up – for example within one's own room, within a building or on a campus – which may make this approach more acceptable. Certain users may wish to have the system remind them of objects that they should have with them when they go to certain areas – such as their front door keys or even a coat.

More precise and task-focussed tracking may be useful in the rehabilitation of brain-injured patients. These people often have difficulty remembering to complete tasks, and effectively have to begin again half way through a task. The tracking system may be able to identify characteristic patterns of movement around the topographic map associated with certain tasks, and prompt the user to complete them when the sequence halts or the user indicates they have forgotten what they are doing. A similar approach would generate speech that indicates what the next task is in the sequence as each one is completed.

4. Discussion

In our discussion we will cover the main practical and conceptual design problems that we face in this project.

4.1. Practical Design Problems

In our study the main practical design problems are a function of our COTS approach. That is, they relate to issues around adaptation of existing technology. However, it is useful to report these as they provide guidance for hardware developers, and open avenues for application of RFID other than in the mainstream areas of tracking and traceability.

4.1.1. Size & Weight

One major issue is the size of the 'aura', which is dependent on the read range of the interrogator, and the size and alignment of the tag. We think that the ideal size of the aura is large enough to incorporate the personal space of the user. This is likely to be around 70–150cm circumference. It would be attractive to be able to control this – for example by using tags with smaller antennae in areas such as within cupboards. Tag size is not a particular issue although flag-type deployment gives greater range on small objects. Currently the prototype interrogator is heavy (1.6kg) and about the same size as a desktop phone – and the antenna presents some problems in terms of size and rigidity.

4.1.2. Privacy Issues and Autonomy

There have been some privacy concerns, however all of the data is stored locally and is controlled exclusively by the user. Access to activity data derived from the system is limited to the user of the system unless they choose to share such information. Data coded onto object identification tags could be encrypted to prevent others reading them at a distance. One key element will be to emphasise that the system is a helper and not in charge of the user's life. Thus any reminders will have to be useful and appropriate. A model that treats this system as more like a guide dog than a human associate may be useful.

4.1.3. User Acceptance

We are working on the assumption that many people are accepting of personal electronic devices (iPod, mobile phone, personal organiser – for example). The public are also generally quite accepting of various types of tags on merchandise that they purchase – e.g. barcodes or tags on clothing. However, usability testing is a major feature of the final stages of our work and findings have not yet been collected.

4.1.4. Health

As all the devices used in our prototype are licensed for use without restriction, there is thought to be no risk associated with the RF energy. Moulder et al. (1999) have conducted a comprehensive study of the risks associated with exposure to radio frequency (chiefly cell phone) and risk of developing cancer. They find no proof of a link, but also conclude that proof of health hazards from cell phone exposure is impossible because of the wide range of contexts and areas of investigation possible.

4.1.5. Multiple Users (Multiple Interrogators in the Same Environment)

Major work is needed on ways to deal with multiple users and occupants operating in the same environment. If multiple users are moving objects, their individual annotated maps will have to be collaboratively updated. Our proposed system does have some inbuilt robustness in that each time losable objects come within the aura of the user, they are recorded and so our system should recover from object misplacement rather quickly.

4.1.6. Other Tags in the Environment

Our system has an initial set-up procedure to register tags in the system and the system 'ignores' tags that are not registered.

4.1.7. User Interface

The user interface is a critical success factor. Following design of current personal consumer devices such as mobile phones, iPods and PDAs, the keypad/screen interface is probably not the best communication approach. Voice recognition could be helpful, but some limitations in the technology might mean that a combination of voice and menu selection might be most practical at the moment.

4.1.8. Antenna Design

The current loop antenna is designed with manufacturing applications in mind. The antenna is rigid and is of an inconvenient shape. In our proof of concept experiments, we have used the antenna in a backpack configuration placed with the top edge just under the shoulder blades and on a 'shield' attached to the user's forearm. Ideally, it would be better to be able to design the antenna to be inserted into a cuff or watchstrap for the forearm.

4.2. Conceptual Design Problems

The chief conceptual design problem that we have encountered is that the aura concept has the potential for false readings in a multi-room environment. That is, because the tags can be read through some building materials that would be used in the home, there are possibilities for a landmark to be associated with the last known location of an object when the tag is on the other side of an internal wall from the landmark. There are a number of ways that this problem could be addressed:

1.   hardware
2.   tag placement
3.   database stored information, and
4.   software intelligence

4.2.1. Hardware

One possible solution to the problem of false reads would be to shield the tag from being read through walls. We thought about using tin foil, which is a very good shield for RF signals, to shield the tag from being read through objects. In our tests we found that it was impossible to shield the tag from only one direction – that is, the foil stopped the signal from all directions even though applied only to the back of the tag. We also experimented with a thickness of card to separate the tag from the foil at the back. While this did allow the tag to be read from one direction, the signal was severely weakened and this seemed like a poor solution since an efficient read range for the tags is so important for our system.

4.2.2. Tag Placement

Another possible solution to the problem is tag placement. It is possible to generate a set of rules about tag placement that would limit the potential for false results. For example, there could be a rule that all tags must be placed at least 70cm from walls. However, this could become quite complex and require expert installation of the tags in the final system, and could restrict the performance of the object location system. Therefore, it does not seem to be a viable solution to the problem.

4.2.3. Database

It is also possible to add some fields to the database tables in the application to allow a room location to be stored. These locations could then be checked using a simple SQL query to ensure that the tags on the object and the landmark are in the same room. This solution will work quite effectively once the system is set-up, but does complicate the registration process and would limit the plug and play capability of the system. For example, it would be difficult to ship the application with a set of pre-set tags and objects if you had to also store the room location, since these will differ from environment to environment.

4.2.4. Intelligent Software

It is possible for the software to implement a type of topological logic inherent in topological mapping (see Section 2). That is, not only does the system feedback and track landmarks that are within the user's aura, the system also applies a sensibility test using a known topological route to check that the items are not in a different room of the house from the user before storing the information. This seems the most sensible solution and is the one that we are trying to implement in our software after initial proof-of-concept experimentation.

5. Conclusion

Earlier in our paper we put forward seven criteria for the success of the assisted living environment system design. In this section we address each in an attempt to evaluate our progress.

Relatively cheap
Essentially, the topological approach to the system, with the reader on the user, makes our system relatively cheap when compared with systems that follow the topographical approach to object location.

Low modification of objects
Placement of tags on the outside of losable objects means that they do not need to be modified greatly to be part of the system, and if the system came with pre-registered tags, this would limit the amount of setting up needed in the system before initial use.

Multiple search methods
We intend to allow the system to use a 'roam' search option as well as the historical object tracking system to allow the system to support multiple ways of searching. There are other possibilities – such as using a grid for searching – but this is outside the scope of this paper.

Intuitive user interface
We recognise that the current prototype interface (which uses the menu of a Pocket PC) is limited in terms of usability. We hope to integrate some level of voice recognition or perhaps touch screen graphics to address this limitation. However, for the purposes of proof of concept of the topological approach, the user interface is not crucial.

Survive home rearrangement
The topological approach to finding lost objects copes quite well with the prospect of home rearrangement, especially if locations of objects are not stored in the database tables. After landmarks and objects have been moved and the first instance of their location has been stored in the database, effectively a new virtual topological map is cre-

ated. The only limitation would be that the user would need to check that the placement of the tags was not affected, such as not being shielded by metal or water.

Not interfering with other occupants lifestyle

The ultimate goal is to develop a system that will not interfere with other occupants' lifestyle. Presently, the size of the prototype is an obvious limiting factor. We also need to develop a sensible cuff/strap embedded antenna to allow usability trials to test for problems with it interfering with daily life. Certainly, something on the user's arm seems less restricting than a glove that would restrict washing up, food preparation and toileting.

Single system

For obvious reasons, a single, well-integrated system is preferable to the complications of combining disparate systems. By associating the system with the user rather than the house, the paradigm of the mobile phone or PDA can be used, thus making it a personal system. This removes the need to interface multiple sensors, or make the user learn multiple interfaces. As a side effect of this, many homes or spaces, such as hotel rooms or public transport, could be fitted with the RFID tags even if the occupants do not currently need the system.

References

[1] UK Audit Commission. Assistive Technology Independence and Well-being 4. 2004 12th Feburary 2004 [cited 2006 1 November 2006]; Available from: http://www.audit-commission.gov.uk/reports/NATIONAL-REPORT.asp?CategoryID=&ProdID=BB070AC2-A23A-4478-BD69-4C19BE942722.

[2] Stauffer, H.B., Smart enabling system for home automation. IEEE Transactions on Consumer Electronics, 1991. 37(2): p. xxix–xxxv.

[3] Helal, S., et al., The Gator Tech Smart House: a programmable pervasive space. Computer, 2005. 38(3): p. 50–60.

[4] Stefanov, D.H., Z. Bien, and W.-C. Bang, The smart house for older persons and persons with physical disabilities: structure, technology arrangements, and perspectives. IEEE Transactions on Neural Systems and Rehabilitation Engineering, 2004. 12(2): p. 228–250.

[5] Jonker, C., M.I. Geerlings, and B. Schmand, Are memory complaints predictive for dementia? A review of clinical and population-based studies. International Journal of Geriatric Psychiatry, 2000. 15(11): p. 983–991.

[6] Holbrook; Paul Robert , L.D.R.G.B.S., Born; Joseph , Hurtado; Raquel Elizabeth , Buczkiewicz; Robert Thomas, Object finder. 2004, Digital Innovations, L.L.C.: USA.

[7] Gillespie, L., et al., Interventions for preventing falls in elderly people. 2006, Cochrane Database of Systematic Reviews.

[8] Suzuki, R., et al., Rhythm of daily living and detection of atypical days for elderly people living alone as determined with a monitoring system. Journal of Telemedicine and Telecare, 2006. 12(4): p. 208–214.

[9] Doughty, K., R. Lewis, and A. McIntosh, The design of a practical and reliable fall detector for community and institutional telecare. Journal of Telemedicine and Telecare, 2000. 6(Supp. 1): p. S150–154.

[10] Altus, D.E., et al., Evaluating an electronic monitoring system for people who wander. American Journal of Alzheimer's Disease and Other Dementias, 2000. 15(2): p. 121–125.

[11] Ni, L.M., et al. LANDMARC: indoor location sensing using active RFID. in Pervasive Computing and Communications, 2003. (PerCom 2003). Proceedings of the First IEEE International Conference on. 2003.

[12] Smith, J.R., et al., RFID-based techniques for human-activity detection. Communications of the ACM, 2005. 48(9): p. 39–44.

[13] Quan T. Tran, E.D.M. The Aware Home – Memory Mirror. 2005 [cited 2006 1st December 2006]; Available from: http://www-static.cc.gatech.edu/fce/ahri/projects/Memory_Mirror.pdf.

[14] Mihailidis, A., B. Carmichael, and J. Boger, The use of computer vision in an intelligent environment to support aging-in-place, safety, and independence in the home. Information Technology in Biomedicine, IEEE Transactions on, 2004. 8(3): p. 238–247.

[15] Adam, S., et al., Tracking moving devices with the cricket location system, in Proceedings of the 2nd international conference on Mobile systems, applications, and services. 2004, ACM Press: Boston, MA, USA.

[16] Prashant Solanki and Huosheng Hu, Techniques used for Location-based Services: A survey. 2005, University of Essex.

[17] Paric Limited. Paric homepage. 2006 [cited 2006 1st December 2006]; Available from: http://www.paric.co.nz/.

[18] Monkhouse, F.J. and H.R. Wilkinson, Maps & Diagrams: Their Compilation and Construction. 1978: Methuen & Co Ltd.

[19] Basrur, P. and D. Parry, "Where are my Glasses?": An Object Location System within the Home. . Bulletin of Applied Computing and Information Technology 2006. 4(2).

[20] Satoh, I. A location model for pervasive computing environments. in Third IEEE International Conference on Pervasive Computing and Communications. 2005.

[21] Michahelles, F., et al., Applying wearable sensors to avalanche rescue. Computers and Graphics, 2003. 27(6): p. 839–847(9).

[22] Molnar, D. and D. Wagner, Privacy and security in library RFID: issues, practices, and architectures, in Proceedings of the 11th ACM conference on Computer and communications security. 2004, ACM Press: Washington DC, USA.

Medical and Care Compunetics 4
L. Bos and B. Blobel (Eds.)
IOS Press, 2007

Safe Pill-Dispensing

Massimiliano TESTA and John POLLARD[1]
Department of Electronic and Electrical Engineering, University College London

Abstract. Each patient is supplied with a smart-card containing a Radio Frequency IDentification (RFID) chip storing a unique identification code. The patient places the Smart-card on a pill-dispenser unit containing an RFID reader. The RFID chip is read and the code sent to a Base-station via a wireless Bluetooth link. A database containing both patient details and treatment information is queried at the Base-station using the RFID as the search key. The patient's treatment data (i.e., drug names, quantities, time, etc.) are retrieved and sent back to the pill-dispenser unit via Bluetooth. Appropriate quantities of the required medications are automatically dispensed, unless the patient has already taken his/her daily dose. Safe, confidential communication and operation is ensured.

Keywords. RFID, patient-identification, Bluetooth, medication database

Introduction

A *safe* pill-dispenser system uses transparent software technology to protect people who are taking prescription drugs. It has the following features:

- Patients and carers are provided with a timely reminder to administer prescribed pills,
- On presentation of a patient identification card (Radio Frequency IDentification, RFID card) the prescribed type and quantity of medication is made available,
- Once pills have been removed from the pill-box during a particular epoch, further supply of these same drugs is prevented together with a warning message that the medication has already been delivered,
- Carers and nurses who supervise the ingestion process are supplied with detailed information about quantity and type of pills supplied. This gives them the opportunity to report to the doctor any noted effects, e.g., contra-indication symptoms to the drug's efficacy.
- The prescription process (doctor), pill-loading (pharmacist) and supervision (nurse) are password-protected for each role.

The consumption of prescription pills continues to increase yearly as the mean age of the population rises. In addition, people are becoming more aware of health issues and the role of pharmaceutical products to alleviate them. Many of these medications may constitute a health hazard if not taken as prescribed.

---

[1] Corresponding Author: Department of Electronic and Electrical Engineering, University College London, Torrington Place London WC1E 7JE; E-mail: jp@ee.ucl.ac.uk.

Demographic studies show a notable growth in the population of elderly people in the UK, so that by 2025 nearly 27% of the population (14.8 million) will be over 60 years old [1]. In addition, the 75–84 and 85+ age groups are predicted to expand by some 30% and 60% respectively over the next 20 years. In comparison, the proportion of people over 60 years of age in 2001 was 20.4% (10.2 million).

There will be a significant responsibility on society to look after the higher numbers of mature and infirm citizens. Logistically, it will become more difficult to provide the health and social care required and the burden on carers, nurses, doctors and administrators may increase substantially.

There is, therefore, a need for a new approach to healthcare whereby it is possible to deploy care and services strategically to where they are most needed. It is hoped that the medical monitoring system to be described in the next section may help to achieve this. Additional benefits are likely to result from improved personal security, efficient energy usage, automated facilities and enhanced maintenance management [2].

Governments are looking for alternative means of care and see the domiciliary care market as the cost effective solution. Dr. Stephen Ladyman, former Minister at the Department of Health said "we need to ... provide simple, low-cost solutions for ... relatives of older people... that can be purchased through high street vendors ... and which they can fit themselves" [3]. It is also recognised that elderly people wish to continue to live independently as long as they are physically and mentally able to do so. The Anchor Trust (a UK charity) commissioned a survey that found 80% of people over 65 wished to remain in charge of their own life. Another survey by BT put this figure nearer the 95% mark.

The success of any home-care solution will depend on the peace of mind it delivers to the individual and their carers. Care is primarily provided by friends or family. They expect to be able to check up frequently on their loved ones and to be contacted immediately when something goes wrong [4].

The proposed pill-dispenser system is suitable for individuals in a variety of home-care situations, residential-care, nursing-homes and hospital use. It utilises inexpensive and unobtrusive technology such as short-range wireless (e.g. Bluetooth [5]), cellular mobile telephones and wired World-Wide Web access. The data communication system is made reliable by using a backbone wireless network with redundancy [6].

1. Healthcare System

It is envisaged that the pill-dispensing system to be described is one element of an integrated healthcare system that is suitable for the home as well as institutions. All individual features of the system have been built in prototype form and an integrated, fully-fledged system remains to be completed.

The generic healthcare system uses Bluetooth-enabled devices to exchange data and to control applications such as pill-dispensing.

Bluetooth is a low power, medium data-rate (700 kbps) wireless transceiver technology that has a voice capability and operates license-free at 2.4 GHz. It is the short-range radio with greatest resilience to interference because of its Hopping Frequency Spread Spectrum characteristic [7].

It is a mature product that has found a mass market in some 700 million mobile telephones. Bluetooth devices are cheap to produce and to buy. Devices differ in functionality by internal software only and the same hardware may act as a Bluetooth Base-

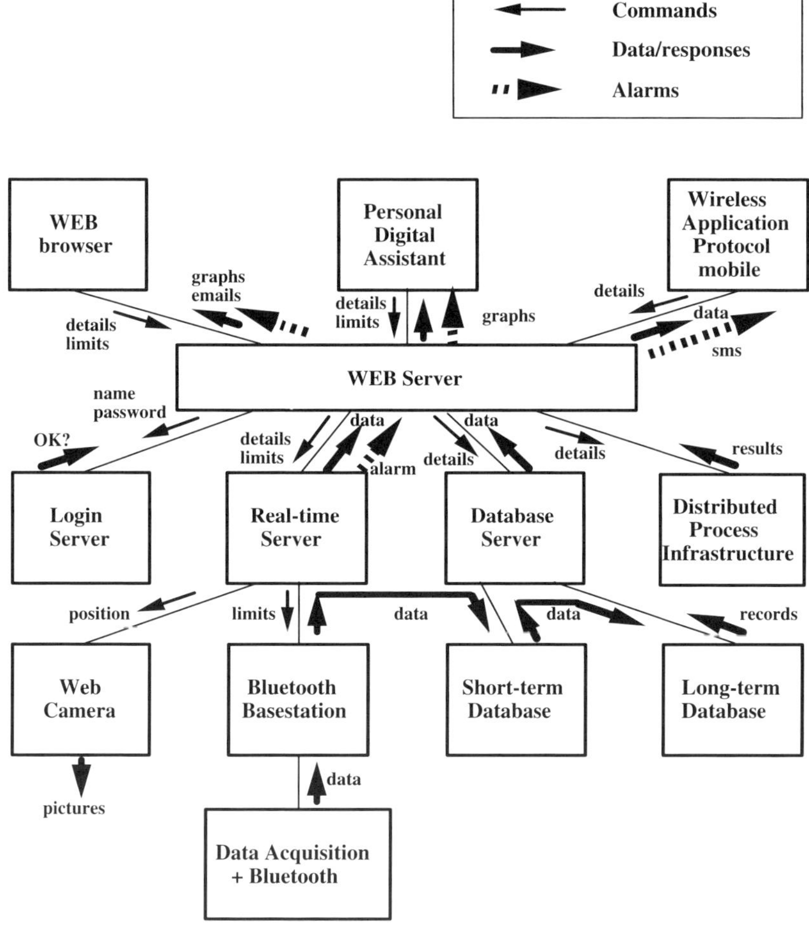

Figure 1. Medical Supervisory Control And Data Acquisition, SCADA.

station (or a Network Access Point) for Sensor Area Networks. Applications using medical-sensors may have a low duty-cycle and so consume little battery power. They create negligible electro-magnetic interference for sensitive medical equipment [8].

The generic medical supervisory control and data acquisition system is shown in Fig. 1. The information flows from the data acquisition unit (e.g. RFID card reader + Bluetooth) to the Base-station that may contain a Short-term Database. It verifies patient identity and prescribed medication.

The Base-station is controlled by a Real-time Server that also controls a (optional) Bluetooth-enabled, stand-alone camera to provide visual communication between doctor and patient [9].

As Fig. 1 illustrates, patient records are stored in a Long-term central Database that is accessible over the wired network. The Database Server controls the movement of data between local Short-term and remote Long-term Databases. This enables health trends and medication needs to be continuously monitored in a more complete system. This monitoring software can be done remotely on a distributed computer system.

The coordination amongst the carers, nurses, doctors and administrators in this medical system is accomplished via the World-Wide Web. These people use Web-browsers, Personal Digital Assistants and Wireless Application Protocol telephones to assist their work of unobtrusive tele-medicine and inter-personal communication about patients under their care. A Login Server authenticates users with different roles. Encryption of communicated data is possible.

In general, medical sensors can be configured with thresholds that trigger alarms, should unusual values of sensor parameters be detected. However, human carers are the usual (and more reliable) agency to warn of medical problems.

1.1. How the System Will Benefit Healthcare Services

The system minimises unnecessary house calls to the elderly and hospital out-patients. The immediate impact is to deploy services efficiently to where they are most needed. Additional benefits to geriatric medicine may accrue from analysing field data, in order to study the correlation between lifestyle and health of the patient. Features of this system are to:

- Provide automatic, verbal or visual medication reminders [10],
- Store and maintain medical data in a private, secure and protected manner and yet allow authorised users to access the system remotely,
- Use technology that is comfortable, convenient, easy to use, and flexible so as to accommodate it to the patient's lifestyle.
- Be useable by non-technical operators (after some training) with the aid of online documentation (e.g. Help menu),
- Cater for system evolution: expansion and technology updates,
- Be based on a full user-needs assessment: how a user is to interact with the technology from a psychological, emotional, physical and social perspective,
- Assist all stakeholders in cost or labour saving,
- Receive regular maintenance and checks, to ensure correct functionality as designed,
- Provide training and interactive modification from the outset, driven by the operators' feedback.

2. Pill-Dispensing Technology

Patients are supplied with a wristband (to wear all the time) that is fitted with a small-sized Radio Frequency Identification Smart-card tag (Fig. 2). This tag contains a Silicon chip with a unique identifier – a combination of letters and numbers. The Smart-card tag also has a conducting coil antenna that provides power to activate the chip when voltage is induced by an external magnetic field, which is produced by an RFID reader.

The pill-dispenser sub-system is shown in Fig. 3.

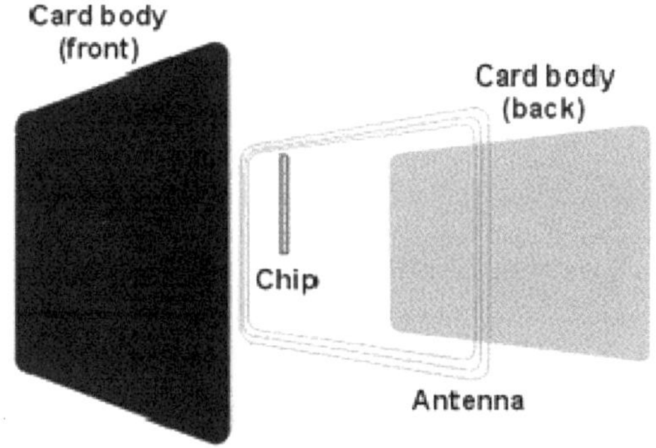

Figure 2. Smart-card Tag.

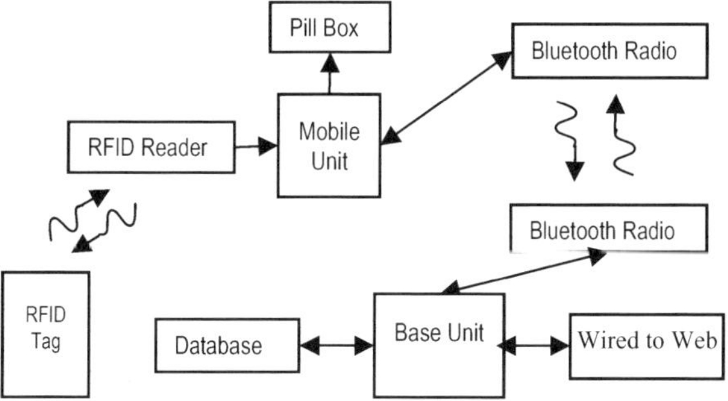

Figure 3. RFID-Based Pill Dispenser System.

A mobile unit consists of an electro-mechanically operated pill-box, a display and associated control circuitry, together with a RFID reader and a Bluetooth radio. When it is time for the patient to take the medication, the pill-dispensing unit reads the patient ID (12-byte alphanumeric code number) from the RFID tag that is placed upon it. This ID is sent to a Base-station computer via wireless Bluetooth technology. The Base-station includes a Short-term database with patient and medical-drug information.

The database is queried using the tag value as a search key, the ID is validated and the pill types and quantities to be dispensed are sent back to the pill-dispenser mobile unit. The dispenser makes the relevant medications available unless it finds that the patient has already taken his or her daily dose. Messages to the user/carer are displayed.

The overview of the software is shown in Fig. 4 as a Use Case diagram.

The Smart-card tag contains patient's information which can be read (displayed/modified/deleted) with appropriate authorisation. The remote mobile unit contains software to connect and send data such as the patient-ID number to the base-station via Bluetooth. The Base-station accepts and records the request for data that is kept in the Short-term database.

A database called *hospital* is created in the ("MySql") Short-term Database Server. The database structure is based on two tables, called *patient* and *medication* (Fig. 5).

     M. Testa and J. Pollard / Safe Pill-Dispensing

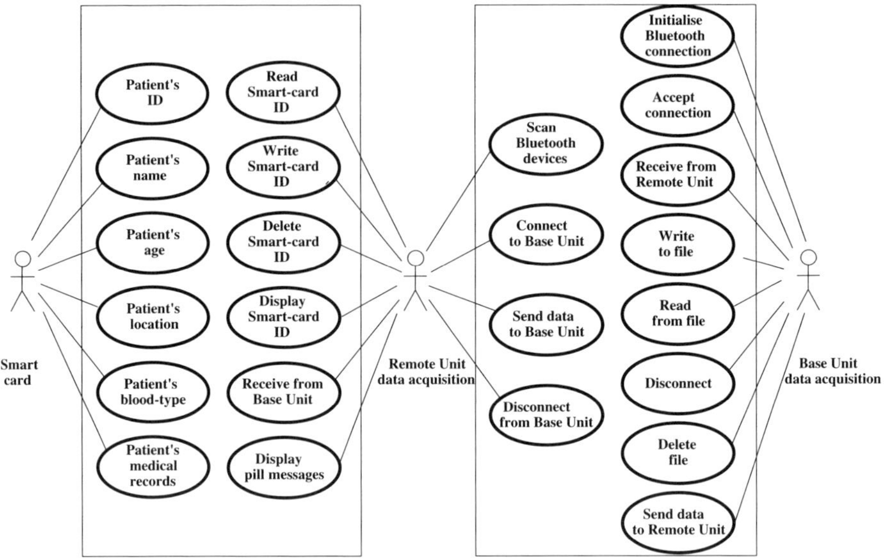

Figure 4. Smart-card ⇔ Remote Unit ⇔ Base Unit Use-Case Diagram.

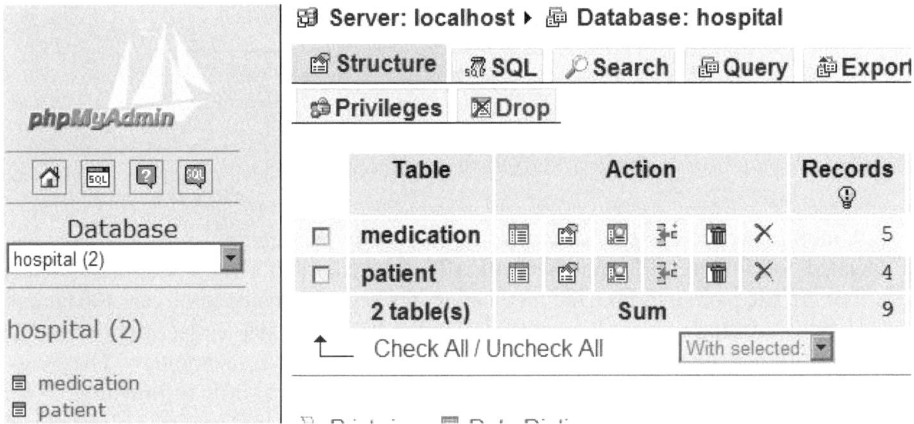

Figure 5. *hospital*-Database Schema.

The *patient* table contains personal information necessary to identify the patient: name, age, address, RFID-tag code and treatment information. The *medication* table contains details of all medications available at the hospital, nursing home or pharmacy.

The patient's tag identifier is the primary key of the table *patient*. The Base-station program sends commands to the database in order to query for the list of relevant medications. The details are found in the *medication* table as illustrated in Fig. 6.

The patient's treatment information (e.g. drug names, quantity and time to be taken at, whether already dispensed, pill photograph, etc) is sent back to the mobile unit for display and to be processed to drive the pill-box mechanism in order to dispense the appropriate medications.

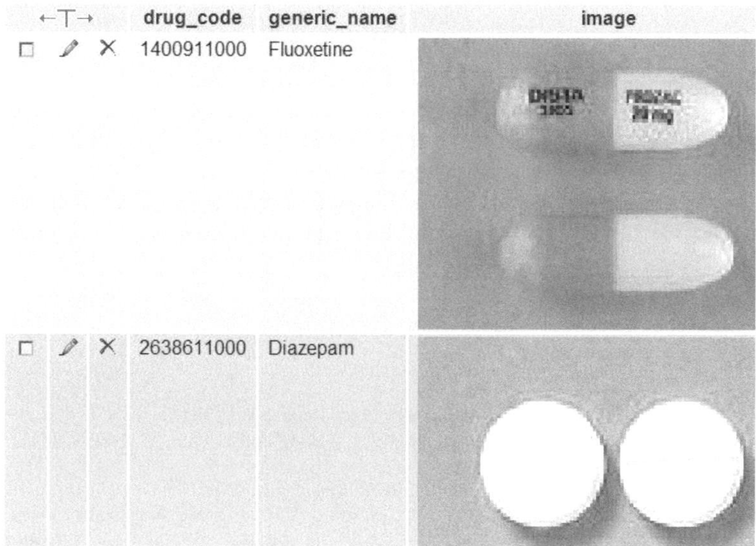

Figure 6. "medication" Table.

```
Patient: John Brown

Drug Code     Generic Name    Quantity    Time To Take It    Already Taken?
1400911000    Fluoxetine      2.0         12:00:00           No
5568111000    Gabapentin      1.0         15:00:00           No
Press any key to continue
```

Figure 7. Example Text Message from Base-station to Dispenser.

An example text message from the base-station to the pill dispenser is shown in Fig. 7.

The dispenser software controls the electro-mechanical pill-box so that the correct medications are made available. If some of the medicines have already been taken by the patient in the prescribed period, this is noted in the message and the pill box does not activate to dispense pills.

3. Conclusion

A pill-dispenser system has been described that uses a software **system** in conjunction with a **reliable** wireless data communication system to ensure patient safety. The system correctly delivers prescribed medication at the appropriate times.

Safety features include patient reminders about type and time for pills to be dispensed. These messages could be verbal (via telephone) or visual (via television). If pills have already been delivered, an informative message is supplied.

Carers, nurses, pharmacists and doctors are provided with password-protected and encrypted facilities to monitor patients, including wireless cameras (if appropriate). Doctors prescribe the medication to be taken at specified times.

The facilities of the World-Wide Web, in conjunction with Web-browsers, Personal Digital Assistants and mobile telephones, are used to assist communication between all parties.

Prototypes of all software and communication elements have been built and tested but the electro-mechanically operated pill-box remains to be bought and integrated in the system.

References

[1] Housing Corporation, "Housing for older people", 2001, London W1T7BN.
[2] D. Gans, J. Barlow and T Venables, "Digital Futures: making homes smarter", Joseph Rowntree Foundation/Charted Institute of Housing, York, 1999.
[3] Bridging the Gap – Participation in Social Care Regulation, Sept., 2004.
[4] R.G. Curry, M.T. Tinoco and D. Wardle, "Telecare: Using ICT to support independent living by older, disabled and vulnerable people, July, 2003 (DoH), www.independentliving.org/docs2/enilfuture.pdf.
[5] J.K. Pollard, S. Rohman, C. Santarelli, A. Theodorou, N. Mohoboob and M.E. Fry, "Wireless and web-based medical monitoring in the home", *Special Issue Medical Informatics & Internet in Medicine*, Vol. 27(3), (Dec, 2002), pp. 219–227.
[6] J.K. Pollard, "Packet Error Correction in Personal Area Networks", Invited paper accepted for AMS2007, Phuket, Thailand, (March, 2007).
[7] N.P. Kontakos and J.K. Pollard, "Bluetooth indoor channel simulation", *Proc. Conf on Intelligent Data Acquisition & Advanced Computing Systems*, Ternopil Acad. of National Economy, Lviv, Ukraine, (Sept., 2003).
[8] Medical Devices Agency, "Electro-Magnetic Compatibility of medical devices with mobile communications", MDA DB 9702, (March, 1997).
[9] S. Rohman, E. Davis, A. Obhrai, J. Mander, M. Patel and J.K Pollard, "Web-based mobile medical system", *Forum on clinical instrumentation, UCL Centre for Advanced Instrumentation Systems*, (Jan, 2002).
[10] P. Yuvacharuskul, "Texts on video encoder", *BEng Project thesis*, UCL, 2006.

Medical and Care Compunetics 4
L. Bos and B. Blobel (Eds.)
IOS Press, 2007

Wearable Real-time and Adaptive Feedback Device to Face the Stuttering: a Knowledge-based Telehealthcare Proposal

Manuel PRADO[1], Laura M. ROA
Biomedical Engineering Group, Network Center of Biomedical Research in Bioengineering, Biomaterials and Nanomedicine (CIBER-TEC) and University of Seville, Spain

Abstract. Despite first written references to permanent developmental stuttering occurred more than 2500 years ago, the mechanisms underlying this disorder are still unknown. This paper briefly reviews stuttering causal hypothesis and treatments, and presents the requirements that a new stuttering therapeutic device should verify. As a result of the analysis, an adaptive altered auditory feedback device based on a multimodal intelligent monitor, within the framework of a knowledge-based telehealthcare system, is presented. The subsequent discussion, based partly on the successful outcomes of a similar intelligent monitor, suggests that this novel device is feasible and could help to fill the gap between research and clinic.

Keywords. Adaptive stuttering therapy, Multimodal monitoring, Wearable intelligent device, Multitier architecture, Telehealthcare, Model-based knowledge discovering

1. Introduction

Stuttering is a disorder that affects approximately 1 % of world adult population, with men prevalence higher than women (1/4) [1]. Formal definitions of the disorder stated by official organisms like WHO (ICD-9-CM) or the American Psychiatric Association (DSM-IV-TR) are complexes and very controversial because they describe the perception of the perturbed speech pattern by an external listener, and lack the knowledge regarding the internal perception of the stuttering subject as well as the etiology of the disorder. For example, according to the ICD-9-CM the stuttering "*is a disturbance in the normal fluency and time patterning of speech that is inappropriate for the individual's age. This disturbance is characterized by frequent repetitions or prolongations of sounds or syllables. Various other types of speech dysfluencies may also be involved including interjections, broken words, audible or silent blocking, circumlocutions, words produced with an excess of physical tension, and monosyllabic whole word repetitions. Stuttering may occur as a developmental condition in childhood or as an acquired disorder which may be associated with BRAIN INFARCTIONS and other BRAIN DISEASES. (From DSM-IV, 1994)*".

---

[1] Corresponding Author: Manuel Prado, Escuela Superior de Ingenieros, Camino de los descubrimientos s/n, 41092, Sevilla, Spain; E-mail: mpradovelasco@ieee.org.

This paper is about permanent developmental stuttering (PDS), which starts during the childhood and develops during the maturation and evolution of the subject that suffers the disorder. This is the most usual type of stuttering. Despite the article is not devoted to the analysis of PDS, we must expose several relevant historical and biomedical issues that help to clarify the current knowledge concerning its etiology and associated therapies.

First references to this disorder appear in ancient Egyptian and China civilizations, and it has been recurrently cited by Greek writers. The strange and variable speech patterns associated with stuttering has challenged to researchers on the discovering of the causal underlying mechanisms since ancient times up to now. This way, from the perturbed state of the famous body humors of Hippocrates and his prescription with sticking blistering substances to the tongue to drain away the dark fluid (4th century BC) up to the surgical resection of tongue's chunks by the reputed Prussian surgeon Johann Friedrich Dieffenbach to prevent its hypothetical spasms, at half of 19th century, many other incredible hypothesis and related therapies were invented, with traumatic and even mortal consequences [2, 3].

After the unsuccessful outcomes of organic hypotheses, and pushed by the emergence of psychoanalysis at the end of 19th century and beginning of 20th century, a great number of psychoanalytical theories were proposed [3, 4]. A parallel line was led by logopedic conceptions, pointing to nervous system and breath affections as the cause of the disorder [5].

These two lines, together with a third one founded on neuromuscular and other neurogenic-approaches were coupled in different manners along the 20th century, providing logopedic-centered conceptions [6-8], psychoanalytical-centered conceptions [4, 9-11], and organic-centered conceptions [12, 13]. Interesting reviews of these theories can be read anywhere [2, 14-16].

The demands and capacities model of Starkweather in 1987 [17] starts a strong tendency to integrate external (environmental) with internal (innate or biological) factors. This model combines concepts from the diagnosogenic theory of Johnson [11] with the inability of the child to respond properly to external demands. Among other subsequent models that follow this integrative line can be cited [18, 19].

This integrative conception and multicausal origin of stuttering provides support to current holistic therapies, which combine direct treatments (logopedic) with indirect treatments (psychological). A review of the current scenario around the world can be seen in [20].

A new branch of stuttering research appeared at the second halt of 1990s, with the well-known work of Fox et al. [21]. By contrasting stuttering with fluent speech using positron emission tomography (PET), combined with chorus reading for inducing fluency, the authors found a lack of left-lateralized activation of the auditory system, characterized by an underactivation of the frontal-temporal system implicated in speech production (left-side), and a overactivation of the premotor cortex (operculum and insula) with right cerebral dominance. These neuronal abnormalities, as well as the dysfluencies, were remediated by chorus reading. These findings have been replicated with different imaging techniques (fMRI) and with different speech tasks, including imagined speech (covert speech). An updated review of this subject appeared in a special issue of the Journal of Fluency Disorders (2003), entitled Brain imaging Research on Persistent Developmental Stuttering.

However, the origin of stuttering remains unknown, and authors continue the debate concerning the nature, cause or effect (compensatory or other one), of the observed brain images [22]. So far as we know, many of the models fail because they try to shoehorn this new knowledge into previous hypotheses. In words of Fox *what is needed is a new view, a quantum leap.*

This obscurity explains the many, variable and depending on speech language professional, number of stuttering therapies, and the high percentage (very close to 100 %) of relapse in adults with PDS. This lack of success has promoted on the one hand the development of self-help groups, in attendance or virtual, thanks to the new technologies on information and communications (TIC). A pioneer example is the Hispanic language virtual forum of stuttering originated in 1998 through the research study of Rodríguez-Carillo [23]. On the other hand, it has promoted studies that negate the biomedical existence of the disorder, with asseverations such (translated) *as our framework distances from positivist and essentialist postulates of medicine, which consider the stuttering as an ill, disturbance, dysfunction, disorder, etc, composed of symptoms or syndrome; ... we consider the stuttering as a social deviated conduct because it is minority* [2]. This asseveration is supported by a serious social field study over self-help and toastmaster groups, but although it could be consistent from a social and intercultural perspective, it is inconsistent with objective facts: subjects with PDS have really serious difficulties to communicate orally because they have not a proper control of their speech production.

The importance and awareness of this disorder is growing, as demonstrate the tri-annual world congresses promoted by the International Stuttering Association (ISA) and the European League o Stuttering Associations (ELSA), since 1986, as well as the creation of local associations such as the Fundación Española de la Tartamudez (www.ttm-espana.com), instituted in February 2002, or the recognition of PDS as a disability in the Spanish legislation.

This paper proposes and discusses a new technology founded on a knowledge-based telehealthcare, which seeks to deliver a multimodal, personalized, and adaptive therapy to treat the stuttering, and to help discovering knowledge that throws light on the etiology. As a consequence of the complexity and extension of this research line, the present paper must be understood as an introductory and brief proposal.

The article is structured as follows. The following Section slightly addresses several of the nowadays causal hypotheses, and suggests which is the most plausible according to the best of our knowledge. The Methods Section selects the best requirements that must fulfill a therapeutic proposal based on the aforementioned telehealthcare paradigm and causal hypothesis. These requirements were the basis of the technological proposal presented in the Results Section, which is in finally analyzed in the Discussion.

2. Causal hypotheses

The goal of this Section is justifying the causal hypothesis of stuttering as a basis of the therapeutic solution that we propose. Although the proposed device is not restricted to that model, because it seeks to give support to the research in the etiology of the disorder, the statement of an initial biomedical framework simplifies the criteria on which technical requirements will be based. This is important on account of the limited extension of this initial proposal.

We certainly start from the premise of an organic basis for the disorder. This is not particularly interesting, excepting to those that need a dualist approach to explain human being behavior. Notwithstanding, the organic approach should not be understood in the sense used by the majority of published hypothesis, but in a systemic one, where experience-driven changes in human brain from synaptic to cortical level that can occur throughout the life span, play a key role [24]. The well-known observed neuronal pattern in PDS does not prove any neurological or genetic innate deficiency. In addition, although PDS could emerge from a sum of causes, the similar neuronal patterns of PDS subjects, together with many other demonstrated conducts related to overt and covert speech, suggest a similar final stage.

In a simplistic manner, the potential reasons of differences in neuronal patterns between fluent and PDS subjects can be classified in three types. The first one refers directly to a neuronal flaw in those areas, as is clearly suggested in [25]. A proposed model concerning this possibility suggests that the right hemisphere overactivation is due to a compensatory mechanism associated with a disturbed timing activation in speech-relevant areas [26-28]. Indeed, the majority of current organic etiological models point to a neurological flaw in speech related areas, in the form of anomalous dominance, functional anomalies on motor speech control coordination, etc.

As a second possibility, the pattern differences could be a secondary effect related to anticipation, avoidance or any similar behavior of PDS subjects. In such a case, the stuttering should emerge as a learning behavior, perhaps induced by some minor innate difficulty. This model has acquired many forms in past hypothesis, some of which has been cited above. This line of research suggest that the subject should be able to re-learn to control his speech by means of speech-therapy (direct) and/or psycho-therapy (indirect). However, considering that this approach has been tested from the beginning of 20th century without success, and according to its difficulty as an explanatory theory for some important characteristics of stuttering, this hypothesis seems flawed.

A third possibility is the observed pattern differences are induced by a neuronal distortion or maladjustment in other brain area. This other neuronal maladjustment has not necessary to be innate, neither involves really a flaw. The relevance of brain amygdala in classic conditioning, rapid responses to conditioned stimuli, and its involvement in fear behavior, with diffuse projections to a variety of autonomic and skeletomotor control centers, including the periaqueductal grey, which mediates the freezing response, suggests that this circuit could be responsible of PDS by means of a reactive inhibition. To the best of our knowledge this kind of hypothesis has been only proposed by Dodge [29]. Many more relevant details regarding this model can be seen elsewhere [29]. Moreover, in our opinion this hypothesis could explain other type of dysfluencies that are less known because they do not affect to oral but other communicative tasks, like writing and even playing music.

In summary, we consider such reactive inhibition model as the most plausible hypothesis to explain the stuttering in agreement with Dodge [29]. A more comprehensive description of this asseveration exceeds the scope of this paper.

3. Methods

Any new therapeutic proposal should be based on a causal hypothesis consistent with the well-known characteristic of stuttering. This should allow discovering knowledge to improve, validate, or reject the basis model, in such a way that fills the gap between the clinical application and the scientific research on PDS. This is the first requirement that results from the previous scenario.

Assuming the reactive inhibition model of stuttering, associated with the limbic system, as the underlying mechanism, the therapy needs to be delivered in the usual environment of the PDS subject. These two requirements compel to search a discreet and wearable technological solution with enough processing capacity (intelligence) to extract knowledge concerning a particular subject and context.

The effect that altered auditory feedback (AAF) has on the reduction of severe dysfluencies, and on the normalization of PDS neural patterns [30, 31], together with the feasibility to develop wearable, non-invasive, and discreet AAF devices [32], point to this technique as a good therapeutic proposal.

However, it should overcome limitations of cutting edge AAF devices such as the one presented in [32]. This way, although discretion and wearability have been successfully accomplished [32], the device has an excessive cost for clinical application, and the customization involves only an initial tuning of several parameters, what impedes to explore freely new hybrid feedback mechanisms and adapt them to the evolving nature of PDS subjects. Moreover, there are not AAF devices that allow extracting knowledge in real time to follow up the clinical evolution of the subject.

As a solution to these requirements, we propose a methodology based on the paradigm of knowledge-based telehealthcare, whose foundation was presented in earlier works within the chronic renal area [33, 34]. The main characteristic of this healthcare paradigm is the capability to generate real-time and adaptive knowledge. It is achieved using a multitier processing architecture, where the first (composed) layer is defined by a set of intelligent monitors that send the measured and processed data towards the second layer, based in turn on systemic dynamic mathematical models [35], encapsulated into computational components, called PPI. More details about this architecture can be seen in the cited articles.

A recent study has shown the advantages of that knowledge-based paradigm [36]. An accelerometer-based human movement monitor, compliant with the knowledge paradigm, was used to evaluate the sensor layer [37]. It can be called multimodal intelligent monitor on account of its ability to manage different types of signals. We will refer to the multimodal intelligent monitor along the text to direct the attention to the monitor architecture, but not to the technical solution and particular accelerometer sensors used in [36].

Our therapeutic proposal will use an AAF device based on a multimodal intelligent monitor, real-time adapted to each PDS subject, with the aim of minimizing dysfluencies. The multimodal capacity must allow monitoring other biomedical signals besides vocal sound, such as EEG and human body accelerations, under request of speech language professionals and researchers. Multimodal capacity seeks to optimize the adaptive function of the AAF device, as well as generate a more complete image of the PDS subject evolution, in agreement with the first requirement.

4. Results

This Section describes several relevant issues concerning the technology of the AAF device based on a multimodal intelligent monitor. This one is an extension of the patented accelerometer-based human movement monitor previously cited [36, 37]. The AAF device therapeutic proposal differs from the human movement monitor only in the wireless communication technologies among internal devices and the use of an intelligent headset (IHS). The last element is an extended headset that implements an adaptive AAF algorithm. Therefore, the IHS comprises an intelligent sensor (IS) together with an effector element (headphone). Accordingly, the term monitor refers to both except when the contrary is indicated.

The monitor is composed by a personal server element (PSE) and a set of ISs associated with different biosignals. Last ones communicate with the PSE using a wireless personal network (WPAN), under a star topology (PSE is the center). The monitor architecture involves two layers, set by the ISs and the PSE, respectively. The ISs measure and perform a first analysis of the signals, computing the associated features that are sent to the PSE. This approach reduces the dimensionality of the data to be processed by the PSE, making easier to adopt a real time processing approach. This distributed processing optimizes the resource allocation and reduces the volume of data transmitted between layers, which in turn helps to reduce the power consumption and the device size [37].

This strategy makes easier to fulfill the wearability and discretion requirements. Other details of the intelligent monitor related the healthcare framework can be seen elsewhere [33, 34, 37].

Any IS device includes sensors, a microcontroller for management and signal processing, a wireless transceiver and the associated antenna, and auxiliary circuitry that depends on IS functions. The ability of IS to be adapted to the subject and context evolution is related to processing capacity of the microcontroller. The advantages of this capability were successfully shown with the falling detection function of the human movement monitor [36]. This feature allows a real-time adapting of the AAF parameters to the PDS subject evolution.

Despite the design reduces the IS – PSE (and IHS – PSE) data volume, the maximum channel capacity must allow transferring the complete signals waveforms under special circumstances: tests, research tasks, or around IS detected events. In the case of the human movement monitor, the events alert PSE of possible impacts, whereas in the AAF device based on a multimodal intelligent monitor, the events can be set to detect speech blocking patterns from a multimodal viewpoint, that is, the event can be triggered by an IS different of the IHS.

Most of the biosignals needed in telehealthcare, including EEG, require a sampling rate value lesser than 10^2 S/s approximately. This fact allows the use of very low cost microcontrollers, as the one used in the intelligent acceleration unit presented in [37]. In addition, these signals can be transmitted by means of low data rate communication protocols like the modern Zigbee [38], which has a maximum data rate of (2.4 GHz) 250 Kbps. The maximum signal sampling rate depends on the required accuracy and overhead, but signals with sampling rates up to 10 KS/s, approximately, can be transmitted. This value includes accelerometer signals associated with high energy human physical activities.

However, the IHS needs a channel with capacity to transmit audio signals, and a processing capacity higher than normal ISs. With that objective, the communication technologies used between PSE and ISs within the multimodal intelligent monitor have been extended, taking advantage that the earlier PSE [36] used Bluetooth (BT) to link with the healthcare center via a remote access unit.

Accordingly, the PSE of the AAF device based on a multimodal intelligent monitor implements a new single Wibree/BT solution. This one takes advantage of the lower consumption of Wibree compared with BT 2.0, despite the lower data rate of Wibree (1 Mbps vs. 3 Mbps) (www.wibree.com). High speed IS and effectors-IS devices will use BT or Wibree, as a function of the availability.

The proposed IHS is based on the BlueCore™ 5-Multimedia single-chip solution (http://www.csr.com/products/bc5range.htm). This integrated circuit (IC) is a programmable single-chip Bluetooth 2.0 (and v 2.1 ready) solution with on-chip and specialized Digital Signal Processor (DSP), stereo CODEC, and Flash. The chip includes also a lithium battery charger & switch-mode DC-DC converter. It is a low cost circuit designed for headsets whose DSP will execute the AAF algorithm, besides to calculate the signal's features for sending to the PSE. The adaptive capacity of the AAF algorithm is supported on the distributed processing of the audio signal between IHS and PSE.

The IHS can be worn partly or fully into the ear canal, with or without the pinna support, depending of the discretion level. A more detailed technological description of the remaining elements exceeds the scope of the present work.

5. Discussion and conclusion

The feasibility of the proposed device is associated with the ability to accomplish the requirements of functionality, cost, size, wearability, autonomy and discretion, which in turns depends on the state of the art in electronic technology (e.g. sensors, microprocessors and communications) and signal processing techniques for speech, EEG and accelerometers.

Previous works have shown the feasibility of an accelerometer-based human movement monitor, compliant with the same requirements of the AAF device based on a multimodal intelligent monitor [36, 37]. Current advances in microprocessors, Micro-Electro-Mechanical System (MEMS) sensors, communications, signal processing and embedded devices should make easier to keep those specifications despite the higher data rates and processing capacity required for the IHS.

The processing capacity and functionality of embedded current headset solutions such as the BlueCore™ 5-Multimedia IC seem to provide a proper hardware basis for the IHS, overcoming the limitations in cost, real-time adaptability and knowledge extraction of the AAF device published in [32].

Other issues of the IHS refer to the speech processing technique. The ability to recognize speech, and voice impairments has been widely demonstrated [39-41]. Moreover, recent works have achieved success even on pervasive speech recognition [42]. Accordingly, the architecture of our proposed AAF device seems able to support real-time speech processing algorithms, dividing the task between the DSPs of IHS and PSE, and focusing the DSP of IHS mainly to alter the auditory feedback in a monaural way.

Regarding the feasibility of the EEG-IS, the acquisition of EEG signals needs scalp electrodes, which could require an electrolyte gel for electrical conductivity, and as little hair as possible in the target zone. This is a limiting factor in our proposal. Ideally, the electrode elements would be inconspicuous and be wearable as easily as clothing. However, there is a strong interest to develop electrode sensors that will be friendly to use and inexpensive. This is pushing this research line with successful results [43]. Regarding the possibility to monitor EEG of speech related brain areas during stuttered speech, a recent work has demonstrated that EEG artifacts associated with the speech musculature and ocular activity can be removed in stutterers [44].

It is relevant to remark that the AAF device proposed in this work is considered a therapeutic system and not only a prosthetic device, in opposition to current AAF devices. This is based on the assumption that stuttering is caused by a reactive inhibition supported by the brain amygdala, and there are many cues that point to the possibility to remodel weights of diffuse projections associated to fear conditioning and similar emotional states [26, 45, 46].

According to this analysis and to the best of our knowledge, this is the first therapeutic proposal able to be used at the same time as a full and real-time prosthetic aid in the usual environment of the PDS subject, in opposition to other research or commercial AAF devices [32, 47].

Acknowledgements

This work has been partly supported by the Spanish National Board of Biomedical Research (Fondo de Investigaciones Sanitarias, Instituto de Salud Carlos III), under Grant PI040687, as well as by the Dirección General de Investigación, Tecnología y Empresa de la Junda de Andalucía, under Grant EXC/2005/TIC-314.

References

[1]   A. Craig, K. Hancock, Y. Tran, M. Craig, and K. Peters, "Epidemiology of Stuttering in the Community Across the Entire Life Span," J Speech Lang Hear Res, vol. 45, pp. 1097-1105, 2002.

[2]   C. L. Zamora, "(Stuttering as a sociocultural phenomenon: an alternative to the biomedical model) La tartamudez como fenómeno sociocultural: una alternativa al modelo biomédico," in Department of Sociología I (Teoría, Metodología y Cambio social): UNED, Spain, 2006, p. 628.

[3]   B. Bobrick, Knotted Tongues: Stuttering in History and the Quest for a Cure: odansha Amer Inc., 1996.

[4]   C. V. Riper, The treatment of stuttering. Englewood Cliffs, New Jersey: Prentice Hall, 1973.

[5]   A. Chervin, (Suttering and other pronunciation defects) Tartamudez y otros defectos de pronunciación. Paris: Société d'Éditions Scientifiques, 1896.

[6]   G. A. Lewis, The origin and treatment of stammering. Detroit, Michigan: Photometer Press, 1906.

[7]   J. Ordoñez, (Stuttering) La tartamudez. Madrid: Studium, 1956.

[8]   J. Parellada, (Causes of stuttering. Paths towards the correction) Las causas de la tartamudez. Vías hacia su corrección. Barcelona, Spain: Jims, 1978.

[9]   D. Barbara, Stuttering: a psychodynamic approach to its understanding and treatment. New York: Julian Publishers, 1954.

[10] O. Bloodstein, A handbook of stuttering. Chicago: National Easter Seal Society, 1981.

[11] W. Johnson, "A study of the onset and development of stuttering," Journal of Speech Disorders, vol. 7, pp. 251-257, 1942.

[12] L. E. Travis, "The cerebral dominance theory of stuttering: 1931--1978," J Speech Hear Disord, vol. 43, pp. 278-81, 1978.

[13] B. S. Lee, "Artificial stutter," J Spech Hear Dis, vol. 16, pp. 53-55, 1951.

[14] C. Büchel and M. Sommer, "What Causes Stuttering?," PLoS Biology, vol. 2, p. e46, February 01, 2004 2004.

[15] A. Craig, "The Developmental Nature and Effective Treatment of Stuttering in Children and Adolescents," Journal of Developmental and Physical Disabilities, vol. 12, pp. 173-186, 2000.

[16] G. Andrews, A. Craig, A. Feyer, S. Hoddinott, P. Howie, and M. Neilson, "Stuttering: a review of research findings and theories circa 1982," J Speech Hear Disord, vol. 48, pp. 226-46, 1983.

[17] C. W. Starkweather, Fluency and Stuttering. Engleewook Cliffs, New Jersey: Prentice Hall, 1987.

[18] B. Guitar, Stuttering: An integrated approach to its nature and treatment. Baltimore, Maryland: Williams y Wilkins, 1998.

[19] O. Bloodstein, "Genes Versus Cognitions in Stuttering: A Needless Dichotomy," Am J Speech Lang Pathol, vol. 9, pp. 358-359, November 1 2000.

[20] F. P. Limongi, U. Subramanian, B. Prabhu, R. Ezrati-Vinacour, O. Amir, M. Kenjo, C. Lundström, M. Garsten, S.-l. Yang, W. Botterill, and J. Fry, "Stuttering Research and Treatment Around the World," The ASHA Leader, pp. 6-41, 2005.

[21] P. T. Fox, R. J. Ingham, J. C. Ingham, T. B. Hirsch, J. H. Downs, C. Martin, P. Jerabek, T. Glass, and J. L. Lancaster, "A PET study of the neural systems of stuttering," Nature, vol. 382, pp. 158-162, 1996.

[22] P. T. Fox, "Brain imaging in stuttering: where next?," Journal of Fluency Disorders, vol. 28, pp. 265-272, 2003.

[23] P. R. Rodríguez Carrillo, "(Stuttering under the stutterer perspective) La tartamudez desde la perspectiva de los tartamudos," Caracas: Universidad Central de Venezuela, 2002.

[24] C. Kelly, J. J. Foxe, and H. Garavan, "Patterns of Normal Human Brain Plasticity After Practice and Their Implications for Neurorehabilitation," Arch Phys Med Rehabil, vol. 87, pp. S20-29, 2006.

[25] A. L. Foundas, A. M. Bollich, D. M. Corey, M. Hurley, and K. M. Heilman, "Anomalous anatomy of speech–language areas in adults with persistent developmental stuttering," Neurology, vol. 57, pp. 207-215, 2001.

[26] K. Neumann, C. Preibisch, H. A. Euler, A. W. v. Gudenberg, H. Lanfermann, V. Gall, and A.-L. Giraud, "Cortical plasticity associated with stuttering therapy," Journal of Fluency Disorders, vol. 30, pp. 23-39, 2005.

[27] M. Sommer, M. Koch, W. Paulus, C. Weiller, and C. Buchel, "Disconnection of speech-relevant brain areas in persistent developmental stuttering.," Lancet, vol. 360, pp. 380-3, August 3, 2002 2002.

[28] C. Preibisch, K. Neumann, P. Raab, H. Euler, A. von Gudenberg, H. Lanfermann, and A. Giraud, "Evidence for compensation for stuttering by the right frontal operculum.," Neuroimage, vol. 20, pp. 1356-64, October 1, 2003 2003.

[29] D. M. Dodge, "A Reactive Inhibition Model of Stuttering Development & Behavior: A Neuropsychological Theory Based on Recent Research," http://telosnet.com/dmdodge/reactinh.html (Last accessed Feb 21, 2006), 2006.

[30] T. Saltuklaroglu, J. Kalinowski, V. N. Dayalu, V. K. Guntupalli, A. Stuart, and M. P. Rastatter, "A temporal window for the central inhibition of stuttering via exogenous speech signals in adults.," Neuroscience Letters, vol. 349, pp. 120-4, Oct 2003.

[31] J. Kalinowski and T. Saltuklaroglu, "Choral speech: the amelioration of stuttering via imitation and the mirror neuronal system ," Neuroscience and Biobehavioral Reviews, vol. 27, pp. 339-47, Sep 2003.

[32] A. Stuart, S. Xia, Y. Jiang, T. Jiang, J. Kalinowski, and M. P. Rastatter, "Self-Contained In-the-Ear Device to Deliver Altered Auditory Feedback: Applications for Stuttering," Annals of Biomedical Engineering, vol. 31, p. 233, 2003.

[33] M. Prado, L. Roa, J. Reina-Tosina, A. Palma, and J. A. Milán, "Virtual Center for Renal Support: Technological Approach to Patient Physiological Image," IEEE Transactions on Biomedical Engineering, vol. 49, pp. 1420-1430, Dec 2002.

[34] M. Prado, L. Roa, J. Reina-Tosina, A. Palma, and J. A. Milán, "Renal telehealthcare system based on a patient physiological image: a novel hybrid approach in telemedicine," Telemedicine Journal and e-Health, vol. 9, pp. 149-165, 2003.

[35] L. Roa and M. Prado, "Simulation Languages," in Wiley Encyclopedia of Biomedical Engineering, M. Akay, Ed.: John Wiley and Sons, Inc., 2006, p. 4152.

[36] M. Prado, L. M. Roa, and J. Reina-Tosina, "Viability study of a personalized and adaptive knowledge-generation telehealthcare system for nephrology (NEFROTEL)," International Journal of Medical Informatics, vol. 75, pp. 646-657, 2006.

[37] M. Prado, J. Reina-Tosina, and L. Roa, "Distributed intelligent architecture for falling detection and physical activity analysis in the elderly," in 24th Annual International Conference of the IEEE-EMBS and Annual Fall Meeting of the BMES, Houston, TX, USA, 2002, pp. 1910 - 1911.

[38] "ZigBee Specification," ZigBee Alliance December 1 2006.

[39] K. Umapathy and S. Krishnan, "Feature analysis of pathological speech signals using local discriminant bases technique," Medical and Biological Engineering and Computing, vol. 43, pp. 457-464, 2005.

[40] M. Piccioni, S. Scarlatti, and A. Trouve, "A Variational Problem Arising from Speech Recognition," SIAM Journal on Applied Mathematics, vol. 58, pp. 753-771, 1998.

[41] J. I. Godino-Llorente and P. Gomez-Vilda, "Automatic Detection of Voice Impairments by Means of Short-Term Cepstral Parameters and Neural Network Based Detectors," IEEE Transactions on Biomedical Engineering, vol. 51, pp. 380-384, 2004.

[42] N. Alewine, H. Ruback, and S. Deligne, "Pervasive speech recognition," Pervasive Computing, IEEE, vol. 3, pp. 78-81, 2004.

[43] V. Stanford, "Biosignals offer potential for direct interfaces and health monitoring," Pervasive Computing, IEEE, vol. 3, pp. 99-103, 2004.

[44] Y. Tran, A. Craig, P. Boord, and D. Craig, "Using independent component analysis to remove artifact from electroencephalographic measured during stuttered speech," Medical and Biological Engineering and Computing, vol. 42, pp. 627-633, 2004.

[45] C. Herry, P. Trifilieff, J. Micheau, A. Luthi, and N. Mons, "Extinction of auditory fear conditioning requires MAPK/ERK activation in the basolateral amygdala," European Journal of Neuroscience, vol. 24, pp. 261-269, 2006.

[46] A. Gruart, M. D. Munoz, and J. M. Delgado-Garcia, "Involvement of the CA3-CA1 Synapse in the Acquisition of Associative Learning in Behaving Mice," The Journal of Neuroscience, vol. 26, pp. 1077-1087, January 25, 2006 2006.

[47] "Electronic speech therapy devices for stuttering and Parkinson's, http://www.casafuturatech.com/Catalog/index.shtml, (Last accessed Feb 27, 2006)," Casa Futura Technologies, 2006.

Medical and Care Compunetics 4
L. Bos and B. Blobel (Eds.)
IOS Press, 2007

Innovating *e*Health in the Netherlands

Adrie C.M. Dumay

TNO Quality of Life, Wassenaarseweg 56, 2333 AL LEIDEN, the Netherlands

Abstract. Innovation is essential to improve accessibility, effectivity and efficiency of healthcare delivery. *e*Health promises these improvements provided that it complies to essential requirements with respect to quality and patient safety. *e*Health must be implemented thoughtfully to yield full benefit to the patient. However, there exists no structured framework of essential requirements to guide development, implementation and usage. The scope of application of *e*Health is wide and new technology is introduced continuously. So, the framework of essential requirements must evolve as well to support and encourage innovation. The author proposes a process for continuous verification and validation of *e*Health throughout development, implementation and use and a method to continuously update the framework of essential requirements.

Keywords. *e*Health, innovation, quality, patient safety, essential requirements

1. Introduction

1.1. Driving innovation

Innovation is about the successful exploitation of new ideas. Innovation is often referred to as the process of making improvements by introducing something new. The improvements are changes that create a new dimension of performance. What is new is an unprecedented idea, method or device. Something new must be substantially different, not an insignificant change. Innovations are intended to make someone better off, and the succession of many innovations grows a whole economy [16]. The term innovation may refer to both radical or incremental changes to products, processes or services. The often unspoken goal of innovation is to solve a problem. Innovation is an important topic in the study of economics, business, technology, sociology, and engineering. Since innovation is also considered a major driver of the economy, the factors that lead to innovation are also considered to be critical to policy makers [17]. The need to innovate in healthcare delivery is socially very relevant. Subjects driving the innovation needs are:

1. Increasing demand for healthcare delivery as a result of demographic development: More elderly people will need healthcare for a longer period;
2. Increasing demand for efficiency. Increase in demand must be handled by (relatively) fewer healthcare workers;

3. Increasing patient empowerment. Patients and healthcare consumers will have a stronger influence on healthcare delivery. The patients' needs will get more focus and attention;
4. Increase in the effect of market forces. New markets emerge for health insurance, the healthcare (pre) procurement market and health delivery. More often a careful decision must be made based on quality, patient safety and effectivity of resources in the healthcare delivery market.

*e*Health is an innovation which promises to increase patient empowerment and accessibility, quality, patient safety and effectiveness. It comprises the application of information and communication technology in the healthcare delivery process:

"eHealth refers to the use of modern information and communication technologies to meet needs of citizens, patients, healthcare professionals, healthcare providers, as well as policy makers" [1].

It is expected that *e*Health applications will substantially increase by type, number and volume to the benefit of the patient.

1.2. Market introduction

From the point of view of market introduction, *e*Health can be divided into two groups: *e*Health applications which are not part of the insurance provision (either private or public insurance) and those applications which are. If the *e*Health applications are not part of insurance provision, it can still be marketed if it meets the legal requirements with regard to quality and patient safety (see Section 3.1). In that situation a market price is charged for the innovation, which will tax the budget of healthcare providers, healthcare institutions and/or households. If there is a desire to include an *e*Health application in insurance provision, then the application must be well-considered and it must meet minimum requirements with regard to the desired efficiency and perhaps also with regard to quality and patient safety.

1.3. Research question and commentary

The discussion of admitting an innovation contributing to quality, patient safety and efficiency then leads to the following research question:

Which assessment process should be followed to admit eHeath innovation?

The question of who determines and maintains the minimum requirements and implements them into an assessment process is a political one and is not investigated in this publication. The requirements themselves are the subject of research and also fall outside the scope of this publication. The response to the central questions is given in five steps (section 2). Section 3 gives the results of each step. The publication is concluded with a discussion (Section 4).

2. Approach

The solution to the question has been set in motion in five parts [6] [7] [8]. Firstly, the legal and normative framework for quality and patient safety has been analysed. Secondly, the management of *e*Health is placed in the legal and regulatory context supplemented by current ideas on market operation and supervision. Thirdly, a general model is drawn up for quality improvement in the entire innovation process of *e*Health with attention to process and product specifications. Fourthly, a method is sought for making qualitative aspects measurable. Finally, all this is made operational in a test model on the basis of the so-called **TERTZ®** method[1], also developed by TNO. All steps are evaluated by consulting experts.

3. Results

3.1. Legal and normative framework for quality and patient safety

In the Medical Device Directive 93/42/EEG concerning medical aids, requirements are laid down in legislation with regard to quality and safety. This directive aims to promoting trade within Europe [2]. In this Regulation a medical device is defined as follows:

a) 'Medical device' means any instrument, apparatus, appliance, material or other article, whether used alone or in combination, including the software necessary for its proper application intended by the manufacturer to be used for human beings for the purpose of diagnosis, prevention, monitoring, treatment or alleviation of disease, diagnosis, monitoring, treatment, alleviation of or compensation of injury or handicap, investigation, replacement or modification of the anatomy or of a physiological process, control of conception, and which does not achieve its principle intended action in or on the human body by pharmacological, immunological and metabolic means, but which may be assisted in its function by such means;

b) 'Accessory' means an article which whilst not being a device is intended specifically by its manufacturer to be used together with a device to enable it to be used in accordance with the use of the device intended by the manufacturer of the device.

The directive refers to essential requirements with regard to quality and patient safety of medical devices and has been transformed into the Dutch Decision on Medical Devices [3]. The essential requirements are based on a high level of protection of health and safety and assessing the utility of the device in relation to the possible risk to the patient. If there are risks involved in the use of the device for its intended purpose, the user of the device must be informed of this. The Medical Device Directive lays down strict requirements with regard to safety and quality for admittance to the market,

---

[1] Technologie Effect Rapportage Transmurale Zorg (Technology Effect Report Transmural Healthcare)

including vigilance and post-marketing surveillance and inspection by the Health Care Inspectorate.

The minimum requirements with regard to quality and safety are well summarized in various national and harmonized standards. The ISO standard 9001: *Guide for health care services* defines the requirements with regard to suitability, patient safety, effectiveness and efficiency, care/respect/privacy, continuity of care, patient and customer experience, availability and accessibility. The NEN-EN-ISO Standard 6061 defines the requirements with regard to safety, use and appropriateness of specific devices. The Dutch NEN-EN-ISO Standard 14971:2001 defines the process of risk management for the entire life of the device [18]. Finally, NEN-EN-ISO Standard 6385:2004 defines the requirements with regard to ergonomics and work systems [19]. The author regards an *e*Health application with one or more aims as mentioned in the Medical Device Directive 93/42/EEG a medical device. That provides a clear framework for responsibilities, choice of basic product and process standards and supplementary professional guidelines.

A TNO certification comprising all these aspects for medical information [4] and medical information systems are already available [5].

3.2. eHealth management in context

*e*Health is much more than a technical application. It is a medical service placed on the market by an organization and in which information technology (IT) and/ or medical apparatusses play an important role. An important aspect for assessment is the quality of the management of the service.

In order to implement the qualitative aspects of the organization the following components should be identified, which must be assessed separately:

- The organization;
- The quality management system;
- The front office (helpdesk, for example);
- The back office (including services leased from third parties);
- The equipment used such as medical devices and ICT systems.

Assessment criteria and indicators are widely available in the literature.

3.3. The place of testing in the innovation process

Every product has a life cycle, in which the following stages can be identified:

- The process of technical realization: Specification, design, realization and testing;
- Purchase and implementation;
- Management, maintenance and utilization;
- Removal from use and/ or the market.

The testing has to take place in all phases of the innovation process. Here too the assessment criteria and indicators are widely and readily available. However, a number of *e*Health products and services will make claims which can only be verified and validated in practice.

It is proposed that products and services for which admittance to the market or the insurance provision has been requested, be subject to a Quick Scan. The scan is carried out in four steps:

1. define the context in which *e*Health is being applied;
2. analyse the maturity of the application on the basis of relevant criteria and minimum scores;
3. analyse critical scores in detail, and,
4. describe the socio-technical map.

Step 2 induces a process of standardization of the qualitative aspects (see section 3.4) If the minimum scores are attained (step 2), it can be decided to proceed with a provisional or conditional admittance, whereby it becomes possible in an experimental phase to adjust the service in such a way that it meets the desired requirements. A provisional rate can then be fixed for use in this phase. If the desired effects can be realized in a demonstrable fashion within a previously agreed term, then a definitive admittance and rate can be fixed. If the desired scores are not attained, the product or service should not be admitted to the insurance provision. It will then still be possible to introduce it onto the market, as long as it meets the legal requirements. Acceptance and price of the product or service can then be determined by the market. In this way *e*Health will get a chance to prove itself and to improve during the temporary admittance phase.

3.4. Standardization of the qualitative aspects

The standardization and quantification of the qualitative aspects can be done according to the QUINT method [9] [10] [11]. This method is based on the ISO standard 9126 [18]. The method provides the qualitative aspects of medical software and software-based services and a model for scoring those aspects. The relevant feature within the context of this publication is that five score levels are specified for each qualitative aspect:

1. **Minimum level**: In the case of a criterion reaching a lower score the product is unusable;
2. **Current level**: In general the acceptable level will not be lower than a currently accepted level;
3. **Acceptable level**: If all criteria reach a score at the acceptable level then the innovation is successful;
4. **The target level**: Each criterion can be provided with a challenging target level in pursuance of further innovation;
5. **Maximum level**: This is a theoretical level which indicates what can reasonably be taken as the maximum level which is feasible.

During the application of the Quick Scan, the relevant qualitative aspects are selected and the levels above are scored. The levels are derived from the description, context and socio-technical map. At the end of the temporary admittance phase, the target level must be reached for all criteria. During the operational phase, that level must be guaranteed. It therefore also provides a testable standard to be maintained.

3.5. Assessment procedure in 10 steps

An assessment system which connects the Quick Scan, improvement in the experimental phase and the final assessment for definitive admittance is the so-called **TERTZ®** method. The goal of **TERTZ®** is to enable the organization (producer, management and user organization) to make well-considered choices and implementations [12]. The method was originally developed to make an assessment and the accompanying process of improvement of quality, safety, appropriateness and cost effectiveness of specific medical technology in new healthcare models. The **TERTZ®** method has been adapted to assess and improve *e*Health products and services. The adjusted version is called **TERTZ®** admittance and is carried out in 10 steps.

3.5.1. Part 1: The Quick Scan is carried out in ten steps

Step 1: Description of the context
In this step the eHealth product is described in a standardized manner according to the components mentioned in 3.2. The description also includes the desired user environment, target group and the technical/ organizational/ legal context.

Step 2: Analysis of readiness
The analysis is carried out by determining criteria and scoring levels on the basis of the context description. The analysis provides an insight into which components of the eHealth innovation are new with regard to already existing facilities and to what extent it can fit into existing structures and infrastructures. The analysis will also provide insight into how well-considered and developed the desired context is and whether it is justified to carry out a practical test.

Step 3: Further research of crucial aspects
The components which still require clarification after the analysis, thereby casting doubt on the feasibility, will be further studied or discussed with experts. This can lead to supplementary criteria with which the application must comply.

Step 4: Description of the socio-technical map
The socio-technical map indicates all the parties involved with description of their roles and the influence of these parties on the success and failure of the innovation is analysed and synthesized.

Step 5: Description of the relevant aspects to be tested
After applying the Quick Scan it will become clear which aspects will most strongly influence the success and feasibility of the innovation and which of them require attention in this practical testing phase. This will be incorporated into the work plan for the test phase. Existing legislation, regulations, norms and standards, directives and other documents play an important role. They are often agreements on the basis of consensus which have come into practice via the legislator or the standardizing organizations.

Step 6: Drawing up the testing and evaluation plan
The description includes the research questions, the research plan and the overall work plan for the practical test.

Step 7: Implementation of test and evaluation plan
During the implementation of the test and evaluation plan the *e*Health facility is both tested and improved. It is possible that in retrospect criteria will turn out not to be relevant or that criteria are lacking. It is also conceivable that the levels which the facility must meet need to be assigned a different value. Naturally, in this step adjustment of levels and criteria must be avoided as much as possible, but not ruled out.

Step 8: Standardizing the tested results
The findings of the practical test can be standardized and generalized for similar *e*Health applications and used for future practical tests. It will be clear that the qualitative criteria developed which have been tested in practice will be valid for all comparable facilities in the future.

Step 9: Compiling the admittance recommendation
The admittance recommendation includes a specification of the new *e*Health facility together with the accompanying qualitative criteria, scores and standard values.

Step 10: Documentation and report
During the entire process a product dossier will be built up and modified according to the relevant ISO 9000 qualitative requirements. Finally, a management summary will be drawn up for the organization which determines the admittance to the market.

4. Discussion

*e*Health promises to improve the quality, patient safety, efficiency and also accessibility of healthcare. Whether that is justified or not, is not the subject for discussion here. It can be stated, however, that for many reasons *e*Health is not being implemented on a large scale and that many experimental introductions are not being sustainably implemented. The medical device regime sets strict patient safety and quality requirements for admittance to the market. The rules for market admittance have not been sufficiently operationalized, so that defective products are probably being brought onto the market. The regime also includes monitoring after entry to the market.

The author therefore proposes an assessment process with the aim of promoting a well-considered introduction and application of *e*Health and to develop testable rules (criteria and standard values). So, *Which assessment process should be followed to admit eHeath innovation?*

One problem in addressing this question is the very fact that *e*Health is under development and that it can adopt many forms and sizes. It is therefore hardly possible to formulate all requirements in advance. For each service offered to the market, it is probable that different aspects will have to be assessed. A strict programme of requirements will make innovation impossible. In every case the legal requirements must be met in order not to endanger patient safety.

The **TERTZ®** admittance makes it possible to test the quality and patient safety of each type of *e*Health product and service in a structured fashion during its development. The method also makes it possible to formulate testable criteria and standard values with regard to the characteristic parts of the service. On the basis of a Quick Scan it can be determined whether the *e*Health application meets minimum requirements and which criteria are not met. On the basis of such analysis a provisional admittance must be possible with accompanying rates. During the temporary, provisional admittance the application must be adjusted so that all criteria are scored at standard level. This approach produces much information, lending a new impetus to innovation. In addition, it makes the criteria for supervision transparent. The requirements can be maintained in two ways, i.e., new products which seek entry as provided for by **TERTZ®** admittance or by vigilance and post marketing surveillance.

Vigilance, post-marketing surveillance, incident report and research and regular inspection by the Health Care Inspectorate [13] [4] are important instruments for scoring the testable standards and the degree to which they are being met. Central registration of the set of testable standards and the five quantitative levels within this provides a basis for the state of art quality, patient safety and efficiency of *e*Health. Another condition is that a standardized nomenclature be developed and used for *e*Health. [15]. A European approach is the obvious solution.

References

[1]　*e*Health Ministerial Declaration, May 22, 2003, Brussels. http://ec.europa.eu/information_society/eeurope/ehealth/conference/2003/doc/min_dec_22_may_03.pdf

[2]　European Council Directive 93/42/EEC of 14 June 1993 concerning medical devices, OJ L169, 12/07/1993

[3]　Wet op de Medische hulpmiddelen, Besluit 243 van 30 maart 1995, gewijzigd 30 augustus 2001

[4]　T. Lopes, R.G.M. van Melick and M.W.M. Oostenbrug, "TNO QMIC® Essential Requirements for European Medical Web Applications," TNO-PG/TG/2002.101, 2002

[5]　Dumay, A.C.M., G. Freriks & M.W.M. Oostenbrug, "TNO QM-ICT Essential requirements for the electronic healthcare record and semantic system to system interoperability," TNO-PG/TG/2002.181, 2003

[6]　Dumay, A.C.M. and G.Freriks, "Quality management issues for medical ICT," The Journal on Information Technology in Healthcare 2004; 2(4):225-235

[7]　Freriks G., M .Schoone en A.C.M. Dumay, "Aspecten van kwaliteitscriteria van *e*Health zorgdiensten en zorgproducten," TNO KvL/KZ/2005.051, 16 maart 2005

[8]　Dumay, A.C.M., G.Freriks en M.Schoone, "Pakketeizen voor telemedicinevoorzieningen in verzekerde zorg," TNO KvL/KZ/2005.96, 2 mei 2005

[9]　van Zeist, 1996a, "Kwaliteit van softwareprodukten", B. van Zeist, P. Hendriks, R. Paulussen en J. Trienekens, 1996, Kluwer Bedrijfswetenschappen, Deventer, Holland, ISBN 90-267-2430-6

[10]　R.H.J. van Zeist, 1996b: *"Specifying Software Quality with the Extended ISO Model"*,. In: Software Quality Management IV Improving Quality, M. Bray, M. Ross, G. Staples (editors), pages 145 - 159, Mechanical Engineering Publications Limited, London and BurySt Edmunds, UK, 1996

[11]　R.H.J. van Zeist, 1996c: *"Specifying Software Quality with the Extended ISO Model"*. In: Software Quality Journal, part 5, number 4, pages 273 - 284, Chapman & Hall, 1996

[12]　van Boxsel, JA.M. en M. Schoone, "Nieuw zorgproduct? Toets met **TERTZ®**," TNO PG/TG/99.107 Leiden, november 1999

[13]　IGZ 04-67, 2004. "ICT in ziekenhuizen. Beveiliging van informatie nog onvoldoende voor een betrouwbare papierloze patiëntenzorg. Een inventarizerend onderzoek bij twintig ziekenhuizen, uitgevoerd in najaar 2003"

[14]　Dumay, A.C.M. en M.Schoone, "Assessment of a baseline of ICT related quality measures in health care institutions," ISQUA International Conference, Vancouver: Conference Proceedings, pp.7-8, 2005

[15] van Nimwegen, Chr. en A.C.M. Dumay, "Global Medical Device Nomenclature. Een nieuw classificatiesysteem voor medische hulpmiddelen," Technologie in de Gezondheidszorg , nummer 12, Jaargang 17, pp. 6-8, 2001
[16] Hesselbein F., M. Goldsmith and I. Somerville (eds.), Leading for innovation: and organizing for results, New York: Jossey-Bass, ISBN 0-7879-5359-8, 2001
[17] J. Ettlie, Managing innovation, Butterworth-Heineman, an imprint of Elsevier, 2nd edition, ISBN 0-7506-7895-X, 2006
[18] http://www.iso.org/
[19] http://www2.nen.nl/

Contact information: adrie.dumay@tno.nl

Medical and Care Compunetics 4
L. Bos and B. Blobel (Eds.)
IOS Press, 2007

COGKNOW
Development and evaluation of an ICT-device for people with mild dementia

F.J.M. MEILAND [a], A. REINERSMANN [a], B. BERGVALL-KAREBORN [b],
D. CRAIG [c], F. MOELAERT [d], M.D. MULVENNA [e], C. NUGENT [e], T. SCULLY [b],
J.E. BENGTSSON [b], R.M. DRÖES [a].

[a] *Dept. of Psychiatry, Alzheimer Centre, VU University medical centre/GGZ
Buitenamstel, Valeriusplein 9, 1075 BG Amsterdam, The Netherlands
fj.meiland@vumc.nl*
[b] *Centre for Distance-Spanning Healthcare, Luleå University of Technology, Sweden*
[c] *Division of Belfast City Hospital/ Queen's University, Division of Psychiatry and
Neuroscience, Belfast, Northern Ireland*
[d] *Telematica Instituut Brouwerijstraat 1, 7523 XC Enschede, The Netherlands*
[e] *University of Ulster, Shore Road, Northern Ireland*

Abstract. Dementia is a progressive, chronic disease affecting 5% of all persons above 65 and over 40% of people over 90. The aim of the COGKNOW project is to achieve a breakthrough with research that addresses the needs of those with dementia, particularly those with mild dementia living in the community. This entails cognitive reinforcement in four main areas: helping people to remember, helping to maintain social contact, helping with performing daily life and recreational activities and finally enhance feelings of safety. Based on a sound foundation of needs reported in dementia literature, workshops and individual interviews have been carried out with dementia sufferers and their carers in three European countries. A ranked analysis of information from workshops and interviews, and the state of the art of successful ICT solutions will be the basis for formulating the functionalities of the technical solution and for the development of a cognitive prosthetic device with associated services for people with mild dementia. The research and evaluation will be conducted from human factors, technology, and business perspectives in three phases of one year each.

In this paper we discuss the design of the COGKNOW project, the first results of the user needs inquiry workshops and the ICT solutions the COGKNOW project will focus on in the first year.

Keywords. Dementia, ICT, Needs, User-centered, Business models

Introduction

Studies in which people with dementia themselves describe their needs indicate that the most frequently identified unmet needs are in the areas of information (on treatment, care and support, appointments), memory problems, communication, meaningful activities during daytime, and psychological distress [1-4].

The challenging aim of COGKNOW is to perform breakthrough research that addresses the needs of people with dementia, particularly those with mild dementia in Europe [5]. Our vision is to help people navigate through their day, by providing cognitive reinforcement. The social objectives of our research for the needs of people with mild dementia is, helping people to remember, maintain social contact, perform daily life activities and enhance their feelings of safety. The technical objective is to research and prototype a portable, remotely-configurable, user-validated cognitive prosthetic device, together with associated services for people with mild dementia.

The COGKNOW project started in September 2006 and will end in August 2009. It is supported by the European Commission and eleven participating organisations from eight countries[1].

1. Persons with dementia and their needs

Dementia is a progressive, disabling, chronic disease affecting 5% of all persons above 65 and over 40% of people over 90 years [6,7]. The term dementia refers to a combination of symptoms involving impairments of memory, speech, thought, perception and reasoning. Early impairments in performing complex tasks lead to an inability to perform even the most basic functional activities such as washing and eating. Often there are changes in personality, behaviour and psychological functioning, such as depressive symptoms, apathy and aggression. These neuropsychiatric symptoms appear to afflict the overwhelming majority of sufferers and are reported to be particularly potent precipitants of institutionalisation [8, 9].

The most prevalent type of dementia in the elderly is Alzheimer's Disease (AD). Two thirds of older people and one-third of younger patients (50-65 years old) with dementia have AD. The clinical course is typically only slowly progressive. Demographic changes mean that the countries of Europe can expect a massive rise in the number of older people and a corresponding increase in the number of dementia sufferers. If one considers the associated costs of community-based caring strategies and the emotional and economic burdens associated with institutionalisation, it is clear that these unfortunate individuals must be considered in the context of both national and European healthcare strategies, as well as social and economic policies.

Until recently, these strategies and policies were based on what other persons considered important for persons with dementia. Relatively few studies exist in which persons with dementia were surveyed and allowed to describe their own specific unmet needs. Aside from physical problems such as loss of eyesight and hearing and incontinence, the most frequently identified unmet needs are in the areas of information (on condition, treatment, care and support possibilities, appointments with care services etc), memory problems, and communication and psychological distress (anxiety) [3,10-12]. A report examining quality of life issues of dementia sufferers has recently identified seven key domains [2]: physical and mental health, social contact with

---

[1] Participating organisations are: Telefónica (Spain), University of Ulster (Northern Ireland), Luleå University of Technology (Sweden), Telematica Institute (The Netherlands), VU University medical centre (The Netherlands), AcrossLimits Ltd (Malta), Groupe des Ecoles des Télécommunications – Institut National des Télécommunications (France), University Hospital of North Norway/Norwegian Centre for Telemedicine (Norway), Belfast City Hospital/Queen's University of Belfast (Northern Ireland), Mobi Solutions OÜ (Estonia), Norrottens Läns Landsting (Sweden).

family and friends, being useful to others, enjoyment of activities, self-esteem (being respected by others), and self-determination and freedom.

A different personal perspective and lack of insight into their predicament causes patients to report fewer needs, and in some cases different needs, than their carers [1,3]. In one study the needs identified by the informal carers were associated with their own mental health [1] suggesting that the greater need of the carers could also be related with the mental health problems of the carers themselves. Unmet needs mentioned both by patients and carers include: information (on the disease, prognosis, care policy, possible care and support services, appointments), memory problems of the person with dementia; communication; (enough) meaningful activities during daytime; and feelings of safety.

If we analyse these needs as described above from various studies, we can see the importance of various strands of the person's life. This includes feeling of autonomy, that needs reinforcement of orientation in space and in time, of topographic memory and of (auto-) biographical memory. Also included is the ability for the person to maintain contact with their social environment and improve their relationship with it and their peers. This involves not only reinforcement of identity, episodic memory, and assisting the fight against apathy, but also facilitation of all aspects of communication and motivating people to express their opinions and thoughts, wishes and fears and reinforce their feelings of social belongingness.

In the COGKNOW project, field work and literature reviews will be performed to formulate functionalities of a multimodal technical solution that addresses those needs, and to develop a cognitive prosthetic device for people with dementia.

2. Method

The user needs will be further analysed by means of workshops and interviews with persons with dementia and their carers. Furthermore, a literature search will be performed on the state of the art of helpful ICT solutions for persons with dementia, healthcare models, technological infrastructures and existing standards in EU member states. This information will enable us to formulate functional requirements of a prototype that will be developed and tested in three iterations in the three countries (The Netherlands, Sweden, and Northern Ireland). The COGKNOW device will be developed in a user-centred approach, each field trial will be performed with a maximum of 18 persons with dementia and their carers (6 dyads per test site).

The study has been approved by the relevant Ethical Commission of each test-site.

2.1. Workshops and interviews on user needs

The workshops and interviews will take place in Amsterdam (The Netherlands), Belfast (Northern Ireland) and Luleå (Sweden), with a maximum of 6 persons with dementia and their carers at each site.

The target group of patients involved in these workshops will be suffering from mild dementia of the Alzheimer type. They are recruited from memory clinics at the different test sites and meeting centres for people with dementia and their informal carers. To operationalise the stage of severity of dementia the Global Deterioration Scale of Reisberg [13] is used. Only patients with moderate cognitive decline (late confusional stage) and moderately severe cognitive decline (early dementia stage) are invited to participate in the workshops and the field studies. The (confirmation of the) diagnosis of Alzheimer's Dementia and the stage assessment is obtained from, or performed by, clinicians in the different sites (neurologist/psychiatrist/geriatrician from the memory clinic and programme coordinators of the meeting centres) based on the DSM-IV-TR criteria [14] and by using the Global Deterioration Scale (GDS). Besides information on the diagnosis and severity of dementia, data are obtained in individual interviews with patients and carers. Due to the deteriorative nature of the condition of the users, it is to be expected that only one or two persons will participate three years in the project, therefore new participants will be recruited for each test phase. In every test phase a maximum of 6 user dyads will be recruited on every test site (country). This means that a maximum of 54 patient-carer dyads will participate in the project. Informed consent will be obtained from all participants.

Separate workshops are carried out with persons with dementia, and with informal carers and professional carers who are involved in the care situation. At least two project members will be present. One leads the discussion, the other fills in when necessary and makes notes and observations. The workshops are organised following a set of guidelines. The workshop starts with an introduction of the project, the aims and structure of the workshop, and an introduction of all participants. Then, needs, wants and demands [15] are discussed in the four COGKNOW areas in relation to improvement of the Quality of Life (QOL) and experienced autonomy of the persons with dementia. This way data can be gathered on how people think that their QOL and experienced autonomy would improve for every COGKNOW area. The needs, wants and demands that are mentioned within each domain are outlined on a flip-over. The priority of needs, wants and demands is discussed with the participants in the context of the importance for their quality of life and experienced autonomy.
A list with explanations of the four COGKNOW areas is made beforehand to standardise the method in the workshop among the test sites, which will increase the comparability of the results. In the discussion we conceptualise and verbalise going through the day from awakening in the morning until going to sleep at night. To focus on different time frames during the day, time-specific pictures are shown in a slide show. Next, possible ICT solutions for the needs, wants and demands mentioned are discussed. Besides brainstorming with the participants, possible directions of solutions are brought forward to discuss about (what do they think about this idea, do they think they can work with it). For each COGKNOW area some solutions are shown in a slide show. Also, the priority of preference for possible solutions in the different COGKNOW areas will be discussed.

When participants cannot or do not want to join the workshop, interviews are conducted following the same structure as in the workshops.
In separate interviews with persons with dementia and their carers, background characteristics are inventoried (age, education, relation patient-carer, etc.), as well as cognitive disabilities (cognitive section of the CAMDEX [16]), difficulties performing activities of daily living [17], needs, experienced autonomy, coping, informal network, and quality of life.
This will generate relevant information to specify technical requirements of the device that will be developed, and will make the characterization of the user group on which the prototype in the COGKNOW project is tested possible as well as comparisons of the user groups in the different test sites in the three countries. The aim is to contribute to the development of really user-friendly applications, as this is a strong and currently often unmet requirement for persons with dementia.

2.2. Development and evaluation of prototype in three field tests

The prototype will be developed in collaboration among the COGKNOW partners, and it will then be evaluated in three field tests at the same testsites as were the workshops are conducted, that is Amsterdam, Belfast and Luleå. During these field tests (one each project year), people with dementia and/or their carers are provided with the COGKNOW device in their daily life for a period of several days up to several weeks. The evaluation will be performed from three perspectives, identifying critical human, technology and business success factors.

2.2.1. Human Factors

The human factors analysis intends to define the functionality, performance, intended results and other user requirements which the system to be developed must fulfil in order for services to be adequate for testing. The testing will be performed by sufferers of mild dementia and their carers, both informal and professional. There are four evaluation objectives:

1. Obtain better insight into the needs, wishes and demands of the users in the COGKNOW-selected domains of daily life with reference to the key areas of remembering, maintaining social contact, performing daily life activities and enhancement of feelings of safety.
2. Evaluate the user-friendliness and usability (performance, reliability etc) of the device for the users;
3. Evaluate the usefulness (helpfulness in their individual daily life, safety factors, suitability or desirability) of the device for the users;
4. Evaluate the impact of the developed system on functioning of the users in the selected COGKNOW domains, on actual and perceived autonomy and quality of life.

Users collaborate in the development and evaluation process (using a method of "users as designers") and will be asked to make comments on the user friendliness, usefulness and impact of the developed service on their daily life throughout the project.

The prototype will be developed and tested in three phases in three countries in order to investigate the significance of different social contexts on the usability. During each test of the prototype service and device, the data are collected by means of standardized scales and questionnaires, semi-structured interviews and possibly a software platform SeniorXensor which is an extension of SocioXensor [18] (SocioXensor is an extensible toolkit that captures data about human behaviour, their context information and user experience). Based on the outcomes of these tests a further Human Factors Analysis will be performed. This analysis aims to determine the supportiveness of the prototype in enhancing (actual and perceived) autonomy and quality of life of the persons with dementia, as it relates to the four main COGKNOW areas remembering, maintaining social contacts, performing daily life activities and feeling safe.

At the end of the first year a prototype test will be carried out at the three test sites with a maximum of six participants per site. In this first field test, information will be collected on user friendliness and usefulness of the device by means of semi-structured interviews and diaries to inventory user problems. On the basis of that test and the collected data, a Human Factors Impact Analysis will be carried out, in order to feed back information to the developers. At the end of the second year an updated prototype will be tested. Again the focus will be on user friendliness and usefulness of the device by means of semi-structured interviews and diaries to inventory user problems. On the basis of that test and the collected data the second Human Factors Impact Analysis will be carried out to help the developers to fine-tune the prototype service and device.

At the end of the final test in year three, a deep analysis of the results will be carried out and the results from the previous tests will be added. This will deliver the final Human Factors Analysis on the impact of the developed system on functioning in the selected domains of daily life of the person with dementia and on actual and perceived autonomy and quality of life. In this last phase the main focus will be on the usefulness and efficacy of the system.

Concrete questions will be for example:

- Does the device support the memory problems of the persons with dementia?
- Does it help them to communicate and stay in contact with their family and friends?
- Does it help them to execute, or participate in, activities that they enjoy?
- Does it influence their mood and self-esteem positively and does it decrease their feelings of being isolated and unsafe?

To determine the usefulness and efficacy of the device in the user groups at the three test sites a 'pretest-posttest one group' design will be used in this final test. Semistructured interviews and diaries will be used to assess the user friendliness, usefulness and efficacy of the device in the daily life of users. With regard to the efficacy of the device, before and after the third field test data are also collected. This is done by standardized measuring instruments on the person with dementia's severity of dementia, cognitive (dis)abilities, deterioration in daily activities, ways of coping, quality of life, experienced autonomy, contextual information, information on received care and (unmet) needs. The results from this analysis provide crucial insight in user requirements on future products for future exploitation.

2.2.2. Technology Factors

The technical evaluations will focus on technology itself as opposed to the impact it may have on the user. The aim is to advance the state-of-the-art in the following areas:

- Capability of predicting context
- Mobile based delivery of reminding services
- Pervasive and ubiquitous computing, balancing transparency vs proactivity
- Deployment of we-centric services
- Use of multi-modal services

It is necessary, that each individual component be evaluated in terms of integration performance with all other system components in addition to evaluation in isolated terms. Figure 1 provides a general overview of the four proposed main technical components, of the system.

Within each technical component, an evaluation of technical performance aspects will be assessed based on the COGKNOW functional requirements. For the Cogknow Cognitive assistant these are amongst other things, impact of software upgrades, application system crashes, device recall, and battery life; for the Cogknow Server: down time, reliability, response time and delay; for the Cogknow Home Hub: average processing time, aborted connects, uptime and cost-effectiveness; for the Cogknow Sensorised Home: technician call outs, aborted connects, device sensitivity; and for all aspects: interoperability issues, system stability, and ease of integration

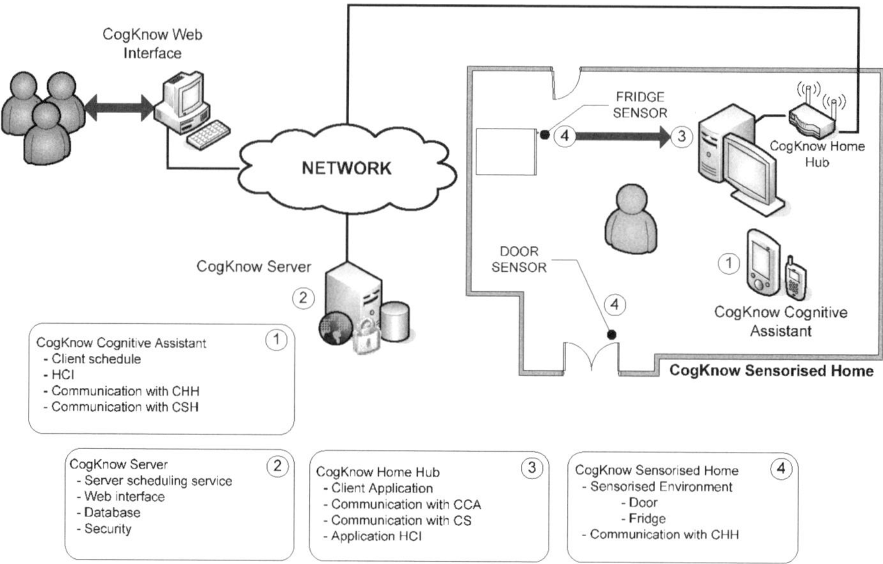

Figure 1: Overview of the four main technical components within the system

2.2.3. Business Factors

Getting innovations from the pilot state to actual innovations in the market is notoriously difficult, especially in health care; as it requires cooperation by multiple parties to provide valuable service offerings. Therefore the evaluation of the COGKNOW device also considers the Organisation and Financial Domains of the developed business models in order to make the business opportunities emanating from COGKNOW innovations sustainable on the market considering potential competition. The main COGKNOW innovation will be a user-validated cognitive prosthetic device with associated services for people with dementia. The aim of the evaluation is therefore: to check the viability of COGKNOW business opportunities, and to identify critical business success factors that feed back into the development of COGKNOW services.

This leads to the following research questions:

- What constitutes a viable business model for the service bundle (four services) that we develop in COGKNOW?
- What are or could be the mentioned services which together form the COGKNOW services? What is the core service or value of the COGKNOW bundle?
- What can we learn from business models for provision/dissemination of other comparable ICT services, or service bundles, for ageing people (with dementia) already on the market
- What roles are needed to deliver the COGKNOW services?
- Which actors could fulfil these roles?
- What are potentially viable business configurations for providing the COGKNOW services?
- What are the critical design factors?

- What differentiates COGKNOW services from other alternatives? How can the COGKNOW services be introduced to the market?"

The critical success factors will be analysed in the financial and organization domains. Those factors are distinguished in: market factors (clear target group, compelling value proposition, non-obtrusive customer retention), business modelling factors (complexity of business model - single-actor vs networked business; profitability potential), and actor viability factors (sustainability of business model, acceptable quality of service delivery - the resources provided by the selected commercial actors, customer reach of the selected actors)

3. First results of the workshops on user needs and possible ICT solutions

The data on user needs and ICT solutions were collected in Amsterdam by means of workshops and one individual interview, in Belfast by means of individual interviews and in Luleå by means of individual interviews and group interviews. In Amsterdam, all participants were willing to participate in the workshop, one couple was on holidays and was therefore interviewed later (separate interview for person with dementia and carer). In Belfast and Luleå, persons with dementia and their carers seemed not familiar with talking about their illness and needs in workshops, and they therefore participated in (small group) interviews. Characteristics of the participants are shown in Table 1.

Table 1. Characteristics of participants at the three test-sites.

	Amsterdam (n=6)	**Belfast (n=6)**	**Luleå (n=5)**
Persons with dementia			
Age	Mean 64.0 (range 56-78)	Mean 72.7 (range 65-86)	Mean 67.8 (range 60-77)
Gender	3 female 3 male	5 female 1 male	3 female 2 male
Civil status	5 married 1 widow	3 married 2 widowed 1 single	5 married
Carers			
Age	Mean 58.5 (range 49-78)	Mean 53.0 (range 40-72)	Mean 61.4 (range 23 – 78)
Gender	4 female 2 male	3 female 3 male	2 female 3 male
Relation to patient	5 spouses 1 daughter	3 spouses 2 children 1 cousin	4 spouses 1 son

In each country reports were made of the workshops and interviews. The most important needs (according to the participants) and the most preferred ICT solutions (according to the participants) were summarized for each COGKNOW area. Based on this overview and on the state of the art of ICT solutions that have proven to be helpful for persons with dementia, a Top 4 list of preferred ICT solutions was made for each test site. This top 4 list is presented in Table 2.

This top 4 list was discussed between the test site leaders and technological partners who assessed the feasibility to implement these ICT-solutions or functionalities in the first field trial. The main functionalities that are proposed to be studied and developed further are: reminding, picture dialling, support for activities for pleasure and safety warnings. The aim is to provide these functionalities as an integrated system. Next, functional requirements will be formulated, based on remarks of persons with dementia and their carers during workshops and interviews, results of questionnaires and scales on (dis)abilities of users, and literature review.

3.1. Examples of the four functionalities of the COGKNOW device in the first field trial

[reminding functionality] At 10 o'clock the COGNOW navigator reminds Martin to take his medicine using a specific sound that is backed up by a written message on the display. Martin reads that it is time to take his medicine.

[picture dialling] To call his son or daughter, Martin has to touch the phone symbol under their photographs. He presses the phone symbol and a connection is made to his daughter, with whom he talks for a while.

[support for activities for pleasure] During the evening Martin frequently uses the COGKNOW navigator to turn on the television because he has trouble finding the right TV channel and programme on his television.

[safety warning] When Martin goes out for a walk and he forgets to take his mobile and/or his keys with him, the front door sensor will always provide a gentle reminder as he passes through it. If he doesn't know where he left his mobile, he can touch a pictogramme of a mobile at the COGKNOW stationary device and a buzzer sound leads him to the place were he left it.

Table 2. Top 4 list of preferred ICT-solutions at the three test-sites.

Amsterdam	Belfast	Luleå
COGKNOW area: Support for memory **Reminding and remembering**		
Reminder for not forgetting activities/appointments/take medicine/to take things outdoors, like key and mobile phone/mobile device. The solution should preferably be stationary with touch screen as well as mobile: f.i. Neuropage [19-21]	Item locator, misplacement of items is a key early, and almost universal, symptom of a dementing illness – reflected in BCH workshops and literature review (see SMART home, BIME (Bath Institute of Medical Engineering))	Activity reminder/electronic calendar, stationary device with touch screen

| **COGKNOW area: Support for social contacts** | | |
Enable communication with family and friends		
Picture dialling function on touch screen integrated within the screen of the stationary device of the reminding system (thus not as a separate pictophone)	Electronic calendar with emphasis on appointments and social activities pending. Usefulness emphasized in workshops and within research community; see Forget-me-not http://www.ihagen.no/english.htm	Picture dialling function on touch screen integrated within the screen of the stationary device of the reminding system (thus not as a separate pictophone)
COGKNOW area: Support with daily activities		
Help executing activities that provide pleasure, recreational acitivies, useful activities		
Support for activities for pleasure: f.i. picture gramophone ENABLE-project (Adlam et al., 2004; ENABLE site) integrated within touch screen of activity reminder or picture of TV on touch screen that starts the TV when touched	Pill dispenser – medication management issue identified as an important "daily activity" particularly within workshops and concerning elderly persons generally [22]	Support for activities for pleasure: f.i. picture of TV on touch screen of the stationary device of the activity reminder that starts the TV when touched
COGKNOW area: Enhance feelings of safety		
Prevent people with dementia from experiencing anxious or dangerous situations		
Support during cooking f.i. Cooker usage monitor ENABLE project [23] (ENABLE site). Signal on stationary and mobile activity reminder device. or Warning to close door/ take things outdoors such as keys or simple mobile phone with or without GPS: f.i. Mobile Coach [24]	Picture telephone identified in workshop discussions and see Mobile Telecoach [24]	Reminder to turn devices of on stationary device, for example the stove (not as a separate artefact, but as a function within the activity reminder system) or Direct or easy contact possibilities to a service or emergency line (not as a separate artefact, but as a function within the reminder system)

4. Conclusion

The COGKNOW approach is anticipated to result in a cognitive prosthetic device and associated services for elderly people with mild dementia, with a focus on the real needs and wants of users. This solution will help this group of people to navigate through their day; improve independence and quality of life; and also improve infrastructure and processes for professionals in dementia care.

The identified services, requirements and technical vision will be further developed within the COGKNOW project, and the results will be published in reports and articles in scientific and professional journals, and presented at national and international symposia and congresses.

For more information, visit the project website, http://www.cogknow.eu.

Acknowledgement

The COGKNOW project is mainly funded by the European Commission's Information Society Technologies (IST) programme under grant 034025.

References

[1]   G.A. Hancock, T. Reynolds, B. Woods, G. Thornicroft, M. Orrell. The needs of older people with mental health problems according to the user, the carer, and the staff. *Int J Ger Psychiatry* **18** (2003), 803-11.

[2]   R.M. Dröes, E.J. Boelens, J. Bos, L. Meihuizen, T.P. Ettema, D.L. Gerritsen, F. Hoogeveen, J. de Lange, C. Schölzel-Dorenbos. Quality of life in dementia in perspective; an explorative study of variations in opinions among people with dementia and their professional caregivers, and in literature. *Dementia: The International Journal of Social Research and Practice* **5** (2006), 533-58.

[3]   H.G. van der Roest, F.J.M. Meiland, R. Maroccini, H.C. Comijs, C. Jonker, R.M. Dröes. Subjective needs of people with dementia: a review of the literature. *Int Psychogeriatr.* **4** (2007), 1-34.

[4]   H.G. van der Roest, F.J.M. Meiland, H.C. Comijs, E. Derksen, A.P. Jansen, H.P.J. van Hout, C. Jonker, R.M. Dröes. What do you need? That's the question. *Submitted 2007*

[5]   *COGKNOW – Description of Work.* Proposal no. 034025, Accepted EC 19-04-2006.

[6]   L. Fratiglioni, L.J. Launer, K. Anderson, et al. Incidence of dementia and major subtypes in Europe: A collaborative study of population-based cohorts. Neurol Dis Elderly Res Group. *Neurology* **54** (2000), 10-5.

[7]   L.J. Launer, A. Hofman. Frequency and impact of neurologic diseases in the elderly of Europe: a collaborative study of population based cohorts. *Neurology* **54** (2000), 1-3.

[8]   D. Craig, A. Mirakhur, D.J. Hart, S. McIlroy, P. Passmore. A Cross-Sectional Study of Neuropsychiatric Symptoms in 435 Patients With Alzheimer's Disease. *Am J Geriatr Psychiatry* **13** (2005), 460-468.

[9]   A. Mirakhur, D. Craig, D.J. Hart, S. McIlroy, P. Passmore. Behavioural and psychological syndromes in Alzheimer's disease. *Int J Geriatr Psychiatry* **19** (2004), 1035-9.

[10]   K. Walters, S. Iliffe, S. See Tai, M. Orrell. Assessing needs from patient, carer and professional perspectives: the Camberwell Assessment of Need for the Elderly people in primary care. *Age and Ageing* **29** (2000), 505-510.

[11]   A.M. Beattie, G. Daker-White, J. Gilliard, R. Means. Younger people in dementia care: a review of service needs, service provision and models of good practice. *Aging & Mental Health* **6** (2002), 205-212.

[12]   A.M. Beattie, G. Daker-White, J. Gilliard, R. Means. 'How can they tell' A qualitative study of the views of younger people about their dementia and dementia care services. *Health and social care in the community* **12** (2004), 359-68.

[13]   B. Reisberg, S.H. Ferris, M.J. de Leon, T. Crook. The Global Deterioration Scale for assessment of primary degenerative dementia. *Am J Psychiatry* **139** (1982), 1136-9.

[14]   American Psychiatric Association (APA). *Diagnostic and Statistical Manual of Mental Disorders (DSM-IV-TR)*, Fourth ed., 2000.

[15]   P. Kotler. *Principles of marketing.* Englewood Cliffs, NJ: Prentice-Hall, inc., 1980.

[16]   M. Roth, E. Tym, C.Q. Mountjoy, F.A. Huppert, H. Hendrie, S. Verma, R. Goddard. CAMDEX. A standardized instrument for the diagnosis of mental disorder in the elderly with special reference to the early detection of dementia. *Br J Psychiatry* **149** (1986), 698-709.

[17]   S. Teunisse, M.M. Derix. The interview for deterioration in daily living activities in dementia: agreement between primary and secondary caregivers. *Int Psychogeriatr* **9S1** (1997), 155-62.

[18]   G.H. Ter Hofte, R.A.A. Otte, A. Peddemors, I. Mulder. *What's Your Lab Doing in My Pocket? Supporting Mobile Field Studies with SocioXensor*, Extended demonstration abstract accepted for the CSCW2006 Conference Supplement, Banff, Alberta, Canada, 2006.

[19]   B.A. Wilson, H.C. Emslie, K. Quirk, J.J. Evans, et al. Evaluation of Neuro Page: a new memory aid. *J Neurol Neurosurg Psychiatry* **63** (1997), 113-15.

[20]   B.A. Wilson, H.C. Emslie, K. Quirk, J.J. Evans. Reducing everyday memory and planning problems by means of a paging system: a randomised control crossover study. *J Neurol Neurosurg Psychiatry* **70** (2001), 477-82.

[21]   N. Hersh, L. Treadgold. Rehabilitation of memory dysfunction by prosthetic memory & cueing. *Neurorehabilitation* **4** (1994), 187-97.

[22] C.D. Nugent, D. Finaly, R.J. Davies, M.D. Mulvenna, J.G. Wallace, C. Paggetti, E. Tamburini, N.D. Black. The next generation of mobile medication management solutions. *International Journal of Electronic Healthcare* **3** (2007), 7-31.

[23] T. Adlam, R. Faulkner, R. Orpwood, K. Jones, J. Macijauskiene, A. Budraitiene. The installation and support of internationally distributed equipment for people with dementia. IEEE Transactions on *Information Technology in Biomedicine* **8** (2004), 253-57.

[24] S. Kort. *Mobile Coaching. A pilot study into the user-friendliness and effects of Mobile Coaching on the wellbeing of people with dementia and their informal caregivers.* MSc thesis, Faculty of Psychology, Vrije Universiteit, Amsterdam, 2005

Medical and Care Compunetics 4
L. Bos and B. Blobel (Eds.)
IOS Press, 2007

Web-based or paper-based self-management tools for Asthma – patients' opinions and quality of data in a randomized crossover study

Ricardo CRUZ-CORREIA [a,b,1], João FONSECA [a,b,c], Luís LIMA [a], Luís ARAÚJO [c], Luís DELGADO [c,d], Maria Graça CASTEL-BRANCO [c], Altamiro COSTA-PEREIRA [a,b]

[a] *Department of Biostatistics and Medical Informatics*
[b] *CINTESIS – Center of Research in Health Information Systems and Technologies*
[c] *Division of Immunoallergology, Hospital S. Joao*
[d] *Department of Immunology*

Faculty of Medicine of University of Porto
Al. Prof. Hernâni Monteiro, 4200-319, Porto, Portugal

Abstract. The use of communication technologies may overcome some of the difficulties of conventional, paper-based, self-management of chronic diseases. This paper aims to describe and evaluate the use of P'ASMA – a web based asthma self-management support tool regarding the opinion of patients and their adherence to monitoring in comparison to standard paper-based tools. System description: P'ASMA allows the collection of asthma monitoring data and provides, to both patient and doctor, immediate feedback about patient's condition. For each patient a set of forms and scheduling options can be chosen. Evaluation methods: Twenty-one adults with previous medical diagnosis of asthma were included in an exploratory randomized crossover study. Patients used P'ASMA or a paper asthma diary and action-plan each during 4 weeks in a random sequence. Results: The number of patients who wrote negative remarks regarding P'ASMA was 2 and regarding paper-tools was 11; positive comments were 6 and 1 respectively for P'ASMA and Paper-based. Twelve patients were very interested to continue to monitor their asthma using P'ASMA whereas only 2 with Paper-based (p=0.002). Of the 19 problems reported with P'ASMA, 9 were related to the Internet connection, 5 to the user interface, 3 to internal system errors and 2 to the questions interpretation. The completeness of paper diary records was better; however, 10 patients reported filling it several days at once which was not allowed in P'ASMA. Conclusions: The intervention was feasible, safe and the problems detected in the web-application can be corrected. With P'ASMA data quality improved as the integrity features increase the reliability of the data. Moreover, patients preferred the web-based application to monitor their asthma.

Keywords. Asthma, self-management, monitoring, respiratory function tests, health technology assessment, personal health record

---

[1] Corresponding Author: Ricardo João Cruz Correia; E-mail: rcorreia@med.up.pt

Introduction

Chronic diseases are now the leading cause of disability, mortality and health-related costs in adulthood. Clinical practice and health care organization must react to the change from the predominance of acute health problems to chronic diseases. Within the approaches currently proposed for improving health care outcomes in chronic diseases, patient and information-based strategies are predominant as both clinical decisions and the organization of delivery of care depend heavily on the availability and quality of information. In chronic diseases with fluctuating courses, regular monitoring of the disease status is necessary to capture the actual burden of the disease in patients' lives. Between contacts with health care providers, the patient is the observer and the decision-maker.

Amongst chronic diseases, asthma is a variable disease with high prevalence, and personal and societal costs. In recent decades, impressive scientific advances in asthma pathogenesis and pharmacologic treatments have occurred. However, asthma burden remains exceedingly high. Although a small proportion, patients with more severe asthma are responsible for the majority of asthma's morbidity and costs. Improving the availability and quality of clinical information may be needed for a better care of patients with more severe asthma. Patients may provide valuable information for asthma management, if simple and valid self-assessment tools are made available.

A web-based application named "Portal for Assessment and Self-management of Asthma" (P'ASMA), accessible at http://www.pasma.med.up.pt, was developed in the Faculty of Medicine of the University of Porto. The application was designed to support asthma self-management, improve medical assessment and records and strengthen patient-doctor communication. It is accessible via Internet through a web-browser allowing its use both at medical facilities and during patients' daily life.

This paper aims to describe and evaluate the use of P'ASMA – a web based asthma monitoring tool, namely the opinion of users (patients) and adherence to monitoring in comparison to standard paper based tools.

1. System architecture

The implemented web-based system is installed in a server running Red Hat Linux operating system, Apache web-server and Oracle 9i Relational Database Management Server (Figure 1). Dynamic web pages are implemented in PHP 5 and templates using PEAR (PHP Extension and Application Repository).

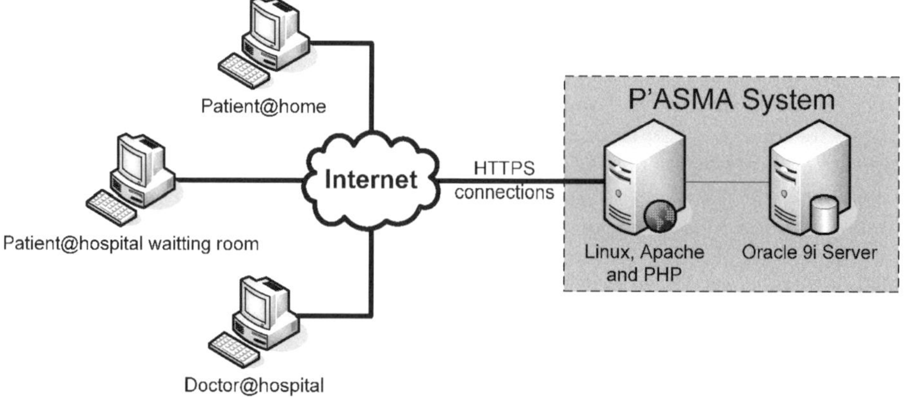

Figure 1: General system architecture describing how users access P'ASMA System.

P'ASMA complies with European standards for security ENV 12251 [1]. The confidentiality of patient related information is assured by controlling access to the system and encrypting all information in transit using the security standard TLS/SSL V.3 [2]. This standard allows for client/server authentication via a web-browser and also for the creation of a tunnel where all information in transit is encrypted during connection. It uses a Role-Based Access Control platform for access control (named Web.care) previously implemented in our department [3].

P'ASMA allows the collection and central storage of an electronic patient record and provides, to both patient and doctor, immediate feedback about patient's condition helping the therapeutic decisions. It also allows patient access to asthma educational materials, including an original manual about asthma self-management and a "Frequent Asked Questions" list. Furthermore, a secure, non-intrusive messaging system and the customized, interactive action plan were developed to strengthen communication between patient and doctor.

The Internet application includes restricted areas for asthma patients and for doctors. For each patient a program consisting of a set of questionnaires and scheduling options can be chosen (e.g. monitoring symptoms once a week and quality of life before medical visits).

The charts summarizing patient data are GIFs generated using PHP's Image Functions and the GD library (Figure 2). These charts illustrate the patient evolution regarding the asthma condition.

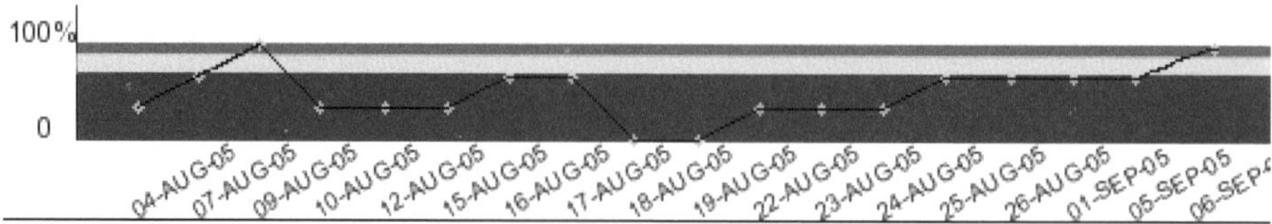

Figure 2: Chart representing patient evolution

2. System use

At home the patient records monitoring data (PEF - Peak Expiratory Flow, FEV1 - Forced Expiratory Volume in one second, symptoms and exacerbations) and receive immediate graphical and written feedback based on the action plan recorded at the medical consultation visit. Automatic messages and alerts are triggered when pre-defined conditions are met (e.g. a red color in the action plan or a scheduled consultation). Additionally, the patient can answer self-administered questionnaires (e.g. asthma control and ALQ - Asthma Life Quality test) at specified times (e.g. before medical visit).

Doctors have complete access to their patients' medical record, including the monitoring and questionnaires data, enabling a thorough assessment. Based on data recorded by the doctor at the consultation, classifications of asthma control, severity, and high-risk for near fatal asthma classifications are shown. Summaries of the monitoring data and questionnaire scores are also provided. Figure 3 illustrates using UML the use cases describing three different stages in P'ASMA use – Patient registration in P'ASMA (top left); P'ASMA use with patient at home (bottom left); and P'ASMA use just before clinical consultation (right).

3. Study design

In this exploratory randomized crossover study, patients used a web-based monitoring and decision-support tool or a paper asthma diary and action plan, each during 4 weeks, in a random sequence (Figure 4). In both periods patients monitored PEF/FEV1 once daily using a Piko-1® [4]. Randomization was performed using a computer generated algorithm.

Patients' physician was allowed to schedule regular medical appointments along with study visits. However, no asthma follow-up visits were scheduled during the period patients participated in the study. The treatment action plan that was prescribed by the patients' physician was used to adjust regular treatment at the end of visits two and three and recorded in the web application and in the written action plan.

Participants were instructed on how to use the monitoring instruments in each period of the study, the Piko-1®, the Internet application and the paper-based diary and action plan.

Patients used the Internet application or the paper-based tools during their daily life. Patients were asked to use the monitoring instruments, including the Piko-1®, once per day just before taking their inhaled medication.

Local research ethics commission approved the study. Patients were given oral and written information about the study and gave written informed consent. The database was registered in the "Comissão Nacional de Protecção de Dados" (National Commission for Data protection). The project design and procedures complied with the recommendations of the Declaration of Helsinki and followed the CONSORT statement (Consolidated Standards of Reporting Trials) where applicable.

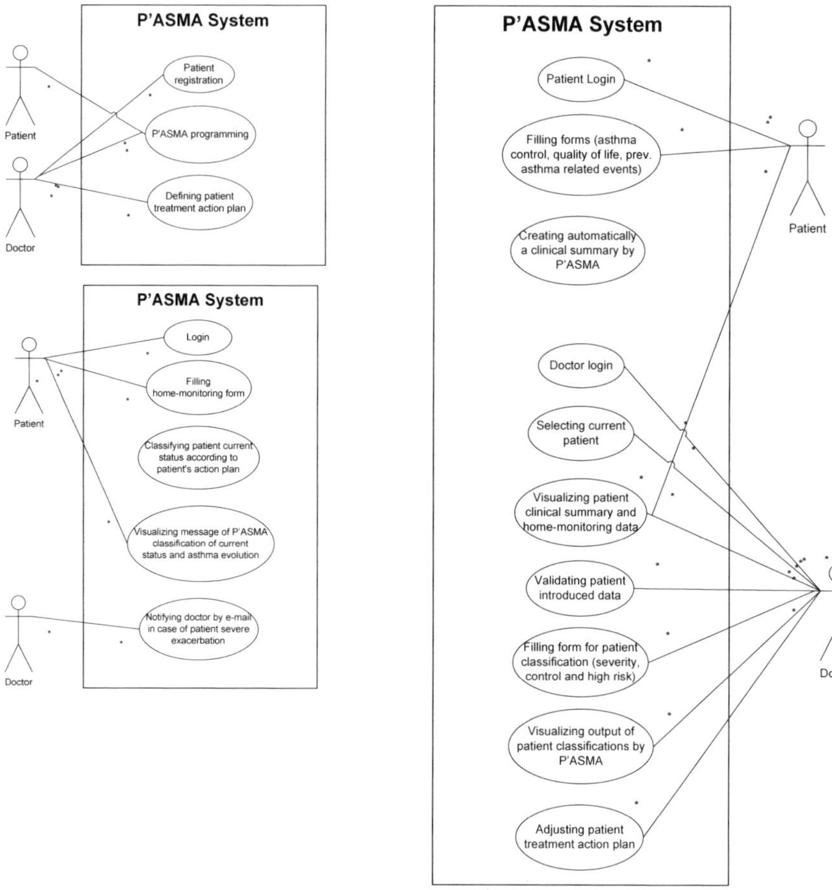

Figure 3: UML use cases describing three different stages in P'ASMA use – Patient registration in P'ASMA (top left); P'ASMA use with patient at home (bottom left); and P'ASMA use just before clinical consultation (right).

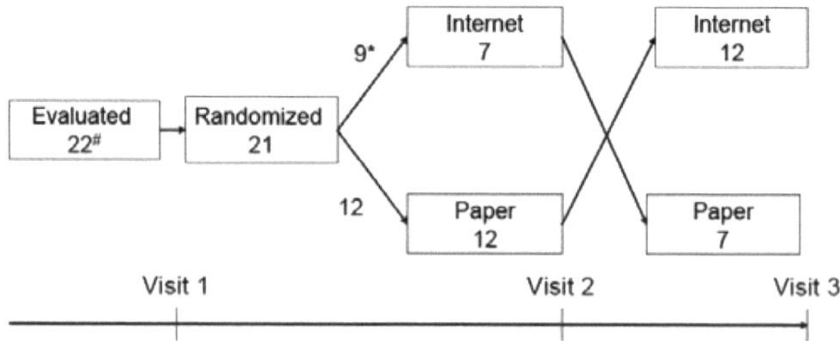

Figure 4: Study design and patient's flow chart. Visits were scheduled at 4 week intervals. # One patient did not fulfill the treatment inclusion criteria; * two patients randomized did not start the intervention – one lost access to the Internet during the study period; the other moved to another city and would not continue in the study.

4. Evaluation methods

The messaging system, the educational content and the features designed to be used by doctors were not evaluated in this study.

Paper-based tools were as follows: an asthma symptoms diary adapted from Juniper et al [5] that had the same questions of the web symptoms monitoring form. Patients were given a hand-written asthma action plan similar to the one generated by the web application. Piko-1® was used for monitoring lung function parameters.

4.1. Selection of participants

Patients could be included in the study if aged between 16 and 65 years old, had a medical diagnosis of asthma for more than 6 months, were treated with inhaled budesonide (400-1600 mcg/day) and formoterol in a single inhaler and had a prebronchodilator FEV1 over 50% of predicted. Patients were excluded if they had a severe psychiatric, neurological, oncologic or immunologic disease or could not use the Internet during the study period. Twenty one patients from the Immunoallergology outpatient clinic of Hospital S. João were included from 28 patients assessed.

5. Results

5.1. Participants characteristics

Patients were between 18 and 62 years old with a mean (sd) age of 29 (10) years old and 15 (71%) were women. The median number of years of school education was 11 (range 4-18). Two thirds used the Internet daily, while one quarter only used it less than once a week. Lung function parameters were mostly within normal range with 5 patients below 80% predicted; Mean (sd) FEV1 90(21) percent of predicted values. Asthma control score ranged from 0 to 3.5 with 5 patients below 0.75 (well-controlled asthma) and 7 patients above 1.5 (uncontrolled asthma). The two groups, internet→paper and paper→ internet, were not significantly different.

Four patients had previously monitored their asthma symptoms or PEF, none had done self-monitoring in the previous month.

5.2. Patients' opinions

Sixteen patients provided their opinions about the monitoring instruments used in the study. The number of patients who wrote negative comments was 2 regarding Internet application and 11 regarding paper diary; for positive comments the numbers were six and one respectively.

Nine patients reported problems related to the use of the Internet application, summing a total of 19 problems. Of these 9 were related to Internet connection, 5 to graphical user interface, 3 to internal system errors and 2 were difficulties in the interpretation of questions. Two patients stated they were unable to use the Internet application because of technical problems. Five patients reported problems with Piko-1®, mostly related to the batteries, with two of them being unable to do PEF/FEV1 monitoring because of technical problems. Five patients report problems related to paper diary, however only one was of technical nature (difficult to read), the other were related to be easy to forget to fill in or to lose it or be more difficult to understand how asthma was changing.

The median (p25-p75) time to fill in the Internet and paper diaries was similar (p=0.675), respectively 3 (2-6) and 3 (1-4.8) minutes, and significantly more than PEF/FEV1 monitoring 2 (1-3) minutes (p=0.028 and p=0.036 respectively).

Table 1 summarizes the opinions of patients regarding the monitoring tools. When looking at positive and negative answers there were not many differences in opinions regarding the different tools. However, in comparison to paper diary, more patients considered the Internet very useful (p=0.038) and liked it very much (p=0.030). Viewing previous data on the Internet was more frequently considered much easier than in the paper diary (p=0.038).

Most (12) patients were very interested in continuing to monitor their asthma using the Internet application, whereas only 2 answered the same for paper diary (p=0.002). When asked what instruments would they choose to do self-monitoring in the future (alone or in combination with others), only one patient chose exclusively the paper diary, 4 chose paper diary with other instruments and 12 patients did not chose paper diary at all. The most frequent choices were Piko-1® in 6 (38%) patients, Internet in 5 (31%) and Piko-1 ® together with Internet in 5 (31%).

Patients considered the more important features of the Internet application the asthma diary (93%), the educational content (82%) and the questionnaires to self-assess asthma status done just before the medical consultation (79%). Receiving information about asthma and exchanging messages with their doctor (both 85%) were more frequently considered interesting features than receiving messages about medication (69%) or about consultations (67%).

None of the patients referred unwillingness to monitor their asthma in the future and half stated they were willing to do it always. Furthermore, one third of patients were happy to monitor their symptoms daily, whereas 20% preferred to do it less than once a week and another 20% weekly.

Table 1 – Patients' opinions related to the different monitoring instruments used in the study. Valid percentages are shown, n varied from 13 to 16

	Paper n (%)	Internet n (%)	Piko-1 n (%)
I am very interested in using it for monitoring asthma	2 (12)	12 (92)	14 (80)
It was easy to record data	14 (93)	14 (93)	13 (93)
Very easy	10 (67)	11 (73)	10 (67)
It was easy to view data	13 (81)	14 (93)	10 (67)
Very easy	10 (63)	14 (93)	13 (93)
I liked to use it	12 (80)	13 (93)	14 (100)
Very much	7 (47)	13 (93)	11 (79)
Takes too long to use	5 (31)	5 (33)	4 (27)
It was easy to forget	7 (44)	7 (47)	6 (40)
Very easy	4 (25)	2 (13)	1 (7)
It may be useful to me	13 (87)	15 (100)	14 (93)
Very useful	9 (56)	13 (87)	11 (73)
It may contribute to improve:			
Asthma Control	15 (93)	16 (100)	13 (97)
A lot	8 (50)	11 (73)	7 (50)
Treatment adherence	12 (87)	14 (100)	12 (92)
A lot	8 (53)	9 (64)	7 (58)

Asthma care	14 (87)	15 (100)	8 (89)
A lot	11 (69)	12 (80)	5 (56)
How many days you did not register symptoms (during 4 weeks)?			
None	6 (38)	0 (0)	2 (13)
1-2 days	2 (13)	2 (14)	3 (20)
More than 3 days	8 (50)	13 (86)	10 (66)

5.3. Adherence to monitoring tools

The number of monitoring data values was 1044, during paper diary periods 526 (50%) were registered and during Internet diary 518.

Table 2 – Mean percentage of adherence to the monitoring tools in the different weeks and in the two sequence groups.

%	Total	Week number				$p^{\#}$	Sequence		p^*
		1	2	3	4		P-I	I-P	
Piko-1 ® during paper	45	51	47	47	35	**<0.001**	58	25	**<0.001**
Piko-1 ® during Internet	46	38	50	46	49	0.090	44	48	0.451
Paper Diary	92	89	95	95	91	**0.012**	96	85	**<0.001**
Internet Diary	41	32	48	44	39	**0.017**	36	49	**0.004**

Friedman test; * Mann-Whitney Test; P-I Paper before Internet; I-P Internet before Paper sequences. Significant differences between groups are in bold.

Adherence to the monitoring tools used between the second and the last visit was significantly lower than to those tools used first, except for Piko-1 ® when used with Internet monitoring. For the different tools, the first or the forth week had the lowest proportion of recorded values (Table 2). The first day after the study visits had a mean percentage of recordings of 53.

Figure 5 represents the adherence to monitoring tools as a proportion of the number recorded data and the number of data values that should have been recorded during the 4 weeks between study visits. Four patients stated that they did not use monitoring tools because of technical problems with instruments. The adherence of Piko-1® and Internet diary were not significantly different (p=0.289). Adherence to paper diary measured by registered values was significantly higher than adherence to other Internet diary (p <0.001) and to Piko-1® (p <0.001). However, these written recordings seem to overestimate the adherence to paper symptoms diary. Ten patients reported filling in the paper diary several days at once, whereas on the Internet diary only one set of data could be recorded per day. The difference between paper diary and Piko-1® was not expected as patients' were instructed to do both instruments at the same time. In addition, at least 7 patients reported more days without recording symptoms in the questionnaire (Table 1) than the number of missing values in their paper diary, e.g. 3 of the 8 patients who reported not recording at least 3 days the symptoms in paper had no missing values in the actual paper diary.

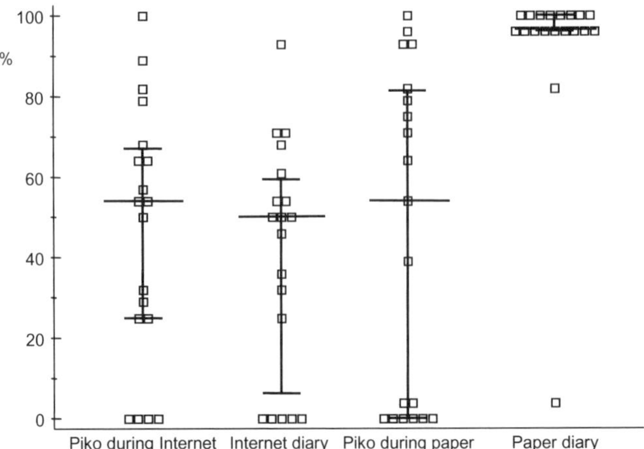

Figure 5: Adherence to monitoring with different instruments. Each square represents the percentage of recorded data values of one patient, horizontal lines represent the 25, 50 and 75 percentiles.

6. Discussion

Home monitoring asthma supported by the web application was feasible and well accepted by patients. After using paper-tools and the Internet application, patients preferred the latter for supporting asthma self-management. No adverse effects related to the interventions were observed.

Patients' adherence to home monitoring was quite variable. Overall, around half of the scheduled measurements were recorded. This is similar to the study by Turner and co-workers where adherence to the self-management plans was only 65% in the PFM group and 52% in the symptoms group [6]. The completeness of home monitoring records was significantly different between the interventions, with an apparent higher adherence to paper tools. However, the data from Piko-1® and from the patients' questionnaires suggests the paper diaries overestimate monitoring – patients fabricated values or recorded several values at once. In fact, a more careful observation of all the data suggests the frequencies of home monitoring using the paper diary and the Internet application were equivalent. In a chronic pain study, Stone and co-workers used a paper diary bound in a binder equipped with a photo sensor that recorded when the diary was used – while the completeness of a paper diary was over 90%, the binder was opened on 32% of the days [7]. In fact, different studies in the last 15 years suggested electronic, time-coded diaries are more reliable [8, 9]. As previously reported for monitoring of lung function parameters, instruments for symptom monitoring should include integrity features such as time-stamps. Nevertheless, the clinical relevance of low reliability of paper diaries is not known. Furthermore, patients' answers indicate a need for customizing monitoring schedules, agreed between the patient and the physician, taking asthma severity and control in consideration.

This study allowed the identification of several aspects of the web-application that need improvement. The data input should be easier; the language and system errors detected must be corrected and customization tool improved. Moreover, considerable redesign is needed in the tools for graphic feedback, for data summaries and for producing the outputs of information (both electronic and printable) [10, 11].

In the last few years a few randomized studies evaluating Web-based interventions for patients with asthma have been published. Their results are promising regarding feasibility and clinical outcomes [12-15]. Other studies reported exciting results regarding adherence and acceptance by the patients [16-18]. Moreover patients with more severe asthma have expressed strong willingness in using web- and mobile-based technologies for supporting self-management [19].

Only recently a randomized controlled study evaluated a web-based intervention for supporting asthma self-management [15]. In 6-month study with 300 patients, Rasmussen and co-workers reported the treatment and monitoring with an Internet-based management tool. The addition of a web-based self-management application to specialized care achieved significantly better clinical outcomes than specialized care alone and also than follow-up at primary care [15]. The authors conclude that the use of an interactive asthma monitoring tool, improves asthma control. However, as the application used included a guideline-based algorithm to adjust the asthma treatment, the Internet group was treated with a significantly higher mean dose of inhaled steroids. In P'ASMA the treatment action plan was established by the patients' physician and the same for both interventions.

Instead of viewing clinical information systems as an organizational resource for health professionals, P'ASMA aims to be an open resource leading to productive interactions between the patient and the practice team [20]. The clinical information can be provided and received not only by health providers but also by patients. Still, further development is needed for integrating medical records and P'ASMA [11].

6.1. Limitations

The small number of patients and the 4-week duration of each intervention could limit the ability to detect differences. However, the results were very consistent and several results point to a preference for the web-based, and Piko-1 device over the paper-based tools.

To be included in the study the patient had to be able to use Internet, therefore the interpretation of the patients' opinions should be cautions. Nevertheless, with the increasing availability of communication technologies, more and more patients will be able to use the internet. In fact, the proportion of households in Portugal that have Internet access grew from 13% in 2001 to 31% in 2005 [21]; moreover in the year 2005, 31% of Portuguese population had searched for health information and 28% had filled official forms on the Internet. Other types of study should address the problems of the use self-management supported by communication technologies in populations with low literacy and economic difficulties [22, 23].

6.2. Future work

Adherence to monitoring may be improved using automatic email and/or SMS reminders [24]; the messaging system which has already been developed should be further implemented. An additional mobile phone interface would increase the flexibility of data input [25-27]. A flexible algorithm able to adjust monitoring to the asthma status and to the patients preferences would also contribute to the improvement of the web application.

P'ASMA is being re-implemented as a Joomla! [28] extension to be used by all APA (Portuguese Association of Asthma Patients) associates – http://www.apa.org.pt.

This site aims to help the communication between the Association and asthma patients and help patients have better control of their condition. Technically, it is being implemented using Joomla!, an open-source Content Manager System. We expect to improve the usability of the system taking in consideration our previous experience with P'ASMA.

7. Conclusions

To summarize, this exploratory study provided encouraging results. The intervention was feasible, safe and the problems detected in the web-application can be corrected. Moreover, the data quality is improved as the integrity features increase the reliability of the data and patients preferred the web-based application to monitor their asthma.

Acknowledgements

Eng. Maria José Amaro, and Mr. Miguel Nunes for helping the implementation of the system. Dr. André Moreira for providing input during the planning of the system and for revising previous versions of the study report. Dr. Tiago Jacinto, for helping in data collection and revising previous versions of the study report.

References

1.   ENV 12251: Health informatics - Secure user identification managementand security of authentication by passwords.
2.   TLS - Transport Layer Security. RFC 2246. 1999.
3.   Farinha, P., A. Ferreira, and R. Cruz-Correia. Web.care - Gestão de acessos e recursos para estudos clínicos multicêntricos on-line. in 1ª Conferência Ibérica de Sistemas e Tecnologias de Informação. 2006. Ofir, Portugal.
4.   Fonseca, J.A., et al., Pulmonary function electronic monitoring devices: A randomized agreement study. Chest, 2005. 128(3): p. 1258-1265.
5.   Juniper, E., et al., Measuring asthma control. Clinic questionnaire or daily diary? Am J Respir Crit Care Med, 2000. 162(4 Pt 1): p. 1330-4.
6.   Turner, M.O., et al., A Randomized Trial Comparing Peak Expiratory Flow and Symptom Self-management Plans for Patients with Asthma Attending a Primary Care Clinic. 1998, Am Thoracic Soc. p. 540-546.
7.   Stone, A., et al., Patient compliance with paper and electronic diaries. Controlled Clinical Trials, 2003. 24(2): p. 182-99.
8.   Hyland, M.E., et al., Diary keeping in asthma: comparison of written and electronic methods. 1993. p. 487-9.
9.   Tiplady, B., G.K. Crompton, and D. Brackenridge, Electronic diaries for asthma. BMJ, 1995. 310(6992): p. 1469.
10. Sittig, D., Personal health records on the internet: a snapshot of the pioneers at the end of the 20th Century. Int J Med Inform, 2002. 65(1): p. 1-6.
11. Tang, P., et al., Personal health records: definitions, benefits, and strategies for overcoming barriers to adoption. J Am Med Inform Assoc, 2006 Mar-Apr. 13(2): p. 121-6.
12. Homer, C., et al., An evaluation of an innovative multimedia educational software program for asthma management: report of a randomized, controlled trial. Pediatrics, 2000. 106(1 Pt 2): p. 210-215.
13. Krishna, S., et al., Internet-enabled interactive multimedia asthma education program: a randomized trial. Pediatrics, 2003 Mar. 111(3): p. 503-510.

14. Guendelman, S., et al., Improving asthma outcomes and self-management behaviors of inner-city children: a randomized trial of the Health Buddy interactive device and an asthma diary. Arch Pediatr Adolesc Med, 2002. 156(2): p. 114-20.

15. Bernstein, K., et al., Modelling and implementing electronic health records in Denmark. International Journal of Medical Informatics - MIE 2003, 2005. 74(2-4): p. 213-220.

16. Finkelstein, J., G. Hripcsak, and M. Cabrera, Patients' acceptance of Internet-based home asthma telemonitoring, in Proc AMIA Symp. 1998. p. 336-40.

17. Finkelstein, J., G. O'Connor, and R. Friedmann, Development and implementation of the home asthma telemonitoring (HAT) system to facilitate asthma self-care. Medinfo, 2001. 10(Pt 1): p. 810-4.

18. Chan, D., et al., An Internet-based store-and-forward video home telehealth system for improving asthma outcomes in children. Am J Health Syst Pharm, 2003. 60(19): p. 1976-81.

19. Fonseca, J., et al., Asthma patients are willing to use mobile and web technologies to support self-management. Allergy, 2006 61(3): p. 389-90.

20. Bodenheimer, T., E. Wagner, and K. Grumbach, Improving primary care for patients with chronic illness: The chronic care model, Part 2. J American Med Association, 2002. 288(15): p. 1909-14.

21. INE 2006 (http//www.ine.pt). 2006, Instituto Nacional de Estatística.

22. Eng, T., et al., Access to health information and support: a public highway or a private road? JAMA, 1998. 280(15): p. 1371-5.

23. Gustafson, D., et al., Use and Impact of eHealth System by Low-income Women With Breast Cancer. J Health Commun, 2005. 10(Suppl 1): p. 195-218.

24. Neville, R., et al., Mobile phone text messaging can help young people manage asthma. BMJ, 2002. 325(7364): p. 600.

25. Anhøj, J. and C. Møldrup, Feasibility of collecting diary data from asthma patients through mobile phones and SMS (short message service): Response rate analysis and focus group evaluation from a pilot study. J Med Internet Res [electronic resource], 2004. 6(4).

26. Anhøj, J. and L. Nielsen, Quantitative and qualitative usage data of an internet-based asthma monitoring tool. J Med Internet Res [electronic resource] 2004. 6(3).

27. Ostojic, V., et al., Improving asthma control through telemedicine: a study of short-message service. Telemed J E Health, 2005. 11(1): p. 28-35.

28. Joomla! an open-source Content Management System.   [cited 15 Feb 2007]; Available from: http://www.joomla.org/.

Medical and Care Compunetics 4
L. Bos and B. Blobel (Eds.)
IOS Press, 2007

Virtual Reality: Towards a Novel Treatment Environment for Ankylosing Spondylitis

Shijuan LI[1], Stephen KAY and Nicholas R. HARDICKER
SHIRE, Univerisy of Salford, Salford, UK

Abstract. The objective of this paper is to outline the project that eventually seeks to visualize clinical knowledge found within the record; the immediate task being to create a model that can be deployed for therapeutic purposes. How therapies for a certain type of chronically ill patient can benefit from Virtual Reality (VR) tools is investigated. Ankylosing Spondylitis (AS) is selected as a test condition. VR is expected to provide a novel treatment environment for AS sufferers, in which they can relax, manage their pain and take part in the routine exercise more effectively and efficiently by using the VR tools. An integral part of this model's construction will be to elicit evaluative detail from the literature and the patients' perspective. The purpose is to understand the inevitable challenges facing this proposed intervention if the design prototype is to successfully move from the research domain and become an integral part of established therapeutic practice.

Keywords. Virtual Reality, Ankylosing Spondylitis, Therapy, Treatment, Model

1. Introduction

The impact of Virtual Reality (VR) with respect to healthcare has been often claimed as "revolutionary". However, the true reality is that the current state of activity is still primarily research based, extremely localized and often remote from routine practice. This research is directed at understanding the specific contributions of a single implementation of VR to healthcare as an intervention. The research investigates how therapies for a certain type of chronically ill patient can benefit from VR tools. Ankylosing Spondylitis (AS) is selected as a test condition.

1.1. Ankylosing Spondylitis Problem Statement

AS is a painful progressive rheumatic disease, mainly of the spine. It can also affect other joints (such as hips, knees, ankles and shoulders etc), tendons and ligaments and other areas, such as the heart, lung, skin and eye can be involved [1, 2]. It is believed that AS is associated with the gene Human Leucocyte Antigen B27 (HLA-B27), which present in 40-95% of cases [2]. However, the actual cause of AS is not clear. Unfortunately, what is clear is that there is no known cure at this point in time. AS affects approximately 1% of men and 0.49% of women in the Caucasian population [2]. In the U.K., approximately one in 100 males and one in 250 females, according to the

---

[1] Corresponding Author: Shijuan Li, SHIRE, University of Salford, Blatchford Building, Frederick Road, Salford M6 6PU, UK; E-mail: s.li@pgr.salford.ac.uk

information from the National Ankylosing Spondylitis Society (NASS) in the UK, are suffering from this disease (NASS 2004).

The main symptoms are: pain, stiffness and fatigue. Current treatments for AS include regular exercise and medicines, classified as one of the following:

- Anti-inflammatory painkillers.

- Ordinary painkillers.

- Other medicines, including Sulfasalazine, Methotrexate, Anti-TNF, and Glucosamine sulphate. [1, 2]

Side-effects, however, sometimes occur with these medicines, such as stomach pain and bleeding. People with asthma, high blood pressure, kidney failure etc. may not able to take anti-inflammatory painkillers [3]. According to some patients' experience, Patches, Acupressure, Acupuncture, Massage, Heat, and TENS machines can help to relieve symptoms. In serious cases surgical intervention is used for patients with advanced hip involvement. However, other surgery is risky and spinal osteotomy is undertaken rarely and only on those with severe spinal curvature [2].

One of the more important treatments is regular exercise. This can relieve the symptoms and help to slow and even prevent further development of AS [2]. Products related to exercise as part of living with AS can be found from the NASS, these products include paper materials (books), audio materials (cassette tapes) and video & DVD. See **Table 1**. in details.

1.2. Ankylosing Spondylitis Management Paradox

Pain and stiffness are the main symptoms treated. Fatigue has also recently been considered to be a core symptom; indeed in studies fatigue has been reported as the main symptom by up to 65% of patients [4, 5]. Long-standing pain and fatigue may give rise to depression. There is a paradox in the management of AS. AS suffers need to participate in routine exercise in order to retain mobility and prevent pain, stiffness and irreversible deformity. However, AS sufferers have difficulty in taking regular exercise due to fatigue and to the very pain and stiffness they seek to prevent.

VR exposure therapy may have advantages over other approaches in helping AS sufferers to overcome their difficulties through simulation. This article investigates issues around the use of VR as a novel treatment environment for AS and considers its ability to retain mobility, and to prevent irreversible deformity while relieving and preventing symptoms.

Table 1. Example products currently available to AS sufferers

Type	Name
Books	Car Driving with Ankylosing Spondylitis
	NASS 1981 Symposium Book
	Living with Ankylosing Spondylitis
	North America Postage for Guidebook for Patients
Audio	Physiotherapy Cassette Tape
Video & DVD	Fight Back

1.3. VR Projects

The use of VR for therapy has made significant progress, especially in Neuro-Psycho-Physiology and Rehabilitation. Several VR systems have been developed and tested for the physical or mental rehabilitation of patients and to support mental health therapy.

Other examples of the application of VR in therapy include: modifying eating disorders, treating agoraphobia and therapy, treating Iraq War Military Personnel with PTSD (Post Traumatic Stress Disorder), distracting dental patients from work being done, diminishing psycho-ontological symptoms in cancer patients, relieving back pain or pain from burns or injury, and facilitating exercise for people with cerebral palsy.[6-9]

Table 2. lists VR projects that are relevant to our specific research. One example in particular, the fMRI image of the brain taken by Hunter G. Hoffman et al, showed that when people engaged in VR programme during the stimuli, the pain-related activity in five regions of the brain that are known to be involved in the perception of pain subsided. Virtual reality is not just changing the way patients interpret incoming pain signals; the programs actually reduce the amount of pain-related brain activity. [6] Another preliminary study by Karen Grimmer and colleagues from the Women's and Children's Hospital in Adelaide (Australia) reported that Immersion in a virtual world of monsters and aliens helps children feel less pain during the treatment of severe injuries such as burns. [10] Researchers at Emory University School of Medicine and Virtually Better (Inc.) have been trying to test the use of virtual reality therapy to find out if it can help people with lower back pain learn how to relax, breathe properly, and manage their pain. While VR tools have been heavily researched in relation to pain, with impressive results, VR applications to support exercise have not been widely investigated; nor have VR applications for AS. Moreover, the majority of studies look at single applications, rather than taking a holistic perspective which requires a mixture of applications. This study seeks to redress the balance.

Table 2. VR projects relevant to the research

Author	Project	Organization	Year
Albert Rizzo, Jarrell Pair, Peter J. Mcnerney, et al	Development of a VR Therapy for Iraq War Military Personnel with PTSD	University of Southern California, U.S.A	2006
Karen Grimmer et al	In Virtual World Alleviates Pain From Injury	The Women's and Children's Hospital in Adelaide, Australia	2005
Barbara Rothbaum et al	Virtual Reality Therapy For Back Pain	School of Medicine, Emory University and Virtually Better, U.S.A	2005
Hunter G. Hoffman et al	SnowWorld	UW Virtual Analgesia Research Center, U.S.A	2004
Bruce Thomas, Emily Steele	Alleviate Pain in Cerebral Palsy Patients	University of South Australia, Australia	2004

1.4. Aim of the Research

This project seeks to create a VR model that can be deployed for therapeutic purposes for this type of chronically ill patient. In particular it attempts to address the management paradox by looking at an environment that is a holistic one. An integral part of this model's construction will be to elicit evaluative detail from the literature and the patients' perspective. The purpose is to understand the inevitable challenges facing this proposed intervention if the design prototype is to successfully move from the research domain and become an integral part of established therapeutic practice.

2. VR Therapy Model

The aim of the research is to specify and design a single virtual environment, in which AS sufferers can relax, manage their pain and better deal with their pain while taking exercise.

According to the therapy information surveyed from Ankylosing Spondylitis International Federation (ASIF), UK NASS and the Physiotherapy department in hospitals, we have constructed an AS physical therapy model (See **Figure 1**) that will be implemented in the VR environment. The main therapy model has four elements: Relaxation, Pain management, Exercise and Evaluation. Besides these four elements, there is one extra function in the model: the patient literature function. And the Risk and Safety Management should be taken into consideration while the construction of the tools. These support the main therapy model.

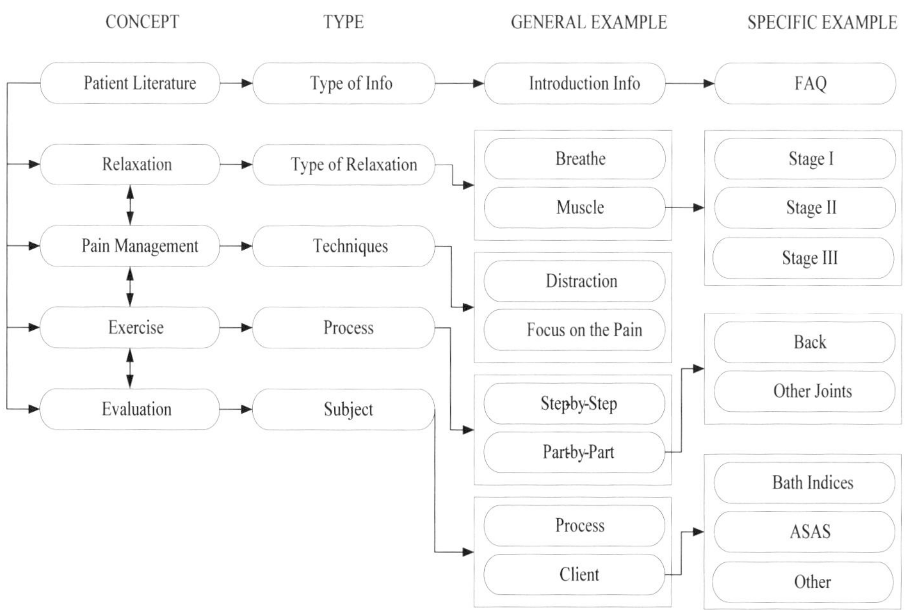

Figure 1. An AS Physical Therapy Model

The four elements Relaxation, Pain Management, Exercise and Evaluation will be implemented in the VR environment. Thus, there will be four VR tools available for AS sufferers: Relaxation tool, Pain Management tool, Exercise tool and Evaluation tool. The four tools comprising the environment are discussed:

- Relaxation tool. The users will be immersed in a comfortable VR environment. For example, it may be visualized as a seaside setting, sitting on a reclining chair with the option of listening to music or not. There will be two relaxation programs [11-13], one is to support breathing relaxation, and the other is muscle relaxation which has three stages to let go of the tension in the muscles of face, neck, shoulders, arms, hands and legs etc. By immersing in a virtual environment, the Relaxation tool is intended to help the user feel comfortable and relaxed.

- Pain Management tool. This tool will include two methods to relieve the pain [14]. One is to distract from the pain by immersing in the VR environment. In contrast, the other is to focus on the pain, viewing and manipulating a simulated image of the pain in order to influence the real experience of pain.

- Exercise tool. This tool will provide the necessary exercise in the form of dynamic 3-D models to users. Users' movements can also be captured and viewed in the form of a dynamic 3-D model, tracking the progress of users and building their confidence.

- Evaluation tool. Besides the measurement of the client by using Bath Indices, instruments from ASessment in Ankylosing Spondylitis (ASAS) and other instruments, a VR evaluation tool will be constructed. The Evaluation Tool is used to assess the other VR tools. By capturing the clients' movements and viewed in the form of a dynamic 3-D model, the usability and efficiency of the other VR tools can be evaluated.

The proposed combination of the four tools (Relaxation tool, Pain Management tool, Exercise tool and Evaluation tool) is important. Each tool will represent a different proportion of the whole therapy process. The Relaxation tool should support the Pain Management tool and the Exercise tool, and the Relaxation tool with the Pain Management tool together support the Exercise tool, and the Evaluation tool should improve the usability and efficiency of the other three tools. The six boxes (Distraction, Focus on the Pain, Breathing Relaxation, Muscle Relaxation, Exercise Part-by-Part Exercise Step-by-Step) in **Figure 1** are the various functions that are to be implemented in VR. The treatment process in VR is described as in **Figure 2**. In the VR environment, the client can choose one VR tool (Relax or Pain or Exercise) at a time or choose to use the tools in order (Relax-Pain-Exercise) or choose the specific tools according to their requirements. Within each tool, there are different functions that can be chosen as well. The Evaluation tool is to provide feed-back showing progress or lack of deterioration.

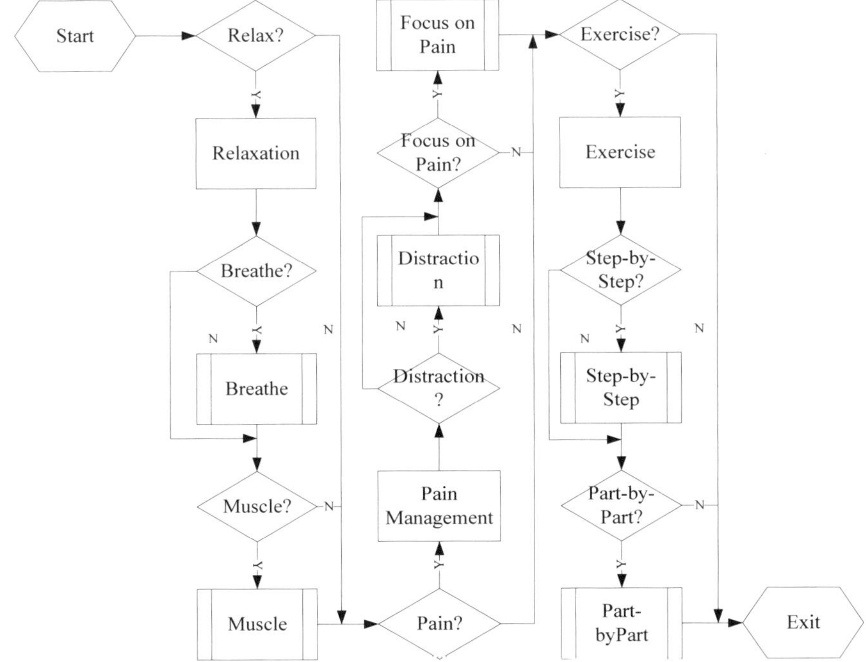

Figure 2. VR therapy process model

3. Discussion

Routine exercise is an essential component in the treatment of AS. The initial symptoms can be prevented and relieved by regular movement of the areas involved. If this is not done, the formation of new bone can lead to increased stiffness, and to deformity with stooping posture in the spine. Eventually the stiffness and deformity become irreversible. Routine exercise is an important treatment for AS. The simulation part of VR could alter perception in an imaginary environment, then successfully distract and reduce the pain of AS sufferers, allowing them to take exercise more efficiently and effectively. This novel approach will not only do well to the patient but may also facilitate the home-based self-care of AS sufferers. Home-based self-care is essential for the successful management of AS. The use of VR tools may help to achieve the ultimate goal of enabling clients to more fully participate in 'real' environments.

Positive outcomes have been reported for the use of VR in the management of the pain and in the facilitation of exercise. This study seeks to combine three aspects of therapy into a single environment: Relaxation, Pain management and Exercise, and to permit Evaluation as part of a holistic approach to the management paradox. The current work has scoped the problem space and identified a preliminary model for AS therapy. The specification of the whole environment is underway.

To apply the VR application into the therapy of chronic illness, such as AS, will face many challenges. There are many parameters that will affect the effect. It is helpful to view the VR experience as a multidimensional model that appears to be influenced by many parameters, such as the selection of VR platforms or the consideration of the client's personal factors (age, sex, etc.). Given the variety of VR platforms, the comparison of different VR platforms is beneficial. Because of the diversity of the population, the client's personal factors should be taken into consideration as well.

Eventually, the goal will be to integrate the VR therapy model into the Electronic Health Record to enhance the continuity of care from diagnosis to therapy and can support the development of a Personal Health Record that can be used in the home rather than laboratory or clinical settings.

References

[1]   Walker J: Ankylosing Spondylitis. *Nurs Stand* 2006, 20(46):48-52.

[2]   Canlin A: Ankylosing Spondylitis. *Medicine* 2006, 34(10):396-400.

[3]   Warrell DA, Cox TM, Firth JD, Benz E: The Oxford Textbook of Medicine, 4 edn. Oxford: Oxford University Press; 2004.

[4]   Jones SD, Koh WD, Steiner A, Garrett SL, Calin A: Fatigue in ankylosing spondylitis: its prevalence and relationship to disease activity, sleep, and other factors. *J Rheumatol* 1996, 23:487–490.

[5]   Wolfe F, Michaud K, Pincus T: Fatigue, rheumatoid arthritis, and anti-tumor necrosis factor therapy: an investigation in 24831patients. *J Rheumatol* 2004, 31:2115–2120.

[6]   Hoffman HG: Virtual-Reality Therapy *Scientific American Magazine* 2004(August).

[7]   Pair J, Allen B, Dautricourt M, al e: A Virtual Reality Exposure Therapy Application for Iraq War Post Traumatic Stress Disorder. In: *IEEE Virtual Reality 2006: 2006*; 2006.

[8]   D. A. Das KAG, A. L. Sparnon, S. E. McRae, B. H. Thomas: The efficacy of playing a virtual reality game in modulating pain for children with acute burn injuries: A randomized controlled trial [ISRCTN87413556]. *BMC Pediatr* 2005, 5: 1.

[9]   Moline J: Virtual Reality for Health Care: A Survey. In: *Virtual Reality in Neuro-Psycho-Physiology: Cognitive, Clinical and Methodological Issues in Assessment and Rehabilitation*. Edited by Riva G. Amsterdam: IOS Press; 1997: 3-34.

[10]   Das DA, Grimmer KA, Sparnon AL, McRae SE, Thomas BH: The efficacy of playing a virtual reality game in modulating pain for children with acute burn injuries: A randomized controlled trial. *BMC Pediatrics* 2005, 5(1).

[11]   Pasero C, Smith N, Christine L: Using Breathing to Supplement Pain Control. *Am J Nurs* 1997:16.

[12]   Bernstein DA, Borkovec TD: Progressive Relaxation Training: A Manual for the Helping Professions. Champaign, IL: Research Press; 1973.

[13]   Wolpe J: Psychotherapy by Reciprocal Inhibition. Stanford, CA: Stanford University Press; 1958.

[14]   Raj PP: Practical Management of Pain, 3rd edn. London: St. Louis; 2000.

Behavioral Compunetics

Medical and Care Compunetics 4
L. Bos and B. Blobel (Eds.)
IOS Press, 2007

Empowering the Patient with ICT-Tools: The Unfulfilled Promise

Wouter J. MEIJER M.D.[a] and Peter L. RAGETLIE M.Sc.[b]
[a]*Partner ICTUS Netwerk*
[b]*Partner ICTUS Netwerk, member NEN standardization committee in the Health Care Sector*

Abstract. For the patient, ICT is a resource that helps the individual to cope with illness. On the basis of in depth interviews with diabetic patients, their desired coping strategies that relate to communication and information were identified. The strategies fall into the following categories: Contact with fellow-patients, Care (choice of care, control of care and control of information) and social environment. Patient empowerment by ICT means that ICT enables the patient to cope with illness. A number of ICT-tools currently available for patients were analyzed on the aspect of patient empowerment. Findings are that most tools provide little support for patients' coping behaviour in choice (of treatment and caregiver), control of care and control of information (by the patient).

This lack of effective instrumental support for a patient's coping and empowerment is not explained by technical restraints, but by the dominance on the supply side in healthcare. To meet the neglected needs of patients, caregivers would have to adapt the organisation of their work. Examples of success in applying ICT/Telemedicine are given. The structural impediments for patient empowerment must be further clarified and removed or minimised.

Keywords. Digital homecare, Self-management, Electronic records and patient record access, Monitoring

1. Introduction

The advancement of ICT (Information Communication Technology) in society implies promising possibilities for patient empowerment in Health Care. This leads to the question: what is the connection between patient empowerment and ICT?

Patient empowerment has to do with people, their lives, needs, goals, achievement and fulfilment. ICT is a technique, and from the patient's view an instrument. This leaves us with 2 questions: Firstly, what are the needs, perceptions and behaviour of patients with respect to communication and information (Section 2) and; secondly how far do available ICT-instruments fulfil the needs of patients (Sections 4–8)? This paper also introduces a method to translate 'patient empowerment' and its conditions into functional requirements for ICT (Section 3).

2. Needs of Patients

2.1. Patient Empowerment Is: Enable Coping

ICT produces instruments that a patient can employ in coping with his own situation, his disease.

'Coping' in the context of patient empowerment: *'Coping is more than simple adjustment; it is the pursuit of human growth, mastery and differentiation allowing us to evolve in an ever changing world'* [18]. Thus, patient empowerment can be considered as enabling the patient in successfully coping with disease. The original question of this paper can now be reformulated as: 'How can ICT contribute to successful coping?'

Coping can be categorized into two types: problem-focused and emotion-focused coping. In problem-focused coping, an individual approaches the problem and makes active efforts to resolve it. For instance, 'seeking information' is a coping strategy of problem-focused coping.

In emotion-focused coping, the individual tries to avoid the problem and focuses mainly on managing the emotions associated with it. Examples of emotion-focused strategies are diversion, resignation and withdrawal.

Diabetes is an interesting case for two reasons. Firstly, it is relevant to problem-focused coping. Diabetes is one of the rare chronic diseases that allow patients to control their own well-being to a greater extent. Patients must comply with the extremely demanding requirements of their regime. Many diabetic patients fulfil these demands by coping in a problem-focused way.

Secondly, emotion-focused coping is equally relevant for diabetes patients. The demanding tasks of self-management can be too high. In addition, despite their efforts, they will possibly encounter complications (e.g. heart disease, blindness or foot amputation). A mental escape can be to ignore the possibility of complications.

Emotion-focused coping is illustrated by the perceptions of the interviewed patients concerning the foot sole scanner. This home based scanner sends the data of the foot sole to a centre every day where the scan is analyzed. If necessary, there is immediate follow-up with early treatment of the infection. (Diabetic patients are at risk of infections on the sole of a foot; such infections must be treated within 24 hours since they can lead to serious complications, including foot amputation). Most of the eight people interviewed would not use the foot sole scanner at home. They explained that in their perception they were not explicitly preventing complications, but instead they are engaged in healthy behaviour and reaching the targets of regulating blood sugar levels. As one participant said: "Speaking about the chance of getting a complication, is as though you will get it".

2.2. Scope

A patient's coping needs, perceptions and behaviour with respect to communication and information are not limited to the health care problem alone, but are related to the three areas of daily life: private life, work and healthcare problem. The reason is that a chronic disorder is of influence on all three areas of life and self-management of patients is not restricted to contacts with care professionals alone.

Health Care in this study is limited to:

- Professional care: Patients participate in professional care, i.e. care given by qualified practitioners.
- Self-care: Patients perform a number of care activities within an agreed treatment. Patients participate in the co-creation of care.

The so called Daily Care, in which a 'patient', without contact with a qualified care-giver attends to their own health, is not part of this study.

2.3. Target Group

In this study the needs of diabetic patients with respect to information and communication were identified by undertaking in-depth-interviews, based on an established methodology [10,30]. The deeper motivations, perceptions and values of people are explored, the more similarities they will show. For this reason a small sample group of approximately eight participants can be sufficient, provided that the participants are sufficiently different from each other [10,30].

From the thirty six people who responded to an advertisement in a local daily newspaper, eight people were selected, using the following criteria:

- Equal numbers of men and women.
- Employed as well as unemployed.
- Participants with both type one and type two diabetes.
- All had diabetes for at least five years.

In the last quarter of 2005 in depth interviews of the eight people took place in the Philips HomeLab.

2.4. Coping

From the interviews the actual or desirable coping strategies with respect to communication and information were deduced and categorised into four areas: daily life, contact with fellow-patients, choice of care and collaboration with caregiver(s).

In their daily life, the interviewed persons experienced discomfort and conflicts due to ignorance of the people in their social environment (private life, work). They thought it a public task (government, insurer) to inform people about diabetes and what it means for daily life.

Contact with fellow-patients brings support and information.

Choice because primarily the patient should be offered choice concerning a care provider and which treatment to chose. When the patient has made his choice in caregiver(s) and treatment/care including related services this should be the subject of (formal) agreement with the caregiver(s). Such an agreement (or contract) is one of the patient's fundamental rights. The agreement also covers the patients own medical files (Electronic Health Record, EHR and keys for access control). Collaboration with caregiver(s) includes self-care and, for chronic diseases, the process of the patient developing into an informed and motivated self-carer. Also, if family or friends as volunteers take care of the patient during a long period, this 'volunteer-care' must be supported by communication with formal caregivers. Finally, the patient should have the possibility to check whether the provided professional care service is delivered as agreed upon in the contract.

Table 1. Coping strategies and requirements for ICT

Area		Goal	Coping strategies	Requirements for ICT
Concordance in daily life (social environment)	Private life	Good private social environment	Inform relatives, friends etc. about diabetes	Provide information to relatives etc.
	Work	Good occupational social environment	Inform colleagues etc. about diabetes	Provide information to colleagues etc
Contact with fellow-patients		Mutual support and exchange of experiences	Contact others for support and exchange of experiences	Communication platform for patients
Care	Choice	Choice of health insurance	Seek information and compare	Provide information on health insurance
		Choice of care	Seek general information on possible care (e.g. treatment)	Provide validated information on alternatives, not restricted to the own care-organisation
		Choice of professional caregiver	Seek information and compare	Provide information that allows to compare caregivers
		Choice of care-organisation	Seek information and compare	Provide information that allows to compare organisations
	Collaboration with caregiver	Control of care by a Contract with caregiver(s)	Reach informed agreement on care service (e.g. treatment)	Support contract with caregiver(s)
		(Self-)care	Acquire knowledge by applying information	Support acquirement of knowledge
			For self-care: train motivation	Support motivational training
			For self-care rec obtain direct professional feedback	Bidirectional communication device
		Volunteer-care	Communication with informal and formal caregivers	Support communication: atient – family/ volunteers – formal caregivers
		Control of information	Receive and manage personal health and medical information	Patient manages own Electronic Health Record
		Privacy	Control access to personal information	Patient controls the key for record access
		Control of care by checking	Compare provided care to contracted care	Provide necessary information for patient

ICT-tools may enable these coping activities if they support the necessary communication and information needed to perform the activities in one or more of these four categories.

2.5. Coping and ICT

Table 1 summarizes the conditions that must be fulfilled to enable patient empowerment in terms of functional requirement for ICT-instruments. It translates the coping strategies of the patient into functional requirements for ICT.

Having established the requirements for ICT in coping strategies of patients we shall now:

- investigate whether several ICT-instruments at present in use enable these coping activities, and
- explore the factors that could explain why instruments fail to do so: is this due to technical constraints or to the conditions under which care is provided or structure of the healthcare system [2].

First we shall present a method of modelling communication (Section 3) and then we shall demonstrate, by six ICT-instruments, which coping needs are met by these ICT-tools (and which coping needs are not supported in using these ICT-tools).

3. A Method of Modelling the Communication Between the Patient and Caregivers

In this section a method is introduced that was employed in this study to clarify the significance of ICT instruments in relation to coping behaviour of patients.

3.1. Coping, Information and Communication

In the previous section from the patient's view point the need for support in coping activities was demonstrated. ICT-instruments offer support through offering communication facilities and access to information, needed for coping activities.

The patient can use communication and information for support of problem-focused coping, or in emotion-focused coping. In this section we limit ourselves to the communication and information needed in problem-focused coping. The method presented below is aimed to clarify the significance of ICT instruments in relation to problem-focused coping behaviour of a patient in managing their care problem.

For patients problem-focused coping activities be categorised as follows:

1. choice
2. control of care
3. (self-)care.

Each of these activities requires information; communication gives the patient access to this information.

Furthermore the patient has to supply information to third parties, like his caregiver(s) in relation to his health (problem).

Thus, the coping activities are interrelated: information created by one actor is used by other actors. Actors are human beings performing a role in healthcare. Each role has its own competence. For example a general practitioner is allowed to perform medical actions and to diagnose the case. A patient is an actor seeking care and with the competence to make his own choices and to express his symptoms.

3.2. Creation and Exchange of Information

Only authorised actors have the competence to create information. The patient knows which symptoms they have and the general practitioner diagnoses the case. Another example would be that parliament determines the rights of patients by law.

Also, an actor is authorised to use information. The physician needs the patient's information about the presented symptoms to make a diagnosis. Both physician and patient must know about laws on rights of patients when determining a treatment agreement. These examples show that actors create and exchange information, and are interdependent. These examples suggest that coping activities can be modelled in the aspect of communication and information.

3.3. Modelling of Communication

The purpose of this research is to link the use of ICT to patient's coping activities.

However, there is a gap between the physical world (activities) and the informational world (ICT). To bridge the gap two translations must be made. Firstly patient empowerment must be translated into a model of communication and information; this is the subject of the present section. The model must show which information the patient uses for his coping activities, and which communication is necessary to supply that information. Secondly, the model is applied to assess the ICT instruments; this is addressed in the following sections.

A tool for modelling communication and information is the Actor Information Diagram (AID). The AID shows who creates information, in which role, and who exchanges this information.

3.4. Illustration of the Method

To illustrate this, we present the AID that describes the next process (Table 2):

1. Parliament adopts two laws, firstly, on patient rights, and secondly, on privacy; both laws are the framework for the (medical) treatment agreement between patient and caregiver.
2. These laws are accounted for when the patient and his caregiver make a treatment agreement (contract).
3. The patient and his caregiver make efforts so that the intended care (including self-care) is realised; necessary information is created by both the patient (e.g. the medical history) and his caregiver (e.g. diagnostics); this information is exchanged between them.
4. The treatment and the treatment agreement is ended.
5. The patient's personal information must be passed onto a third party; the patient gives his consent (authorisation) to the previous caregiver and the information is provided.

In an AID the following symbols are used:

*   C for creating information
*   E for exchanging information
*   D for deleting information.

This example shows some characteristics of the AID:

*   each row of the table contains an activity of an actor; if an actor occurs more than once in the table, this is indicated by a figure between brackets.

Table 2. The AID of the processes 'establishing patient's rights, treatment and data provision'

Actor	Activity	Information on patient rights	Information on privacy	Information on treatment agreement	Information on treatment, created by patient	Information on treatment, created by caregiver	Information on end of treatment agreement	Request for personal information	Authorisation for data transfer	Requested information
Parliament	Adopts law on patient rights,	C								
Parliament	Adopts law on privacy		C							
Patient (1)	Reach treatment agreement	E	E							
Care-giver (1)		E	E	C						
Patient (2)	Takes part in treatment			E	C					
Care-giver (2)	Treats patient			E		C				
Patient (3)	Treatment			E	E	E				
Care-giver (3)	ended, and treatment agreement ended			E	E	E	C			
Third party	Information request							C		
Patient (4)	Decides concerning request	E	E					E	C	
Care-giver (4)	Provides information to third party	E	E						E	C

- if a cell contains a C (or an E), the actor creates (or exchanges) the information (an empty cell means that the actor does nothing with respect to the concerning information).
- each column describes the communication, related to specific information: it is created, exchanged and can finally be deleted; the passing on of information from one actor to the next is communication.
- Thus, the AID describes the communication in the interaction. In two instances, the creation of information requires more than one actor, for making the contract, and ending it. This is clarified in the model.

Clusters of interactions become apparent by the connections of created and exchanged information. Thus, the actual functions of an ICT-tool can be unequivocally analyzed, irrespective of the claims of ICT-suppliers.

In summary, the method permits us to analyze the complex communication between multiple actors and to identify the functions that are of value to the patient, such as choice and control.

3.5. Activity Oriented Approach

The Actor Information Diagram is different from the C, U – diagram that is current in the object oriented approach. In the AID the vertical columns represent communication (the passing on of information) while in the object oriented C, U – diagram the vertical columns relate to objects. The current object-oriented approach is not suitable for modelling this communication as it departs from objects and object-related activities [7] since the information needed is inherently tied to each object. In the present research the focus is on (coping) activities and not on objects.

3.6. Using the Communication Model

One question in this paper is whether several ICT-instruments, at present in use, enable patient's coping activities. The above communication model was employed in assessing ICT-tools. The model links the coping activities to ICT. ICT-tools are resources in which technology is used, such as email, webcam based communication, telemonitoring applications, EHR files and so forth.

The principle is: coping activities → information and communication (communication model) → ICT (technology used).

4. ICT-Tools

The six instruments selected cover all the relevant coping strategies of patients (Table 3).

The instruments chosen were selected by means of the following criteria:

- An existing ICT application,
- with a communication and information function for patients,
- that at present is in use by care organizations and their patients in the Netherlands,
- and where sufficient experience with the instrument is available to allow description.

Table 3. Selected Instruments and coping strategies of patients

Coping strategy of patient	Chatbox	Function Code Book	Telesens	Health Buddy	InfoDoc	MedLook
Contact	+					
Choice		+			+	
Contract with caregiver		+				
(Self-)care			+	+	+	
Control of 's information and Privacy						+
Control of care by checking		+				

The following were chosen:

Contact with fellow-patients: the Chatbox of the Diabetic Association of the Netherlands (DVN), is used as an example of supporting contact between patients with the same (chronic) disorder.

Contract with caregiver: the Function Code Book of CB2 by the careprovider Attent wwz, is an ICT-tool used in creating an explicit agreement (a care contract) between patient and care provider.

Self care: the Telesens system by the careprovider Sensire, offers patients at home digital home care by means of direct video contact with a qualified nurse.

Self care: the Health Buddy System of the company Sananet demonstrates how a system can – to a large extent – take over the monitoring function of a care provider.

Self care: InfoDoc of the company The Health Agency, uses available medical knowledge and information as a framework for producing a personalised digital brochure tailored to the patient on the treatment by a care provider or hospital.

Control of information: The patients own medical files (EHR and keys for access control): the MedLook File of the company Medlook NV, offers an ICT-tool for patients to manage their own EHR.

No instrument however was found that was primarily aimed at 'informing others in daily private life, social environment, or work environment'.

Data Collection

Data collection took place by approaching:

- Suppliers: Gathering information from the suppliers of each tool: both documentation and interviews with the ICT developers and suppliers of the tool.
- Institutions: Interview the institutions offering these tools to their patient.
- Caregivers: Interviewing caregivers on their experiences with these tools.
- Healthcare insurers: Interviewing insurers on their experiences with these tools.

5. Patient's Needs That Are Met by the ICT-Tools

Here the question, to what extent do the instruments contribute to the realisation of the needs of the patient, is discussed.

Below is an indication, in terms of the aims of patients, which instruments support these aims (albeit partially). In other words: to what extent the patient's activities, as defined above, are supported by the instrument, and which other activities are supported?

5.1. Choice and Control of Care

Choice and control processes by patients lead to autonomy in the use of care, such as:

- patient chooses:

  a care insurer
  treatment/nursing/care care offer of care provider
  a care provider
- patient specifies a contract/agreement with care providers concerning the care to be provided; the agreement is a directive for all actors providing care for this patient,
- patient critically monitors the care received.

Patient contact: the Chatbox DVN of the Diabetic Association of the Netherlands
The diabetic patient, as a member of the DVN, can use the DVN chat box and by means of question and answer can obtain informal information on the choice in institution, care provider and type of care. Members of the DVN can also obtain information on the DVN website concerning the selection of a care insurer.

Contract with caregiver: the Function Code Book or CB2 (Attent wwz) is used as a tool in creating an explicit agreement (a care contract) between patient and care provider.
The control process in self-management is executed both by monitoring and changing engagements made concerning the patient's own care process. These engagements have been specified in an agreement or contract. For such an agreement the patient can make use of the Function Code Book.
Support for the patient: More control concerning the care granted to him/her, and empowerment in both control and choice in degree of care offered.
Limitations for the patient: The Function Code Book is mainly used in the care sector in cases of prolonged illness. An instrument which supports making a care contract in a short term illness has not yet been found. Patients with short term illnesses under medical care have fewer possibilities to monitor and change engagements than those in long term nursing care.

Choice for patient: The personalised digital brochure: InfoDoc (The Health Agency)
The information tailored by InfoDoc gives information on the care offered by a care provider in an institution and personalizes this information based on the patient's profile.
Support for the patient: more knowledge of the possibilities for treatment and better, personalised information on treatments provided by the caregiver to support self-management.
Limitations for the patient: Patients can only chose from treatments offered by the selected care provider.

5.2. (Self-)Care

Self care is achieved when the patient and care provider co-operate within the closed agreement. Co-creation of care takes place. The patient carries out activities which were formerly carried out by the care provider and thereby:

- uses available instruments
- acquires general knowledge concerning diabetes, aimed at self-management of care
- manages information concerning their own diabetes (complete and incorporated information)
- obtains direct and professional responses in the co-creation of care
- develops their own motivation and discipline in self-management of care.

Contact with fellow-patients: the Chatbox DVN of the Diabetic Association of the Netherlands
Patient contacts lead to exchanges in experiences concerning the illness, via the DVN Chatbox. Information on instruments available can also be obtained. The DVN website offers general knowledge concerning diabetes, aimed at self-management of care.

Digital home care: the Telesens (Sensire)
Telesens offers patients face to face contact with a qualified nurse as a 7*24 hour service. In dialogue a direct and professional response is given on questions asked concerning health care and supporting self-management.
For the patient: direct and professional answers by Telemonitoring for the support of self-management.

Monitoring patients: the Health Buddy System (Sananet)
Support for the patient in professional feedback for self-care is achieved with the Health Buddy by analyzing a patient's answers to supplied questions, and by direct contact with the care provider if given answers indicate a possible health problem.
The Health Buddy System also supports training motivation and discipline required for self-management of care.
Limitations for the patient: the feedback is not direct,and the patient cannot ask questions.

Personal digital brochure: InfoDoc (The Health Agency)
Acquiring tailored knowledge on the illness necessary for a patient to improve their own self-management of care. This tailored knowledge is obtained through matching the patient profile (i.e. age, sex, diagnosis) with the general knowledge of the illness. Information is also given on physical exercises for this patient.

Personal EHR: the MedLook File (Medlook NV)
The MedLook File supports medication control (reminder messages), prescription requests and ordering medicine.

5.3. Control of Information and Privacy

Self-management with respect to information relates to the control a patient has over personal medical data, not only in managing a personal medical file, but also controlling authorisation to third parties to use the EHR data.

The patients own medical files (EHR and keys for access control: <u>the MedLook File (Medlook NV)</u>.

The patient can use the MedLook file to exercise control over his own medical data, on condition that care providers are prepared to co-operate.

<u>Support for the patient</u>: better transfer of own medical information from one care provider to another.

<u>Limitations for the patient</u>: In practice care providers are not prepared to co-operate, mainly because they find that the patient's data belongs to the caregiver.

As a consequence the MedLook File does not support the patient effectively in the management of his personal EHR data.

6. Patient's Needs That Are Not Met by the ICT-Tools

The chosen examples provide little support for several of the patients' important coping activities, namely:

- choice of type of care.
- choice of caregiver.
- contract: making an explicit agreement with caregivers on treatment and information management.
- (self-)care: Patients have a need for direct professional feedback in self-care, but this is not supported despite the possibilities of ICT for direct bi-directional communication between patient and caregiver. Instead, ICT supports the caregiver in his task of informing the patient, irrespective of the patient's individual questions.
- Control of care by checking: judge whether the care actually provided conforms with the contract mentioned above and to act accordingly.

A restriction of these systems is that the communication between patient and care provider is unilateral, one-way traffic from the care provider to the patient. The patient cannot ask their own individual questions using the system. The care provider's frame of reference stipulates the limits of the communication. An exception is Telesens: here the system supports the interactive communication between patient and care provider by means of a two way webcam based connection.

7. The Significance of the Instruments for the Care Provider

7.1. Which Activities of the Care Provider Are Supported by the Six Instruments?

From interviews and analysis of the six instruments, based on the care provider's perspective, the following was found:

<u>Chatbox DVN</u> is intended for people with diabetes. It does not support care providers directly.

<u>Function Code Book</u> supports the care provider in:

- giving information to patients (offer of personalised care appropriate to the individual),
- information management (electronic engagements of care contract and the actual care provided),
- efficiency in the business processes by two factors:
  - demand-oriented production, as a result, more efficient commitment of staff capacity,
  - administrative and financial processes are directly linked with care processing.

<u>Telesens</u> supports the care provider in:

- personalised care, leading to patient friendly care (direct return to the patient),
- information management (electronic patient files) and
- more efficient business processing (avoiding unnecessary home visits).

<u>Health Buddy system</u> supports the care provider in training programmes for patients and management of patient medical records HER.

<u>InfoDoc</u> supports the care provider in providing patients with information within the limitations of their services in care.

<u>MedLook File</u> leads to a better quality of care from the care provider by supplying correct and complete information, particularly on medication. For the care consumer an advantage of managing their own medical file is that data cannot get lost when for example, the general practitioner stops practising, and the medical files are not taken over, or get lost in the hospital. For the care provider and the care institution MedLook implies a shift in responsibility for the medical data and the access to this data.

The above description of functions leads to the following classification: 1) giving information to patients, 2) managing business information of the care organisation and 3) supporting business processing.

In Table 4 an overview is given by instrument.

7.2. How Do the Care Providers Make Use of the Instruments in Their Communication with the Patient?

Making information easy to assimilate

Each of these instruments is helping the care worker to handle complex and general information easily. This information concerns:

- Function Code Book: the care offered by their care institution.
- Health Buddy system: general medical information.
- InfoDoc: general medical information and the care offered by their care institution.

Table 4. Significance of the instruments for the care provider

EXAMPLES	Chatbox	Care Service Contract	Telesens	Health Buddy system	InfoDoc	Medlook File
Company/ association	DVN	Attent wwz	Sensire	Sananet	The Health Agency	Medlook NV
Instruments	Chatbox	Function Codebook	Telesens	Health Buddy system	InfoDoc	MedLook File
Information to patient		++ (care given examination) in	++ (answer direct questions)	++ (training with transfer of informa-tion)	++ (infor-mation tailored)	
Business processing		++ (admini-stration, registration, and billing)	++ (electronic patient file)	++ (electronic patient file)		+ (data management and access control)
Management		++ (staff capacity)	++ (staff capacity)	++ (staff capacity)		

Each of these three instruments works as an integrated system. The principle of such a system is:

(1) Breaking down of the general information in smaller, usable pieces of information
Function Code Book : Care subdivided into univocal and planned care compo-nents
Health Buddy system : Training program subdivided into 'dialogues'
InfoDoc   : Text information subdivided into information documents

(2) Combining this information, based on characteristics/data concerning the patient. The information required by the patient is provided by linking specific characteris-tics of the patient with the information:
Function Code Book : Based on the medical indication of the patient and the preferences of the patient
Health Buddy system : Based on answers given by the patient on several questions of the Health Buddy system
InfoDoc   : Based on using so-called patient parameters (sex, age, the stage of the treatment).

In Table 5 below some characteristics of the instruments are indicated, relating to the information of the care provided to the patient. Table 5 contains: target group, the set-ting, the process, the methodology, the patient information, the linking characteristics for selecting and combining the information and the result of the combined information.

The principle is that knowledge/information is subdivided in elementary entities called 'bits'. A number of these 'bits' and made available, depending on what informa-tion is required. In order to make this selection, data concerning the information re-quired must be added to the system then the needed 'bits' are selected and presented to the user.

Table 5. Instruments regarding communication with the patient

EXAMPLES	Care Service Contract	Telesens	Health Buddy	Digital brochure
Organisation	Attent wwz	Sensire	Sananet	The Health Agency
Instruments	Function Codebook /CB2Care	Telesens	Health Buddy System	InfoDoc
Target group: to characterise	Long term care	Long term/short term care	Chronic illness	Chronic Illness
Setting	Initial interview conversation with patient	Patient: home situation Care provider: call centre	Answers given by patient to questions posed	Information from EHR regarding needed parameters patient
Process	Agreement on care to be delivered as stated in a contract between patient and caregiver To be delivered care incorporated in planning process of care provider.	The patient contacts, on their own initiative, a qualified nurse on duty for questions; the nurse has access to the HER patient file	Monitors patient's answers and stimulated intervention at high risk answers	Care provider uses patient's parameters on central document system called InfoDoc. InfoDoc selects documents on treatments relevant given the patient's parameters.
Method: using univocal, recognizable elements.	Care subdivided in many small components (univocal care components to be planned)	Questions and answers are catalogued into a decision tree	Training program subdivided in many small elements (the so-called dialogues)	Treatment documentation subdivided in many small documents
'bits'	'bits' are components of the Function Code Book	'bits' of information (for example question in catalogue)	'bits' of information (for example dialogue)	'bits' are small documents , the so-called Docs.
The linking characteristics for selecting and combining the 'bits', in other words: for personalising	The preferences of the patient	The patient's answers on questions	Selection of new questions based on answers to previous questions	Patient profile: Patient profile, with among other things sex, age context, the stage and the treatment of the disorder (so-called parameters)
Result of combining the 'bits'	Personalised care for patient	Contact with patient, and answers to his questions using relevant information	Personalised training and knowledge transfer with motivating feedback and monitoring risk	Tailored information

7.3. The Need for Adaptation of the Organisational Processes of the Care Provider

The introduction of an instrument has possible consequences on the conditions under which care is provided. The structure of care (Donabedian, 2003) is changing as new material resources such as ICT-instruments are used. This results in changes in the organisation of the daily processes of a care provider. For example, three of the examined instruments in the field of information/education (InfoDoc, Health Buddy System, Telesens) show that higher demands are made on the availability of care providers, as the instruments enable more interaction with patients. Self-management of patients however shifts work from the care giver to the patient. Digital home care for example results in less care being provided by caregivers (see below).

At InfoDoc there is no interaction: the patient can ask no questions, and the parameters supplied are selected by the caregiver independent of the patient.

With the Health Buddy system the patient cannot ask questions either, but the data information is dependent on the answers which the patient has given on earlier questions. Therefore there is more interaction between the patient and the system.

Telesens offers the most interaction the patient can ask questions at any time and these are answered directly.

The effects on staff availability is different for each of the ICT-instruments:

In using InfoDoc the care provider no extra tasks have to be performed; the treating doctor simply clicks on the patient's profile on the display. This actually can save the caregiver time in giving information to patients.

In the Health Buddy System the treating care provider spends time every day at a fixed time answering the questions of patients, who have already been classified by the Health Buddy system and provided with a risk profile. This has consequences for implementation, but the organisation (roles and responsibilities) remains the same.

Finally at Telesens the call centre (with a 7*24 availability) have arranged for a qualified nurse to be on duty available to answer questions and make recommendations, also available to the care worker on a home visit. At Telesens there is not only change in the implementation of the care, but also in the organisation of care: a new function was created, that is a qualified nurse on duty who is contactable by means of Telesens.

7.4. Conclusion

The possibilities which (Internet based) ICT offers the patient, are only partly exploited because the care provider has not changed their condition under which care is provided. The structure remains intact, despite using new resources (ICT-tools). Hence adapting the organisation or partly adapting the organisation.

The conclusion is that the possibilities of ICT are only fully exploited when the care provider adapts the organisation and the patient is given the responsibility which he needs.

8. Applicability of the Results

The restrictions of this study to diabetes lead us to the question of whether the goals and problems of patients with other chronic illnesses are different to the research group with diabetes. The research method used, ZMET, is aimed at establishing the hidden causes that have an effect on people (in Health Care as well as our private lives and work). These hidden causes, as established in research, are similar for many people. This fact indicates that the results of the interviews are rather independent on individual characteristics of the interviewed, like illness and coping style.

For the six selected instruments it was investigated whether they support the patient in coping with illness. It was concluded that important activities of patients were not supported. The question is whether a different selection of instruments would have yielded a different conclusion.

For each of the example instruments the following remarks are made:

DVN *Chatbox* is of course an example of a very general facility on the Internet.

Function Code Book is only applied in nursing and home care surroundings not in curative medicine.

Health Buddy System is an example of training and monitoring, not only applied to patients with diabetes but also for heart failures and respiratory diseases. If a knowledge system for any specific illness is available, monitoring facilities can by supplied by the Health Buddy System.

Telesens is an example of webcam based Telecare. Many systems are available in various care institutions.

InfoDoc is an example of a caregiver giving information concerning treatment for a particular illness.

Many other sources of information are available, but most of these do not cover all possible treatments or they are not validated systems.

MedLook File is one of many digital files available. Most of these files are restricted to a specific illness.

In general, development of these instruments is initiated by care providers. The use of other instruments has not led to any significant change in the structure of health care. As discussed, changes in the organisation of the careprovider are needed to comply with patients demands.

In conclusion, no evidence has been found that a selection of different instruments would lead to different conclusions.

9. Implications for Patient Empowerment: The Unfulfilled Promise

Our research indicates that the needs of patients are not or not fully met by ICT instruments offered by caregivers. From a patient's perspective it means fewer possibilities in self-management of his illness.

The institutionalised care organizations are not equipped to tackle the escalating chronic disease burden or health issues which might prevent such diseases through encouraging different lifestyles [22]. A new approach is needed in the co-operation of caregiver and patient: the co-creation of health.

Co-creation of health leads to a different way in health service delivery. The design of systems, the content needed, the approach in using these resources all have to be changed.

Only by doing all of the aforementioned items one can truly speak of Patient Empowerment as it is meant to be.

10. Recommendations

With respect to daily private life, the social environment of the patient or his/her work environment no instrument has yet been found. In order for a patient with a chronic illness *to* integrate into his direct social surroundings (private and work), related information must be provided by the caregiver.

Contact with fellow-patients brings support people with a chronic illness with information on patient. These experiences must be differentiated into patient groups having corresponding experiences, questions and problems. Aggregation of information on patient experiences loses the relevance of the information for the individual.

The patient should be offered choice concerning a care provider and which treatment to chose. The supply of information by the care provider to the patient must be considered as a necessary and indispensable component of care.

When the patient has made his choice in caregiver(s) and treatment/care including related services this should be the subject of (formal) agreement with the caregiver(s). The agreement also covers the patients own medical files (EHR and keys for access control.)

Collaboration with caregiver includes self-care and, for chronic diseases, the process of the patient developing into an informed and motivated self-carer. In order to do so the care provider has to change his organisation to adapt to the needs of patients in co-creation of care.

The patient should have the possibility to check whether the provided professional care service is delivered as agreed upon in the contract.

Given the needs of patients in the field of daily life, contact with fellow-patients, choice and collaboration with caregivers, a targeted policy is necessary to fully exploit the possibilities, which (Internet based) ICT offers for patients. To achieve this, not only care providers but other stakeholders, in particular the patient should also be involved in designing the (software) instruments. In order to fulfil the needs of patients in using ICT instruments care providers have to adapt their organisational processes.

A component of good care is a product/service to provide the patient with information for:

- making choices concerning care, reaching agreements and the monitoring thereof.
- managing and use of a personal EHR with access control for third parties.
- conducting self-care with feedback of care providers.
- influencing his own social environment in several life areas (private, work).

Patients normally have very individual questions. The instruments described however, do not offer the possibility for patients to ask questions; instruments cannot replace a personal conversation with a care provider.

The Dutch Health Insurance law (ZVW) states that the care consumer has a personal responsibility for his health. To execute this responsibility the <u>position of the patient</u> in care needs to be strengthened. Only then can the patient realise this responsibility in the field of self-management and self-care.

Technology itself cannot improve patient care or make better strategic decisions. It does help to empower the patient with ICT-tools.

The rigidity of traditional organizational models too often limits innovation and learning.

The use of technology to complement and enhance what patients want calls for a very different kind of thinking about the organizational structures that best facilitate the work of the health care professional. Technology and organizational strategies are inextricably co-joined in this new world of patient empowerment.

More information on the empowerment of patients by Tele-medicine can be found on the website of ICTUS: www.ictus.nl.

References

Books
[1] Herzlinger RE editor, Consumer-Driven Health Care. San Francisco (CA): Jossey-Bass; 2004.
[2] Donebedian A, An introduction to Quality Assurance in Health Care. New York (NY): Oxford Univ. Press; 2003.
[3] Kazandjian VA, Healthcare performance Measurement. Milwaukee (WI): ASQ Quality Press; 1999.
[4] Slack WV, Cybermedicine. 2nd ed. San Francisco (CA): Jossey-Bass; 2001.
[5] M Zeidner & NS Endler (eds.), Handbook of Coping: Theory, Research and Applications. (NY): Wiley, 1996.
[6] Dinten W van, Met gevoel voor realiteit. 3de druk Delft (NL): Uitgeverij Eburon; 2006-08-21.
[7] Bots JM, Heck E van, Simons JL, Swede V van. Management en Informatie. Bestuurlijke Informatie-kunde. Schoonhoven: Academic Press; 1999.
[8] Dietz JLG, Introductie tot Demo.Alphen a/d Rijn (NL): Samson bedrijfsinformatie; 1996.
[9] Dietz JLG, Enterprise Ontology, Theory and Methodology. Leusden (NL): Springer; 2006.
[10] Zaltman, G, How customers think, essential insights into the mind of the market. Boston (Ma): Harvard Business School Publishing; 2003.
[11] Institute for the future, Health and healthcare in 2010 2nd ed. San Francisco (CA): Jossey-Bass; 2003.
[12] Foresight, Health care 2020. London (UK): dpt. Trade and Industry; December 2000.
[13] Nitel, Patiënt behoeften onderzoeksrapport. Utrecht; augustus 2005.
[14] Rathenau Instituut, Alledaagse zorg, Den Haag; oktober 2005.
[15] ZonMw, Congres Thuis met Technologie, Utrecht; september 2005,Thesis.
[16] Kleffens T, Aandacht voor het perspectief van patiënten. Amsterdam (NL): VU Medisch Centrum, 26-01-2006, Oratie.
[17] Sprangers MAG, Kwaliteit van leven, Oratie Van zacht begrip naar hard getal. Amsterdam (NL): Universiteit van Amsterdam: 29 September 2006.
[18] Zeidner M, Saklofske D. Adaptive and maladaptive coping. In: M Zeidner & NS Endler (eds.), Handbook of Coping: Theory, Research and Applications. (NY): Wiley, 1996, pp. 505–531.

Articles
[19] Pool A, Van beheersen naar begrijpen. Jaarcongres Nederlands Instituut voor Zorg en Welzijn, 2003.
[20] Slikke JW van der, Kennismanagement vanuit het world wide perspectief: hoe blijven we de patiënt een les voor? Voordracht op congres Infertiliteit, Gynaecologie en Obstetrie Anno 2001, Doelen Congres-centrum Rotterdam, 29 mei 2001.
[21] Blume S, Catshoek G, Patiëntenperspectief in Onderzoek. Dit rapport is een uitgave van de Patiënten-Praktijk, een kennisbureau over onderzoek voor patiënten – en consumentenorganisaties; oktober 2001.
[22] Cottam H, Leadbeater C, Red paper 01: HEALTH: Co-creating Services, Design Council, November 2004.
[23] Meijer W, Ragetlie P, Waar blijft de regie? Professionele drijfveren voor transmurale zorgtechnologie en overheidsbeleid, Health Management Forum, nr 1/2005, Jan 2005.
[24] Succes – en faalfactoren breedbandtoepassingen: een quickscan. Platform Nederland Breed.
[25] Tekst KPMG BEA, Amstelveen, Mei 2004.
[26] Zorgcapaciteit efficiënter benutten met CamCare (uitgevoerd door Senter in het kader van een Projectvoorbeeld Subsidieregeling Elektronische Communicatie, maart 2003).
[27] Vrijhoef HJM, Janssen-Boyne J, Engering W, Gorgels A, Telebegeleiding bij hartfalen: haalbaarheidsonderzoek van de Health Buddy. Universiteit Maastricht & Academisch Ziekenhuis Maastricht (2005).
[28] Het Functiecodeboek in de praktijk. Deloitte, zorgsignalen, 7e jaargang nr 3, oktober 2005.
[29] Cliëntvolgsysteem met Functiecodeboek. Deloitte, zorgsignalen 7e jaargang nr 2, juni 2005.
[30] Stegeman K, diepteonderzoek onder de hersenpan van de consument. Tijdschrift voor marketing/januari 2005 (de cliëntbelevingsmethode Zaltman Metaphor Elicitation Technique).

Electronic sources
[31] Chatbox DVN, www.dvn.nl.
[32] Kraan N, Erik Taal E, Stans Drossaert S, Diana Gosens D, Vegt N van de, Lotgenotencontact via internetdiscussiegroepen. Enschede Universiteit Twente; juni 2005. [Elektronische versie ws5.p.e-vision. nl/congres/files/15%20Nelly%20Kraan pdf].
[33] Digitaal Ervaringen Dossier, TNO; www.dvn.nl (forum, persoonlijke verhalen, chatbox).
[34] MedLook uw medisch dossier via internet https://www.medlook.nl/index.jsp.

[35] Telesens http://www.sensire.nl/.
[36] Functiecodeboek http://www.functiecodeboek.nl; www.cb2.nl.
[37] InfoDoc www.infodoc.nl; www.thehealthagency.nl; www.reumafonds.nl; www.voorlichtingopmaat.nl.
[38] Health Buddy www.sananet.nl.
[39] Telesens Sensire: een nieuwe kijk op zorg: demo dvd (april 2005).

Medical and Care Compunetics 4
L. Bos and B. Blobel (Eds.)
IOS Press, 2007

Empowering Patients and Researchers through a Common Health Information Registry: A Case Example of Adrenocortical Carcinoma Patients and Researchers

Deborah ALLWES[1], BSN, RN, MPH and Michael L. POPOVICH, MS[2]
[1] Senior Public Health Specialist, Deborah_Allwes@stchome.com
[2] CEO, Michael_Popovich@stchome.com
Scientific Technologies Corporation, 4400 E. Broadway, Suite 705, Tucson, Arizona
85711, + 520.202.3333

Abstract: Adrenocortical Carcinoma is a rare malignant tumor that forms in the outer layer of tissue of the adrenal gland, which is a small gland situated on the anteriosuperior aspect of the kidneys. These glands produce steroid hormones, adrenaline, and noradrenaline that control heart rate, blood pressure, and other body functions.

Because this cancer affects a limited number of patients, it is referred to as an Orphan disease, which is defined as a condition that affects fewer than 200,000 people nationwide. Internationally, there are 5,000 – 8,000 such diseases affecting an estimated 55 million people. There is often limited medical intervention for many of these conditions.

With a small number of patients, and a correspondingly small number of providers and researches, this disease is a candidate for establishing a sharable information system that is used by the patient, provider, and researcher. This resource empowers the patient to support their care and treatment while allowing medical providers and researches to have valuable and broad access to patient activities and behaviors that may impact their treatment.

Orphan disease registries are prime candidates for establishing health information resources that support communications between patients, providers, and researchers. As a resource, this information can be used to facilitate treatment protocols to include biomarker identification, testing and monitoring of new drugs. By empowering a common community of individuals that share a common disease, the potential to accelerate research and identify improved treatment options may also increase.

This paper presents a strategic plan and design for implementing Orphan disease registries within an e-health environment that specifically links patients and providers with researchers. The Adrenocortical Carcinoma Registry will be used to demonstrate the implementation and potential of these systems.

1. Background

Disease has been an expected part of human life throughout history. Notable infectious diseases, such as influenza and poliomyelitis affect a large number of populations, and therefore receive a large amount of funding and research for treatment. Emergent diseases in the 20th and 21st Centuries, such as the Human Immunodeficiency Virus (HIV) and the Severe Acute Respiratory Syndrome (SARS) seemingly draw international attention for their rapid spread and widespread reach. Other diseases, such as cancer, are found throughout the world and collectively affect a large number of people. However, although cancer is referred to as a single disease, in actuality, cancer consists of over 100 different forms of the disease. The subsets of cancers differ based on many factors such as geography, age, and genetics. Because each subset of cancer, specifically, each type of cancer, potentially affects a small number of people within a given population, often the time, money, and data to support research, and consequently, treatments for such cancers is lacking or nonexistent.

1.1. Orphan Disease Overview

Some types of cancer, as with many types of diseases affecting a small number of people within a population, are classified under Orphan Diseases. In the United States, these orphan diseases, or rare diseases, affect less than 200,000 people. Generally, an orphan disease is one that has a low prevalence, usually a prevalence of less than 5 cases per 10,000 in a given population. Internationally, there are over 5,000 such diseases affecting an estimated 55 million people.

While some orphan diseases, such as Cystic Fibrosis, have been researched and funded to allow for a greater understanding of the disease, most orphan diseases have not. Patients are often left to collect information and understanding of their condition on their own with limited resources. Their providers, which often lack an in-depth understanding of the disease, have to seek out information based on limited research. Finally, the researchers that dedicate time and attention to the orphan disease often do so with very limited financial incentives and lack of a collective data repository.

1.1.1. Adrenocortical Carcinoma: A Case Study of an Orphan Disease

Internationally, of the over 5,000 orphan diseases, only approximately 1,300 have been well studied from a medical perspective[1]. The remaining orphan diseases have yet to be thoroughly studied and medically understood. In the United States, malignant neoplasm's of the adrenal cortex, such as Adrenocortical Carcinoma (ACC) account for only 0.05% - 0.2% of all cancers[2].

Adrenocortical Carcinoma is a rare malignant tumor that forms in the outer layer of tissue of the adrenal gland, which is a small gland situated on the anteriosuperior

---

[1] Weely, S., Leufkens, H., Priority Medicines for Europe and the World "A Public Health Approach to Innovation", Background Paper, Orphan Disease, 7 October 2004.

[2] Latronico, A., Chrousos, G., Extensive Personal Experience, Adrenocortical Tumors, Journal of Endocrinology and Metabolism, Vol. 82, No 5, p. 1317, 1997.

aspect of the kidneys. These glands produce steroid hormones, adrenaline, and noradrenaline that control heart rate, blood pressure, and other body functions.

ACC has a bimodal age distribution with the first occurrence noted in children and the second occurrence noted in the 3rd, 4th, or 5th decades of life. Although the number of individuals actually inflicted with this cancer is small, its impact is dramatic. The prognosis of ACC is poor, and the survival rate is minimal.

Resources for patients with ACC are scarce, and even scarcer are the medical, historical, and epidemiological data available to researchers. There is no centralized repository that promotes patients to interact. Likewise, there is no centralized database for researchers to query medical information. Consequently, patients have objective and subjective case information that is not privy to the researchers that are attempting to develop treatments for the disease. ACC patients, like many orphan disease patients, are a wealth of information that can provide valuable information on an individual level, and collectively as a group.

Figure 1 represents the current state of information within the ACC patient, medical, and research community.

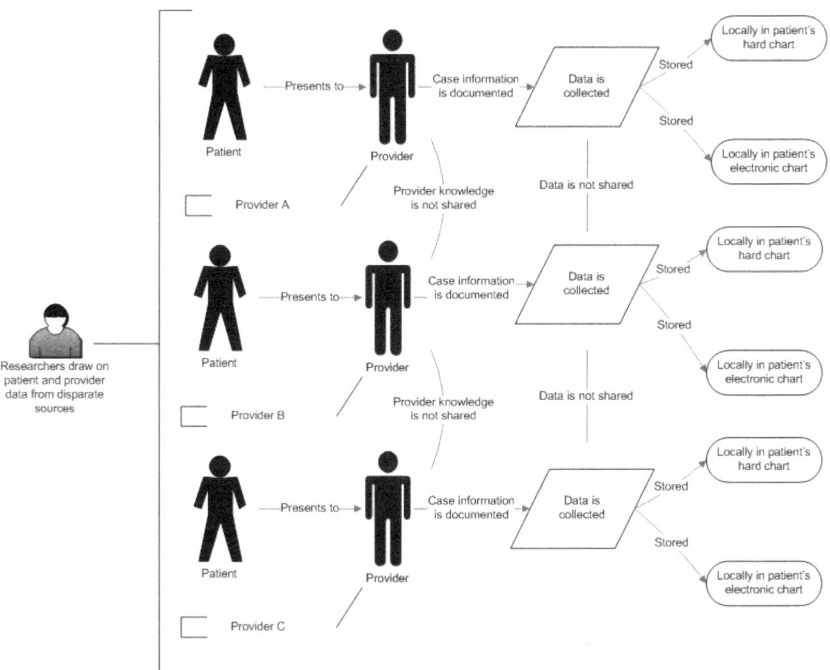

Figure 1. Current State of Information within the ACC Community

Patients are not readily able to find a collective source of information and patients rarely have the ability to exchange archived or real-time information. A new ACC case often presents less than one case per year of a provider's total workload, so knowledge and information for providers is often dependent on the provider's own experience, or research. Because of a lack of a collective data source, researchers have to retrieve data from many disparate sources, leading to time delays and financial burdens.

2. Benefits of a Shared Resource

The benefits to having a shared resource, such as an orphan disease registry application, are immense. In Figure 2, it is demonstrated how patients can interact with each other, either through real-time on-line chat rooms or through archived information. This is a very important aspect to the registry application as it empowers the patients to have control over their disease, as well as allows them to have an active input into their medical case and overall body of knowledge of their disease. Patients can participate in questionnaires and on-line forums that will promote researchers to have a better understanding of the effects a treatment is having on patients as it is happening.

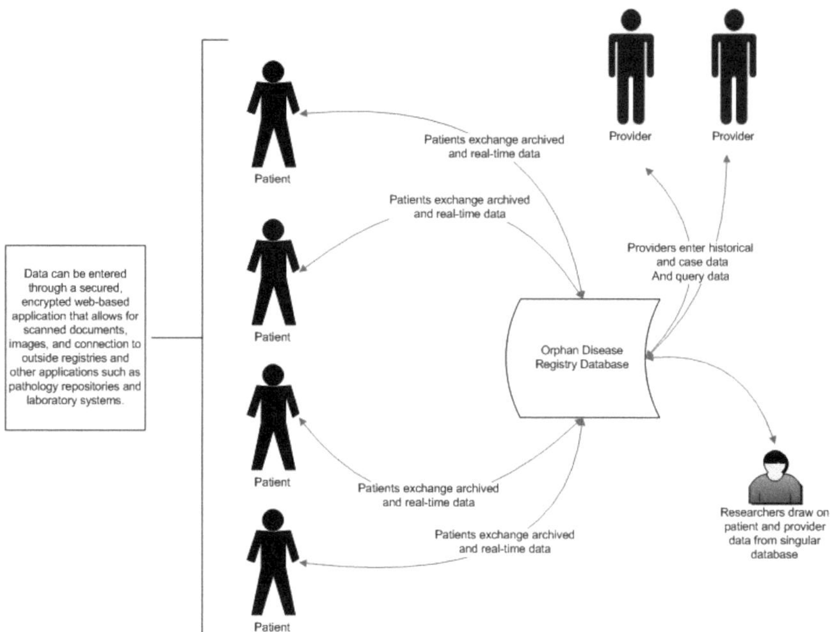

Figure 2. Benefits of a Shared Resource

Researchers have a direct benefit of having all of the data and information of ACC in one secured location. They can extract data through scheduled reports, ad hoc reports, or through extracting the information into SAS, SPSS, Microsoft Access, or other statistical packages. Because patients will have the ability to upload scanned documents into the database, researchers can have access to numerous possibilities of information that they would otherwise not be able to collect. Additionally, researchers can use complex analysis of translational biomarkers and molecular profiling for improved drug therapies and earlier diagnostic testing.

Providers have the benefit of viewing on-line laboratory and pathological information from the database, as well as are able to view what other providers are noting with their patients, and treatment plans.

2.1. Pharmaceutical Industry Benefits

An Orphan Disease Registry Application can provide a common place for the ACC community, and eventually other orphan disease communities, to collaborate, compile, exchange, and analyze information related to generalized disease processes and drug development. Commercial partnerships can be developed to enhance and support this effort, helping to establish links currently missing in overall orphan disease drug development, including those for ACC. Additionally, this collaborative effort can provide the foundation for scientists lacking development expertise and commercial outlets for orphan drug development, testing, commercialization, and marketing.

3. Registry Design for Adrenocortical Carcinoma Case Study

The registry design for ACC, and for all orphan diseases, has to be flexible enough to adapt to evolving disease bodies of knowledge, secure enough to allow patients to know their data is safe, and accessible enough for researchers and providers to query the information they need. Overall, such as design needs to allow for future expansion while allowing for current disease specific information exchange.

3.1. Technical Overview of the Registry

Specific to the ACC Orphan Disease Registry Application, the following criteria must be met. In addition to the criteria is a brief description of the "tools" that should be utilized to measure each criterion.

- **Data entry process:** a data entry process should be established. Data from standard forms should be entered into a web based application/repository. Validations and quality checks should be in place to ensure quality of data.
- **Standardization:** the system should be configured based on accepted standards as defined by clinical data interchange standards consortium (CDISC), health level seven (HL7), and any other designated vocabulary standards.
- **Reporting:** a reporting mechanism should be in place and should provide consistent and ad hoc reports as defined by researchers.
- **Hardware/environment configuration:** required hardware should be procured, and configured (if required) to enable solution delivery.
- **Access to patient data:** providers, researchers, patients, and other authorized users should have online access to patient data via a secure internet site. All patient data should be de-identified, and should follow all security standards, and internal review board (IRB) recommendations, as applicable.
- **Scanner interface:** provide a scanner interface to the orphan disease registry application, to upload and retrieve scanned documents.
- **Help desk:** provide data entry and help line.
- **Training and user manual:** provide user training and user help documentation.

Table 1 is a representation of the hardware/software specifications that should be included in any orphan disease registry application, specifically that of the ACC.

Table 1. Example of Hardware/Software Specifications

Hardware/Software	QTY	Minimum Requirements
Hardware		
PowerEdge 2950 (Database Server)	2	Processor: Dual Core Intel Xeon 5160, 4MB Cache, 3.00GHz
		Memory: 8GB 533MHz (4x2GB Dual Ranked)
		OS: Windows Server 2003 R2 Enterprise Edition
		Hard Drive: 146GB (x5) 15k RPM - RAID 5/i
		Power: Redundant Power Supply with Y cord
		Riser Card with 3 PCIe Slots
		1x6 Backplane for 3.5-inch Hard Drives
		Controller: PERC 5/I, x6 Backplane Integrated Controller Card
		Rack Chassis w/Sliding Rapid/Versa Rails
		Dual Embeded Broadcom NetXtreme II gigabit card
		3 YR Gold Enterprise Support
		24X IDE CD-ROM Driver
		Mouse/Keyboard
PowerEdge 2950 (Application Server)	4	Processor: Dual Core Intel Xeon 5160, 4MB Cache, 3.00GHz
		Memory: 4GB 533MHz (4x1 Dual Ranked)
		OS: Windows Server 2003 R2 Standard Edition
		Hard Drive: 36GB (x4) 15k RPM - RAID 5/i
		Power: Redundant Power Supply with Y cord
		Riser Card with 3 PCIe Slots
		1x6 Backplane for 3.5-inch Hard Drives
		Controller: PERC 5/I, x6 Backplane Integrated Controller Card
		Rack Chassis w/Sliding Rapid/Versa Rails
		Dual Embeded Broadcom NetXtreme II gigabit card
		3 YR Gold Enterprise Support
		24X IDE CD-ROM Driver
		Mouse/Keyboard

Hardware/Software	QTY	Minimum Requirements
Software		
Oracle 10g Standard One	2	
WebSphere 6 Application Server	4	

Primary

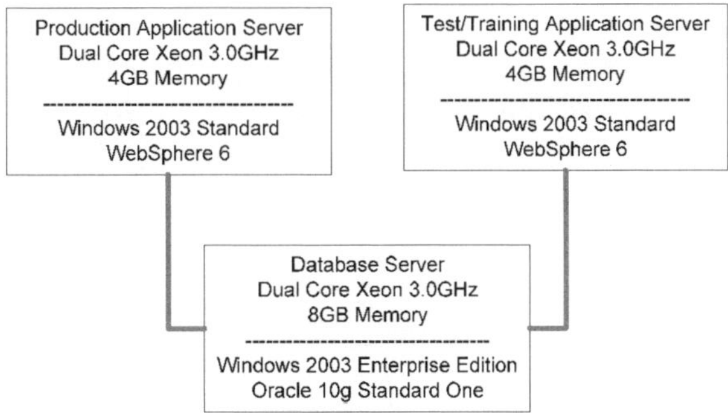

Backup

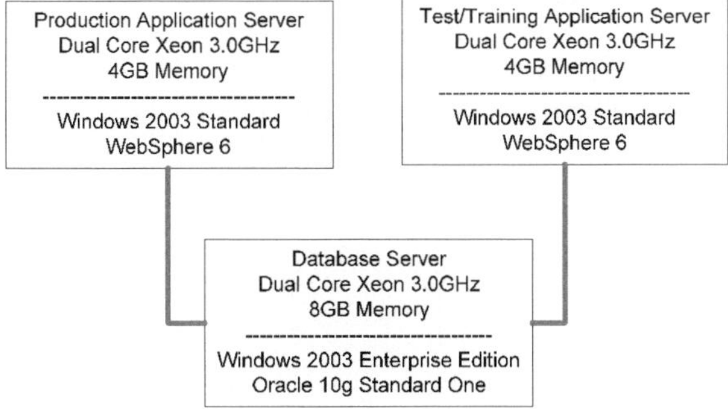

Figure 3. Primary and Backup Systems

A gap analysis will be desirable to ensure that the information that is truly needed to be included in the orphan disease registry application is actually identified and included. Table 2 is an example of a gap analysis matrix.

Table 2. Gap Analysis Matrix Example

Gap #	Gap/Current State Description	System Requirement #	Gap Resolution/Desired State Description
1.00	Disease forms are physically stored in provider offices and providers/patients/researchers currently don't have access to these collective forms	The system must be a web-based application	Online based forms will be established to collect and route the ACC forms from a provider/patient/researcher to a centralized location/database
2.00	Currently there is no electronic tracking of collective ACC data, providers/patients/researchers and other users do not have access to the ACC patient data	The application must have a centralized database	Data from ACC forms will be entered into the Orphan Disease Registry Application for electronic tracking and will be available to authorized users
3.00	Currently there is no validation of provider stored data	To be identified	Incorporate validations required by researchers
4.00	There is no ability to store scanned documents in a centralized location/database	They application must allow for scanning and uploading documents	Orphan Disease Registry Application will have the ability to store and retrieve scanned images
5.00	Currently there is no accepted standards for messaging language	The application must be standards based	Standards will be used in the vocabulary for the Orphan Disease Registry Application

3.2. Example of a Form from the ACC Case Study

The application that is built for an orphan disease registry, such as the one for ACC, is that it is user-friendly. System administrators will need to be able to add, view, edit, and retrieve standard and customized forms. The forms will likely change as time progresses and researchers identify areas of interest for further study. Consequently, the application will need to allow not only the editing and storage of current forms, but archived forms as well. Figure 4 is an example of a partial ACC form that may be used in the application.

1) What is your age? _______

2) What is your gender?
- o   Male
- o   Female

3) What is your race? (Please check all that apply)
- o   White
- o   American Indian/Alaska Native
- o   Asian
- o   Native Hawaiian or Other Pacific Islander
- o   Black or African American

4) Are you Hispanic or Latino?
- o   Yes
- o   No

5) When were you diagnosed with adrenocortical cancer (mm/yy)? __________

6) How was the diagnosis made? (Please check all that apply)
- o   Tumor biopsy
- o   Tumor/adrenal gland removal
- o   Imaging tests such as a CT or MRI scan
- o   Blood tests
- o   Urine tests
- o   Other, please specify:____

7) What symptoms did you experience before being diagnosed? (Please check all that apply)
- o   None
- o   Abdominal pain, date of onset:__________________
- o   Palpable abdominal mass, date of onset:______________
- o   Purple lines on abdomen (abdominal purple striae), date of onset:__________________
- o   Acne, date of onset:__________________
- o   Loss of appetite (anorexia), date of onset:__________________
- o   Weight loss greater than 10 pounds
- o   Weight gain greater than 10 pounds
- o   Excessive accumulation and storage of fat in the central area of the body (central obesity), date of onset:__________________
- o   Cramps, date of onset:__________________ specify cramps, e.g leg or stomach cramps?
- o   Decreased libido, date of onset:__________________
- o   Emotionally unstable (emotional lability), date of onset:__________
- o   Excess blood in the face marked by reddish complexion and swelling (facial plethora), date of onset:__________________
- o   Fatigue, date of onset:__________________
- o   Fungal skin infections, date of onset:__________________
- o   Headaches, date of onset:__________________
- o   Excessive growth of hair of normal or abnormal distribution (hirsutism), date of onset:______________
- o   High blood pressure (hypertension), date of onset:__________
- o   Increased abdominal girth, date of onset:__________
- o   Muscle weakness in upper legs/thighs (proximal muscle weakness), date of onset:__________
- o   Muscle weakness, date of onset:__________
- o   Nausea, date of onset:__________
- o   Kidney stone(s), date of onset:__________
- o   Excessive or abnormal thirst (polydipsia), date of onset:__________
- o   Excessive urination (polyuria), date of onset:__________

If yes, frequency of urination is:
- o   once per 1 hour
- o   once per 2 hours
- o   once per half hour
- o   Other, please specify:__________________________ date of onset:__________

If female:
- o   Deepened voice, date of onset:__________
- o   Irregular menstruation, date of onset:__________

If male:
- o   Impotence, date of onset:__________

8) Have you had a bone scan with abnormal results (for example, evidence of loss in bone volume or mass)?
- o   Yes, date of most recent scan:__________
- o   No

Figure 4. Example of a Partial ACC Form that may be used in the Application

4. Recommendations for Other Orphan Disease Registries

Orphan diseases, when considered individually, are limited by the size of the populations affected and the limited number of cases. Collectively, however, there is an estimated 55 million people affected by one of the 5,000 – 8,000 orphan diseases. As is often the case, there is power in numbers. ACC, in and of itself, doesn't have the large numbers of affected individuals to be sway policy and industry to stop and take notice. However, if taken in whole with the rest of the orphan diseases, there is a strength that all orphan diseases can draw from. Disease processes can be explored for generalization, drug development can be based on the uniqueness of orphan diseases, and patient participation can be capitalized through a common area of shared knowledge.

Many orphan disease registry options can exist. Registries can be built for individual orphan diseases, but are then limited by the lack of ability to draw from all orphan disease processes. By incorporating most orphan diseases, or at least orphan diseases based on commonalities, researchers are not limited to only one set of data and can find common ground among different orphan diseases, thus expanding knowledge and understanding of all orphan diseases.

The Paradigm Change Challenge Towards Personal Health

Medical and Care Compunetics 4
L. Bos and B. Blobel (Eds.)
IOS Press, 2007

Semantic Interoperability of EHR Systems

Dipak KALRA[1,a] and Bernd G.M.E. BLOBEL[b]
[a] *CHIME – Centre for Health Informatics and Multiprofessional Education,
University College London, United Kingdom*
[b] *eHealth Competence Center, University of Regensburg Medical Center,
Regensburg, Germany*

Abstract. This paper describes the challenges that are being tackled and those that remain to be addressed if we are to enable electronic health record information to be shared seamlessly and meaningfully. This goal is known as semantic interoperability, and is needed if computational services are to be able to interpret safely clinical data that has been integrated from diverse sources. Based on sustainable architectural approaches, the paper describes the clinical case for consistently expressed clinical meaning within electronic health records, in particular where computers rather than humans need to be able to process EHR data safely. It outlines the main kinds of information and knowledge artefact that are used to represent meaning within EHRs, and considers for each its role and limitations. The problems that arise with trying to use terminology consistently with EHR reference models is explored, together with the implications for designing EHR archetypes. Examples are given of situations where a diversity of options exists for how to represent compound (multi-part) clinical expressions. Recommendations are made for the kinds of change that are needed both in record structures and in terminology systems to minimise this diversity and thereby aid semantic interoperability.

Keywords. EHR; Semantic interoperability; Terminology; Archetypes

1. Requirements

There are many clinical and health service drivers for integrated electronic health records, in which the cumulative health information of an individual patient can be virtually accessed from any new point of care delivery [1]. All of these, to a greater or lesser extent, contribute to the business case for the present international investment in e-Health:

- Manage increasingly complex clinical care.
- Connect multiple locations of care delivery.
- Support team based care.
- Deliver evidence-based health care.
- Improve patient safety.
    - o reduce errors and inequalities.
    - o reduce duplication and delay.

---

[1] Dipak Kalra, MD, PhD, CHIME – Centre for Health Informatics and Multiprofessional Education, University College London, Holborn Union Building, Highgate Hill, London N19 5LW, E-mail: d.kalra@chime.ucl.ac.uk.

- Support ubiquitous care.
- Empower and involve citizens.
- Enable the move to the Personal Health paradigm.
- Underpin population health and research.
- Protect patient privacy.

In today's health care, some of these, such as the sharing of care within a local health care team, could be served simply by providing access to human readable documents, such as Adobe PDF files accessed via a secure network. Indeed, the authors know a number of clinicians, sceptical of national ICT programmes, who assert that even meeting this basic need seems to date to have defeated the multi-million Euro/Dollar programmes. At the same time, it is now widely acknowledged that the sheer volumes of data accumulated in one patient's record, and the cross-referencing of that data to ever-expanding medical knowledge in a timely fashion, is beyond the realistic expectations of clinical professionals. Just as airline pilots rely upon instrumentation and warning systems to complement their human skills, clinicians will need increasingly to work in partnership with systems that monitor for unusual patterns, interactions, and overdue care interventions.

The wide-scale use of decision support and alerting systems that interact with patient records is an essential informatics contribution to the prevention of errors [2]. An example for this challenge being on the agenda for many countries' eHealth programmes including the Action Plan for eHealth Europe are ePrescribing facilities [3]. Weed has long argued that the expanding wealth of medical knowledge has now exceeded the ability of individual healthcare professionals, however well meaning, to retain and retrieve it appropriately or safely [4]. Straus & Sackett argue that consolidating this vast array of knowledge within evidence based guidelines, developed by trusted organisations, is the only way in which individual clinicians can remain safe and optimally effective [5].

Putting the requirement in more EHR-specific terms, we need guideline and decision support systems, notification and alerting components and analytic tools to be able to process integrated health data in order to improve patient safety, to help deliver evidence based care and to enable clinical audit and research. Even more basic functions such as viewing and searching within a single patient record will increasingly reply upon filters and queries that in turn need to know what every data item means clinically in order to determine if it should be presented to the user in a given context. In terms of EHR semantic interoperability requirements, we need:

- to enable the meaningful sharing and combining of health record data between systems;
- to enable the consistent use of modern terminology systems and medical knowledge databases;
- to enable the integration and safe use of computerised protocols, alerts and care pathways by EHR systems;
- to ensure the necessary data quality and consistency to enable rigorous secondary uses of longitudinal and heterogeneous data: public health, research, health service management.

Many clinical systems can today achieve much of this using data that has been captured within their own applications, because the organisation and meaning of the data can be dictated in advance by each system designer. Semantic interoperability is most needed when EHR data are to be shared and combined from different systems (or across diverse modules within a large system).

For example, it is well recognised that allergy checking by a prescribing module can at times prevent a dangerous prescription from being issued. As such systems become more widely used, clinicians will come to rely upon them. In the vision of e-health, the source allergy list used by such an alerting component might one day be a federated collation of all allergies recorded within a virtual (national) EHR, derived (in real time or by prior caching) from multiple primary and secondary care systems. If allergies are entered in free text in one source system, or are encoded using a non-standard terminology, or in another system are called "medication intolerance" instead of "allergies", will they be missed? What is the clinical utility and safety of performing allergy checking on a list of allergens whose completeness is unknown? Might the result therefore be potentially even more dangerous than when we had no virtual EHR (because at least then we would remember to ask the patient)?

Semantic interoperability ideally requires standards, not just for data to be transferred and structurally mapped into a receiving database, but so that it's clinical content can be mapped to a commonly understood meaning. The goal is to be able to communicate (share) meaning, and in particular, clinical meaning. This is a richer and more complex goal than sharing data structures, data elements and individual values.

A simple answer to harmonising meaning would appear to be to standardise on a precise and comprehensive terminology, in which each clinical concept is clearly defined and has a unique representation. However, this level of standardisation is hard because clinical practice is (and needs to be) inherently diverse. A global and singular representation for each clinical expression is not realistic, and is probably not desirable:

- different levels of detail, different levels of granularity are needed for different clinical settings;
- clinical practice is too diverse and evolving for fine grained standards;
- different cultures, and natural languages need to represent health phenomena and clinical meaning differently;
- patients and carers need a different level of jargon from health care professionals.

Sharing clinical meaning therefore does not automatically imply (and cannot require) identical terms and data structures: different physical or logical EHR representations may have a common meaning i.e. they may be *semantically equivalent*. Therefore the goal of semantic interoperability is:

to be able to recognise and process semantically equivalent information homogeneously, even if instances are heterogeneously represented

i.e. if they are differently structured, and/or using different terminology systems, and/or using different natural languages. This equivalence needs to be robustly computable, and not just human readable, in order for guidelines, care pathways, alerting and decision support components to function effectively and safely across EHRs that have been combined from heterogeneous systems. The EU SemanticHEALTH project has defined this goal as "co-operability": the ultimate level of semantic interoperability [6].

Co-operability is quite a high aspiration, although this is the level of interoperability that is needed in order to realise the benefits of processable EHRs in a distributed e-Health environment. To help make this tractable, at least for the clinical data that computers are useful for, we need still to minimise unnecessary diversity in the ways that equivalent expressions are represented, so that transformation rules can be defined and applied safely to co-process heterogeneous data that are semantically equivalent.

2. Architectural Approaches to Information System Co-Operability

For enabling EHR systems' co-operability, those systems have to be based on an architectural model. The architecture of a system is defined by the structure and behavioural aspects of its components. Following this statement, components, their relationships and their functions define the architecture of a system. The resulting system architecture must be driven by the business processes and the services to be provided. So, the method for designing, implementing and maintaining semantically interoperable health information systems is a service-oriented architecture (SOA) following the Object Management Group's (OMG's) model-driven architecture (MDA) approach [7]. Meanwhile, HL7 slowly moves from a message-based paradigm to an architectural approach, expressed in closer liaison with OMG as well as in the establishment of the SOA SIG [8].

The abstraction body for analysing and designing an information system as described above, the methodology for composition and de-composition of the system defining the appropriate level of system granularity, the focus on specific aspects of system and components as well as the corresponding domain being touched are established by the Generic Component Model [9,10]. Figure 1 presents this model, which is a predecessor of, and extension to, the ISO Reference Model – Open Distributed Processing (RM-ODP) [11]. By that way, the integration of SOA and MDA – mostly considered as incompatible – is enabled. So, the GCM provides an integration of the existing architectural aspects defined in ISO and OMG specifications. It also includes the proposal of an adapted unified process [12].

During the last 10 years advanced health information system architecture development for semantic interoperability, thereby contributing to the establishment of the RM-ODP, a new methodology of the service-oriented and model-driven architecture has been evolved. This methodology is characterised by:

- Component orientation and the distribution paradigm;
- Unified process of definition, design, implementation, evaluation, testing, and maintenance;
- Common reference models for information and processes;
- Common reference terminologies and ontologies;
- Separation of logical and technological views by platform-independent and platform-specific models, respectively;
- Specification of the components' structure and behaviour as well as of the rules being applied based on knowledge, concepts and contexts;
- Enhanced security and privacy services.

For de-composing and composing component-based systems according to the aforementioned principles, the different sub-models have to be transferred into a common environment. To define business processes, domain concepts and user requirements, domain experts must seriously be involved. As these experts' knowledge pres-

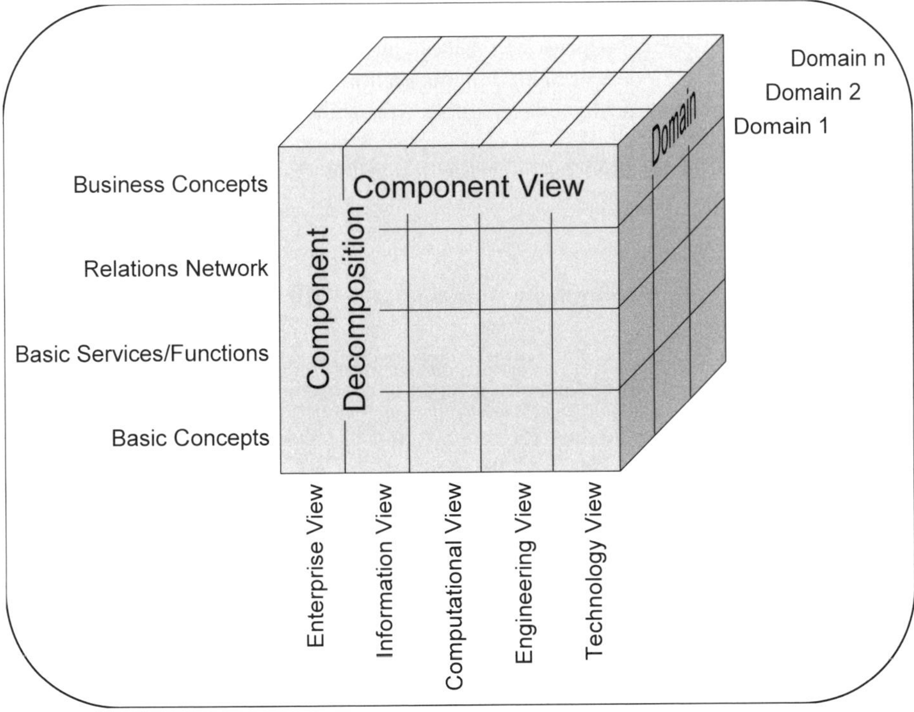

Figure 1. Generic Component Model.

entation is based on their own methodology and grammar, a translation of their domain language into a meta-language must be enabled. Examples for domain-specific grammars are classic workflow models, narrative security policy specification, traditional description of physical or chemical processes in biomedical or laboratory devices, or finally different constraint languages used to represent knowledge in the health care area. Language transformation might be performed, e.g., by tools directly transferring workflow models into XML specifications such as the newest version of the ARIS toolset provided by IDS Scheer [13]. Examples for medical concepts representation are constructs based on the Archetype Definition Language (ADL) [14], Knowledge Interchange Format (KIF) [15], Arden Syntax Medical Logic Modules (MLM) [7], or other knowledge presentation approaches, which have to be preferably transferred into OMG's Object Constraint Language (OCL) [6]. Another challenge, also representing domain knowledge, concerns the composition of components. In that context, the presentation of rules based on reasoning strategies (case-based, spatial, temporal strategies), logics (inductive, descriptive, Fuzzy Logic) but also the combination of different techniques for improving performance or intelligence of algorithms must be mastered.

Also the model exchange between specifications based on different meta-languages such as UML and XML must be supported, which can easily be done using the OMG XMI specification [16] and/or by deploying appropriate tools such as, e.g., Rational Rose® [17].

The sustainable and comprehensive architectural approach discussed in this section and meanwhile standardised in some ISO specifications has not been implemented beyond demonstrators so far. Existing standards and specifications for EHR systems discussed in the following sections are more or less restricted to the medical domain, partially ignoring the important aspects of business modelling and the systems viewpoint focus. So the reference models presented in this section transfers the knowledge needed for performing in a semantically interoperable way without enforcing this behaviour. This enforcement is the issue of GCM characteristics missing in those models. Nevertheless, the GCM can be used as reference for future developments and migration strategies.

3. Current Solutions for Semantically Interoperable EHR Systems

Current attempts to standardise the capture, representation and communication of clinical (EHR) data reply upon three layers of artefact to represent meaning.

1. Generic reference models for representing clinical (EHR) data e.g. ISO/EN 13606 Part 1 [18], HL7 CDA Release 2 [19], the *open*EHR Reference Model [20].
2. Agreed clinical data structure definitions e.g. *open*EHR archetypes [21], ISO/EN 13606 Part 2 [22], HL7 templates [23], generic templates and data sets.
3. Clinical terminology systems e.g. LOINC [24], SNOMED-CT [25], ICD [26].

3.1. EHR Reference Models

The strength of the approach taken internationally on the EHR architecture has been the development of a rigorous generic representation (an EHR Reference Model) suitable for all kinds of entries, even if it does not meet all aspects of a generic comprehensive architecture as presented in the GCM. These reference models, ISO/EN 13606, *open*EHR and HL7 Clinical Document Architecture, each define the high-level logical model for any kind of EHR and the information properties that will be common to all of the entries contained in it:

- dates and times of when observations occurred, health events took place and when information was recorded;
- persons who provided, composed, entered or authorised (signed) particular entries, or who played particular roles in a health care process;
- version management information, including who changed any of the entries, when and why;
- the degree of sensitivity of the information and who should be allowed to access it;
- who the information is about, if not the patient (e.g. if it about a family member, or a third party);
- the ability to label each point in the record hierarchy i.e. to include a name for each folder, document, heading and the parts of each detailed entry;
- a standard way of representing coded clinical terms, measured quantities, dates, times and various kinds of multimedia data.

Provided that the reference model to be used is known by both sending and receiving information systems, any health record extract exchanged between them will contain all of the structure, names and medico-legal information required for it to be represented faithfully on receipt even if the nature of the clinical content have not been "agreed" in advance. This is sometimes termed *structural* or *syntactic interoperability*. The kinds of meaning that are represented using this layer of artefact are predominantly medico-legal rather than related to clinical knowledge.

3.2. EHR Data Structures

The wide-scale sharing of health records, and their meaningful analysis across distributed sites, for example to enable decision support, also requires that a consistent approach is used for the clinical (semantic) data structures that will be communicated via the reference model, so that equivalent clinical information is represented consistently or at least can be mapped to a consistent representation for interpretation.

This principle is not new: the need to define and share clinical data structures is over a century old. However, such definitions have historically been represented in different ways, as paper or electronic forms, templates, tables, spreadsheets, database schemata, etc. Not only has the data on individual patients not historically been shareable, but even the definitions of how the data are to be organised for groups of patients in a given care setting or with a given clinical problem have not easily been shareable. This has resulted in many different professional communities, even in neighbouring hospitals, adopting slightly different templates for similar care scenarios, making it very hard to compare, aggregate or analyse the data.

The solution offered by EHR Archetypes is to provide a generalised systematic approach to representing any definition for a health record data structure. It is important to recognise that the archetype approach is in itself generic, and can represent data structures for any profession, speciality or service, whilst accommodating that the clinical data sets, value sets, templates, etc., required by different health care domains will be diverse, complex and will change frequently as clinical practice and medical knowledge advance.

Individual Archetype instances are knowledge artefacts that each defines how the EHR Reference Model hierarchy should be organised to represent the data for one clinical entry or recording scenario. Because these definitions are each represented as an Archetype, they can be shared and used across record-sharing communities to define how locally-organised clinical data should be mapped to a common form (even if the data originates from many different systems). Archetypes are a clinic-specific alternative to constraint modelling, using OCL or other constraint language in the domain-crossing GCM context, for medical knowledge representation. Thereby, a marketing strategy has been implemented. The GCM offers additionally to the concept representation also constraint models for rule-based component aggregation. In the future, further developments on Archetypes in this perspective can be expected.

Archetypes were developed by the *open*EHR Foundation on the basis of several years of research in Europe and Australia. They are now being adopted (subject to further ballot) by CEN as a European Standard (EN 13606 Part 2) and being considered by ISO for international standardisation.

As already mentioned, HL7 moves with its new Development Framework (HDF) towards an architectural approach and offers some more aspects defined in GCM. In that context, the business perspective that has been provided or will be provided in the future by the EHR-S Functional Model and its refinements. Here, related SOA specifications and interoperability models are important. Such architectural perspective is by nature missing in specifications based on the HL7 Clinical Document Architecture.

HL7 Templates seek to provide a similar knowledge representation framework that can be used to profile HL7 Version 3 Refined Message Information Models (RMIMs) so that conformance to the models can be tested more precisely for particular usage scenarios. In cases where the HL7 RMIM being constrained is a generic clinical model such as CDA, the medical knowledge expressed in an HL7 template might be quite similar to that expressed within an EHR Archetype.

The kinds of meaning that are represented using this layer of artefact are a clinical headings framework, fine grained data structures, and relevant data values, value sets or terminology constraints.

3.3. Clinical Terminologies

The knowledge of clinical concepts and the way in which they inter-relate has traditionally been implemented in healthcare applications through coding systems. These have, at their most basic level, provided nomenclatures, controlled vocabularies and simple hierarchical classifications of diseases, aetiologies and treatments to facilitate the entry and analysis of healthcare data [27]. Examples of this include ICD, ICPC, SNOMED and Read (versions 1 and 2). The coding schemes associated with these terminologies were primarily required to assist with the subsequent analysis and aggregation of the data across clinical systems. Unfortunately many of these terminologies have historically failed to distinguish the requirements of a classification system from that of a clinical vocabulary [28].

A clinical terminology primarily serves to provide a systematised and restricted (controlled) vocabulary of clinically relevant phrases that can be used during data entry to provide a more precise and shareable expression than might be obtained by using free text. By virtue of being controlled expressions, the translation of a terminology to another natural language is moderately scalable, permitting EHRs to be shared across languages. Because the terms are usually arranged in hierarchies, different fine grained (very precise) terms can be cross-mapped to a coarser grained one to permit them to be processed homogeneously. The best-known examples of clinical terminology systems are possibly LOINC and SNOMED.

The use of terms across languages, and the hierarchical organisation of terms are both essential requirements for semantic interoperability.

However, SNOMED Clinical Terms (SNOMED-CT), the newest and largest clinical terminology, has the extra property of term coordination. This means that basic terms can be combined to compose more complex expressions: for example, a "headache" can be stated to be located in the "frontal region" of the head and "left sided" and "severe", all in a single terminological expression. Term coordination is further discussed below.

4. Some Difficulties

Over the past few years it has become clear that some of the greatest challenge areas in semantic interoperability for the EHR lie firstly in the definition and sharing of suitable data structure definitions (e.g. EHR Archetypes) and secondly in the binding of record structure nodes (effectively, Archetype nodes) to terminology.

By binding the nodes of an Archetype to a part of a terminology system (for example, to specify that the value for a node called "location of fracture" must be a term from a hierarchy of bones in the skeletal system) it should be possible to foster consistency and reliability (correctness) in how EHR data are represented, communicated and interpreted.

However, this is only partially true in practice. There are a number of difficulties that mean the binding of nodes of a data structure (Archetype) to a constrained set of terms can be problematic. Record structures and terminology systems have been developed in relative isolation, with very little or no co-operation on their mutual requirements or scope, resulting in overlapping coverage or clumsy fit.

Good information models are designed on the basis of requirements, and provide a usable representation of reality for a clearly defined scope or purpose. However, in the authors experience it is also common for new use cases to be appended to a developing model's scope, as new stake-holders discover the work and wish to take advantage of it. Whilst on one level this can be seen as a measure of success, it results in a model being used beyond its requirements underpinning, and sometimes therefore being a poor fit to those late-addition use cases. This poor fit creates the risk that the Reference Model will be used inconsistently by different vendors within multiple systems because there are multiple ways in which clinical data may be represented in the hierarchy. Context & recursion may be poorly modelled, risking ambiguity or nonsense (for example, being able to define an Entry about a patient's mother but to include within it some data about a different relative, or to instantiate a blood pressure observation with the systolic and diastolic values labelled as being about two different people). Developers of reference models often need to create term lists (micro-vocabularies) for some of the model's attributes, but over time a lack of discipline results in the *ad hoc* proliferation of term lists, maybe introducing multiple scopes for the same attribute, or term lists that are inconsistent with respect to each other.

There are also a number of problems with clinical terminologies. Confusion remains between clinical terminology and classification, such that attempts to classify all terms within disease-oriented hierarchies cuts across the way that terms are used in routine care documentation. Modern terminologies attempt to provide a comprehensive coverage of health care, although many terms cannot be precisely defined, or agreed upon: if many of the terms in a terminology are not used consistently what use is it having them there? SNOMED-CT in particular defines over 1.7 million relationships between its 400,000 terms. The complexity of these relationships may exceed what can be safely implemented and reliably used. We do not yet have enough operational user experience to show otherwise. Terminologies often include multiple representations for the same clinical concept.

Perhaps the most high-risk area of terminology use is *post-coordination*. This is a mechanism to permit users to combine terms (coordination, as described earlier) in an *ad hoc* way during data entry to document a particular situation in a given patient. This seems at first to be appealing, as a scalable way of providing for the complexity and diversity of health and clinical care with a modest number of core terms plus a coordination mechanism. Post-coordination is sometimes inevitable in the context of regional or sometimes even national adaptation (translation) of existing terms. Post-coordination might be adopted by, and integrated in, the terminology system after extended proof. The drawback is that users are relatively free to combine terms in any way they (rightly or wrongly) choose, and it needs to be questioned how much more systematic this will prove to be than writing free text. Post-coordination means EHR systems receiving data from another system have to cater for the unexpected. If 400,000 terms can be combined in many different (and therefore potentially inconsistent) ways, how can semantic equivalence be determined when data are being integrated from another system?

New generation terminology systems, in trying to be a universal replacement for free text, might have lost track of why we needed a clinical terminology in the first place. Our primary need is to systematise the vocabulary for those clinical data items that computers are able to usefully exploit, as discussed earlier in this paper, not for everything. At least, not for the next several years!

Whatever the problems with using reference models consistently, and using large coordinated terminology, the problems become much harder when we try to define EHR Archetypes that use terminology, since each Archetype needs to define the relationship between each part of the Reference Model and an enumeration (list) of terms unambiguously (known as term binding). Because of their overlapping scope, there are often multiple ways of expressing the same information: using a data structure hierarchy or using a single coordinated term. This can best be explained through some examples.

5. Examples of Binding Record Structures to Terminology

In the examples below,

- a coded term is shown as a clinical phrase inside angle brackets,
- a free-text expression is shown in quotation marks,
- a structured hierarchy is represented via indentation to the right: an indented line is a child of the preceding line,
- in a name-value pair, the name and the value are separated by a colon.

```
<Presenting symptom> : <Headache>

<Headaches present?> : <True>

"Have you been getting headaches?": "Yes"

<Headache symptom>
```

Figure 2. Four alternative representations for the presence of headaches.

Each of these ways of representing the information is useful in particular situations, but how are computers to recognise them as semantically equivalent?

The lower, a coordinated term, seems more clinician friendly for data entry and for readability, but is it the best form to store in the EHR for shared care, decision support, analysis?

<Cardiac examination findings>
　<Cardiac auscultation findings>
　　<Murmur description>
　　　　<Phase> : <Ejection systolic>
　　　　<Nature> : <Click>
　　　　<Character> : <Soft>

<Soft ejection systolic click>

Figure 3. A structured representation of a heart murmur, and a coordinated term alternative.

<Discharge Prescription>
　<Prescribed drug>
　　<Drug name> = <Ampicillin>
　　<Strength> = <250>, <units> = <mg>
　　<Formulation> = <Capsules>
　　<Dose> = <3 x daily>

<Ampicillin caps 250mg 3xdaily>

Figure 4. A structured representation of a prescribed drug, and a coordinated term alternative.

The upper structured form is generally preferred for medication and for multi-valued measurements, even for data entry, but the lower version is still more readable when the data are displayed.

A number of options exist for attempting to support semantic interoperability in these situations:

1. Require that coordinated terms are split into a structured form for storage in the EHR (i.e. the coordinated expression is used for data entry, and for display as an "interface term", but is not the stored form); this requires that a structured form is defined for each possible coordinated expression.
2. Create a coarse grained "name" to act as the label or heading for the coordinated term, and store the term faithfully in the EHR as it is.
3. Agree on use cases when highly-structured data or a single coordinated term are each appropriate.

4.   Develop a structure (e.g. Archetype) that could store both, and leave it to each system to populate it with either highly-structured data or a single coordinated term; by being in the same Archetype any subsequent system will be able to infer that they are in a same semantic space.

How shall we choose the right one(s) out of these four options, and for which circumstances?

These options are compounded by the presence in reference models of attributes that explicitly duplicate information that terminology often also covers. For example, the HL7 Procedure Act class includes three attributes (targetSiteCode, approachSiteCode, methodCode) for information that is usually also available as optional qualifiers in a terminology. SNOMED CT expressions will often combine the procedure name, its target site, approach and/or method in a single expression. Even without qualifiers, a term can sometimes indicate the site or method as part of the procedure description e.g. laparoscopic cholecystectomy. In such cases, how should the methodCode be used?

Other examples of such overlapping scope are:

* who the information is about (the subject of the information, as in family history data);
* who provided the information (e.g. reported by the patient, or by a relative);
* when a situation occurred or when it was true (e.g. past or present findings);
* if the care activity was planned, performed etc. (its life-cycle state);
* if a condition is actual, intended, anticipated or to be avoided.

Should methodCode (and other attributes like it) be removed from reference models on the grounds that this is properly the job of terminology? Should terminology remove the terms that specify the subject of information and other terms for "contextual interpretation", on the grounds that this is properly the job of the record structure?

What does it mean if both record structure and terminology indicate negation in the same entry?

* Emphasised negation (really really, no signs of jaundice).
* Double negation (not not jaundiced = was jaundiced).
* Duplication (take either negation, but don't use both).
* Ambiguous (don't trust the data!).
* Error (ignore the data).

Negation really only makes sense for terms, as values, since you would not usually say:

* A systolic BP was not 135 mmHg (i.e. you would not negate a numeric value);
* A date of onset was not 12th July 2002 (i.e. you would not negate a date);
* The patient's relative with asthma is not Jane Smith (i.e. you would not negate a person).

In free text the negation would be part of the text, and negating a whole name-value pair is ambiguous. So, is negation best left to the terminology? This is the view that has now been taken by the *open*EHR and ISO/EN13606 Reference Models.

6. Conclusion

This paper has outlined the main drivers for semantic interoperability, and explained how EHR Reference Models, EHR Archetypes and clinical terminology are each contributors to achieving this. As reference, the Generic Component Model has been used. Archetypes are at present considered to be the accepted approach for expressing clinical concepts and therefore being one key broker for semantic interoperability, since they bind the other two artefacts to each other, hopefully in systematic ways. For meeting the still open challenges of the GCM, Archetypes and related tools will be furthermore developed.

One notable challenge in designing libraries of Archetypes to meet broad areas of clinical practice, for example to cover the complete clinical information needs of a speciality or professional discipline, is to ensure that Archetypes are evidence-based or meet *de facto* established clinical needs. Given that many Archetypes may be needed to cover a given domain, it is also important for them to be mutually consistent and bind to terminology systems in appropriate and consistent ways. EHR Archetypes themselves therefore need to be quality assured, and their authorship and maintenance duly governed, since they will strongly direct the ways in which clinical data is captured, processed and communicated. These processes are progressively being defined by the *open*EHR Foundation.

Given that record structures and terminology systems are, in their present forms, inherently not well made for each other, some general principles for working towards a safer future could be proposed.

1. Generic EHR information models should avoid attributes with explicit semantic roles, although individual qualifiers needed for particular entries might be specified via Archetypes. (When developing the CEN/ISO 13606 EHR Communications Reference Model the approach taken has been to avoid the inclusion of attributes that have semantic roles.)
2. Record modellers should avoid creating or maintaining long attribute term lists. These should ideally be managed by, and be consistent with, terminology systems.
3. Such term lists should make public domain to enable cross-terminology use and to avoid licensing issues, and so that different record structures can adopt common vocabularies where applicable.
4. Negation and uncertainty should be left to terminology or to specific archetypes.
5. Terminology systems should avoid coordinating contextual interpretation terms (e.g. subject of information), but might define term lists that are used by record structures for this.
6. Pre-coordinated terms (i.e. internationally agreed a priori combinations) should each be mapped to an equivalent EHR hierarchy fragment, to permit duplicate storage or dynamic cross-mapping, to support analysis and decision support.
7. Post-coordination without a corresponding record structure (or high-performance and very clever terminology services) seems little better than free text, and maybe should be avoided in most situations.

8.   Whatever decisions are made about the licensing of terminology systems such as SNOMED-CT, the sharing of EHRs requires that terms used within an EHR, and their meaning, can be shared without licensing restrictions.

A set of business rules for how to use SNOMED-CT with HL7 v3 has been produced through an HL7 Committee project known as "Terminfo" [29]. These business rules are themselves surprisingly complex. It remains to be seen if they will prove workable i.e. will they be used consistently enough to support trustworthy co-processing of heterogeneous representations?

As already mentioned in the GCM context, further work is needed to define a generic set of business rules, much simpler than Terminfo, and which will work across multiple record structures and multiple terminology systems.

References

[1] Kalra D. Clinical Foundations and Information Architecture for the Implementation of a Federated Health Record Service. PhD Thesis. University of London. 2002. Available from http://eprints.ucl.ac.uk/archive/00001584/ (Last accessed April 2007).

[2] Bates D.W., Cohen M., Leape L.L., Overhage J.M., Shabot M.M., and Sheridan T. Reducing the frequency of errors in medicine using information technology. J Am Med Inform Assoc. Jul 2001-Aug 2001; 8(4):299–308.

[3] EC eHealth Action Plan.

[4] Weed L.L. Clinical judgement revisited. Methods of Information in Medicine. Dec 1999; 38:279–86.

[5] Straus S.E. and Sackett D.L. Using research findings in clinical practice. BMJ. Aug 1998; 317(7154): 339–42.

[6] Rodrigues J.M., Stroetmann V., Stroetmann K. et. al. Conceptual Framework for eHealth Interoperability, Deliverable 1.1 of the SemanticHEALTH Project. August 2006. Available from http://www/semantichealth.org/deliverables.html (Last accessed April 2007).

[7] Object Management Group, Inc.: www.omg.org.

[8] Health Level 7, Inc. www.hl7.org.

[9] Blobel B. Assessment of Middleware Concepts Using a Generic Component Model. Proceedings of the Conference "Toward an Electronic Health Record Europe '97", pp. 221–228, London 1997.

[10] Blobel B. Application of the Component Paradigm for Analysis and Design of Advanced Health System Architectures. International Journal of Medical Informatics 2000, 60 (3), 281–301.

[11] ISO/IEC 10746 "Information technology – Open Distributed Processing – Reference Model".

[12] Lopez (in this volume).

[13] IDS Scheer AG. ARIS Tool Set. www.ids-scheer.com.

[14] Beale T. Archetypes: Constraint-based Domain Models for Future-proof Information Systems. OOPSLA 2002 workshop on behavioural semantics.

[15] NCITS.T2/98-004. ANSI National Standard (Draft Proposal). Knowledge Interchange Format (KIF). http://logic.stanford.edu/kif/dpans.html.

[16] Object Management group, Inc. www.omg.org.

[17] IBM Rational Software Development Platform. www-306.ibm.com/software/rational/.

[18] Kalra D., Lloyd D. prEN13606 Electronic Health Record Communication Part 1: Reference Model; Final Vote draft. CEN TC/251, Brussels. 2006. [100 pages].

[19] Dolin R. et al. HL7 Clinical Document Architecture Release 2.0. Health Level 7, May 2005.

[20] Beale T., Lloyd D. (editors). The openEHR Reference Model version 1.0.1. Available from http://svn.openehr.org/specification/TAGS/Release-1.0.1/publishing/index.html (last accessed April 2007).

[21] Beale T. (editor). The openEHR Archetype Model (AOM) version 1.0.1. Available from http://svn.openehr.org/specification/BRANCHES/Release-1.0.1-candidate/publishing/architecture/am/aom.pdf (last accessed April 2007).

[22] Kalra, Beale T., Heard S., Lloyd D. prEN13606 Electronic Health Record Communication Part 2: Archetype Interchange Specification; Final Vote draft. CEN TC/251, Brussels. 2006. [143 pages].

[23] Grieve G., Hamm R., Shafarman M., Mulrooney G. HL7 Template Specification (draft). Health Level 7, February 2007.

[24] Logical Observation Identifiers Names and Codes (LOINC). Please see http://www.regenstrief.org/loinc/ (last accessed April 2007).

[25] SNOMED Clinical Terms. Please see http://www.snomed.org/snomedct/index.html (last accessed April 2007).
[26] WHO International Classification of Diseases (ICD). Please see http://www.who.int/classifications/icd/en/ (last accessed April 2007).
[27] Chute C.G. Clinical classification and terminology: some history and current observations. J Am Med Inform Assoc. May 2000–Jun 2000; 7(3):298–303.
[28] Cimino J.J. Desiderata for controlled medical vocabularies in the twenty-first century. Methods of Information in Medicine. 1998; 37(4–5):394–403.
[29] Krog R., Markwell D., Dolin R., Gabriel D., Cheetham E., Spackman K., Hamm R., Rector A., Chute C., Huff S., Klein T., Lynch C., Ryan S. Using SNOMED CT in HL7 Version 3; Implementation Guide, Release 1.2. Health Level Seven, November 2006. Available from http://hl7.org/library/committees/terminfo/terminfo%5Fpublish%5F20061120%2Ezip (last accessed April 2007).

Medical and Care Compunetics 4
L. Bos and B. Blobel (Eds.)
IOS Press, 2007

How to Manage Secure Direct Access of European Patients to their Computerized Medical Record and Personal Medical Record

Catherine QUANTIN [a,1], François André ALLAERT [b], Maniane FASSA [a],
Benoît RIANDEY [c], Paul AVILLACH [d,e], Olivier COHEN [f]
[a] *Service de Biostatistique et Informatique Médicale, CHU de Dijon, France*
[b] *Department of Epidemiology and Biostatistics, Mc Gill University, Montreal Canada*
[c] *Institut National d'Etudes Démographiques (INED), Paris, France*
[d] *LERTIM Faculté de Médecine Université de la Méditerranée, Marseille, France*
[e] *ISPED Université Victor Segalen Bordeaux II, Bordeaux, France*
[f] *HC Forum, Meylan, France*

Abstract. The multiplication of the requests of the patients for a direct access to their Medical Record (MR), the development of Personal Medical Record (PMR) supervised by the patients themselves, the increasing development of the patients' electronic medical records (EMRs) and the world wide internet utilization will lead to envisage an access by using technical automatic and scientific way. It will require the addition of different conditions: a unique patient identifier which could base on a familial component in order to get access to the right record anywhere in Europe, very strict identity checks using cryptographic techniques such as those for the electronic signature, which will ensure the authentication of the requests sender and the integrity of the file but also the protection of the confidentiality and the access follow up. The electronic medical record must also be electronically signed by the practitioner in order to get evidence that he has given his agreement and taken the liability for that. This electronic signature also avoids any kind of post-transmission falsification. This will become extremely important, especially in France where patients will have the possibility to mask information that, they do not want to appear in their personal medical record. Currently, the idea of every citizen having electronic signatures available appears positively Utopian. But this is yet the case in eGovernment, eHealth and eShopping, world-wide. The same was thought about smart cards before they became generally available and useful when banks issued them.

Keywords. Data Security, Electronic Signature, Direct Access, Medical Record, Patient Identifier.

---

[1] Corresponding Author: Catherine Quantin, Service de Biostatistique et Informatique Médicale, CHU de Dijon, BP 1524, 21034 Dijon Cedex, France. E-mail : cquantin@u-bourgogne.fr

Introduction

In an increasing number of countries, patients have a direct access to their medical records (MR) and some countries as France [1] have decided to provide a personal medical record (PMR) to the patient. We define MR as patients' medical information recorded by the medical practitioner under his or own responsibility and ideally electronically signed by him/her in order to authenticate the provider and to prevent any modification of its content.

On the contrary, the PMR is personally supervised by each patient who has the right to mask any information he/she does no not want to be read. According to the Committee on Maintaining Privacy and Security in Health Care Applications of the National Infrastructure [2] patients are very worried about their privacy being disclosed. Such concerns are increased as more sensitive medical details, such as psychiatric records, HIV status, and genetic information, are stored in their EMRs.

Today the simplest solution is to give a paper copy of their medical record to each patient or, if it is computerized, to give him/her a printed record or even a copy on a machine readable storage medium. This arrangement of the communication process can be carried out "without constraint at reasonable intervals and without excessive delay or expense" as required by Article 12 of the Directive "On the Protection of Individuals with regard to the Processing of Personal Data and on the Free Movement of Such Data" (commonly known as Directive 95/46/EC). The time allowed for the provision of access provides the opportunity for ensuring that the individual making the request has be properly authenticated and that, any additional conditions on access, such as those allowed in Article 13 section 1(g) allowed "for the protection of the Data Subject or the rights and freedoms of others" have been correctly observed. This current approach does not involve any particular risk to the information system but, there are already pressing demands from patients to speed up these processes so that the interaction with the delivery of patient care cannot be affected.

Additionally, system designers are willing to provide patients with direct access to the medical record systems of the hospital or to their personal medical record. Actually, it will be very difficult to resist to these pressures due to the fast moving electronic environment. It is thus difficult to imagine that this traditional process will be accepted for much longer. Soon, patients will be expecting to have a direct access to their MR or to their PMR by the intermediary of an electronic transmission through internet or equivalent. Instead or trying to resist this inescapable evolution, it is preferable to seek solutions that provide safety for patients and for the medical record systems while allowing the respect of personal freedoms and human rights.

One of our challenges is that, in healthcare applications, the move towards developing EMRs and linking them to affiliated healthcare databases over a public network brings an urgent issue of patient-identity theft. The mean cause is that, eavesdroppers can intercept the transfer data via a public network on any place at any time, thereby resulting in an increase possibility of improper disclosure of patients' sensitive information and potential abuses of EMRs [3].

The management of a secure direct access of European patients to their computerized medical records and personal medical records requires three conditions:

- unique identifier to have access to his own record and only to this one (availability)

- secure access to the MR or PMR with on line authentication of the patient and a cryptographic transmission of the data (confidentiality)
- digital signature of the MR to protect its integrity against any modification attempt

1. The Creation of a European Family-Based Unique Identifier

The development of medical genetics has pointed out the importance of the familial dimension of the medical information and the need for introducing a familial component in the individual record of the patient [4]. The interest of such familial component is supported by the identification of genetic factors influencing the outcome of some diseases or the therapeutic response to the drugs. In this framework we have set up an Internet application which gives the possibility to authorized geneticians and researchers to gather all the medical data concerning a patient with a genetic disease. By the use of anonymous family-based identifiers, data concerning the patient will be gathered along with the information issued from the medical records of the other members of his family.

1.1. Principle

With the patient's agreement, this anonymous identifier is transmitted by a secured system to the data centre called HC-Forum platform [5] with all his medical data. Thus the patient will benefit from a medical record accessible from any medical centre. This record will be regularly updated with his own information and those of his family. In this data centre, for statistical purpose, this identifier will be rendered anonymous a second time in order to avoid any kind of dictionary attacks [6]. The rules governing the information system are strictly in accordance with the European directive for data protection in order to guarantee the confidentiality of his data and of his relatives, and to grant the subject the right to obtain the rectification, of data. The French National Data Protection Authority (CNIL) validated this aforementioned project in March 2004 (advice n° 04-006). A patent was filed to the French Patent Office in September 2004.

1.2. Composition of the Family-Based Identifier

The choice of the criteria included in the individual part of the patients' identifier (Figure 1 below) is based on a previous work we have conducted, with the French Department for the Modernization of Health Information Systems, which have demonstrated that the key information for patient identification are his first and last names and his date of birth [7], [8], [9].

The first name is the first one recorded in the register of birth and the last name is the family name which means for the women their maiden name and not their marital name for example.

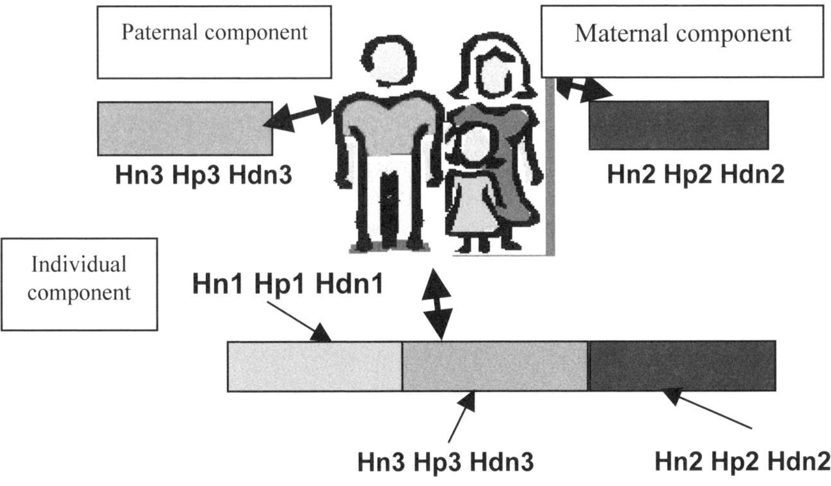

Figure 1. Family-Based Identifier

The familial components (last name, first name and date of birth of the mother and the father) were added to the individual component (Figure 2) following the work conducted by our department on the linkage [10], [11] of the mother and her babies medical records in the Burgundy perinatal network [12] which has pointed out the necessity of introducing the maternal component in the individual identifier of the baby. However, we also need a paternal component to rebuild the genealogic tree.

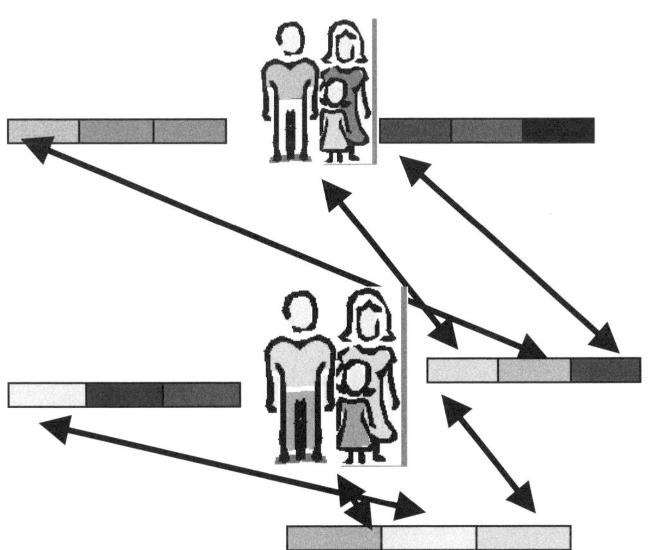

Figure 2. Familial linkage

1.3. Anonymous the Family-Based Identifier

Hash algorithms are not reversible and cannot be deciphered and one of the most reliable [13] and freely available one is the Standard Hash Algorithm (SHA). The three key variables included in the individual part of the patient identifier (Last name, first name and date of birth) are separately hashed in order to maintain a higher security level. For the individual component, we have three variables:

- Hn: anonymous number corresponding to the last name of the subject;
- Hp: anonymous number corresponding to the first name of the subject;
- Hdn: anonymous number corresponding to the subject's date of birth.

The family based identifier includes 9 variables (Figure 2 above). This anonymity is made locally before any kind of data flows in such a way that only anonymous data are sent and made available on the HC forum data centre.

1.4. Familial Linkage

Using the link existing between the identifiers of the subjects of a same family, the genealogic tree of the patient can be described. Based on this linkage, one can thus build the family tree from a "vertical" point of view, i.e. ascending/descending of an individual. This linkage also makes it possible to build the family tree from an "horizontal" point of view, i.e. within the same generation, for the following cases:

- the phratry: by sorting the dates of birth of all the individuals having the same parents;
- halfbrothers and sisters: by sorting the dates of birth of all the individuals having the same father or the same mother.

1.5. A Common Identifier for all European Countries

The great advantage of this European health identifier based on the family component is to be founded on very basic information available for everybody, easily checkable and permanent during all patient's life which is not the case for the social insurance number. To fulfill the rules of the European directive on data protection and of the medical deontology, the use of hash algorithms [14] with different keys would allow to create, from the information of the family-based identifier, different anonymous identifiers for a same patient [15] which could be used in the different countries for different applications i.e. Medical personal record, healthcare network, epidemiological or clinical studies. The fact that all these anonymous identification numbers are issued from the same initial information will facilitate the linkage of the data of a same patient, coming from different health information systems, in a secure environment. If an error occurs on one of the identification criteria (Last name, first name or date of birth) of the patient or of the parents, the use of a probabilistic linkage algorithm could be used to recreate the link with the other parts of the medical information and to rebuild for example the medical record of a patient.

2. Patients' Access to MR or PMR Online

The direct access to the MR or the PMR by electronic media causes many difficulties, more linked to organization than to computer problems. The principal difficulty in this field is to ensure that only the holder of the access rights will be able to access to the Personal Data. This is considerably more complex than ensuring that only the staff will have access to the needed information for their jobs. The first reason is that the number of persons involved in the staffs is very much smaller than the number of patients: this number is multiplied by at least 10 (up to 100 or a 1000 in some cases).

The second reason is that the staff benefits from the organizational management control of the medical team and thus, can be encouraged to participate in relevant training courses. On the contrary, patients would have to be provided with intuitive, foolproof access facilities, without requiring them to participate in any training courses. The difference between "doctor or nurse proof" facilities and "patient or general public proof" facilities is substantial even though the number of applications and functions available to the patient would, of course, be much less than those available to and required by members of staff.

The traditional authentication approach of individuals has two components: assertion of that identity, followed by the proof of that identity. Generally, this proof can be in terms of something that the individual knows or something that the individual has or something that the individual is.

The technical solutions exist to cover any degree of proof in authenticating individuals but many of them would require the establishment of a substantial organization before they could become effective. Even today after so much computerization of Medical Record systems, the simplest and most common authentication mechanism is still that of an "Identifier" together with a "Password". This approach combines simplicity of use and management but it is the weakest and the most unsatisfactory mechanism. There are many examples of password copying, sharing, cracking and other forms of misuse to allow unauthorized access to information systems. Even with this approach, it is possible to improve the security of information systems by the adoption of the CEN Password standard, ENV 12251, for managing passwords [16].

3. Use of Digital Signatures and Smart Card Solutions to Access to Medical records

A brief consideration of the risks associated with unlawful access to Medical Record systems for patients and the healthcare organization makes it clear that a very reliable authentication system will be required before allowing any public access to such systems. The most satisfactory approach would lie on the creation of an individual patient chip card, including the electronic signature cryptographic algorithms. But this will take some time and will cause considerable expenses before becoming the accepted standard. Moreover, due to the legal recognition of the electronic signature, this solution would provide an access follow-up, having value of proof in front of the courts. However, as this more satisfactory electronic solution cannot be implemented now and everywhere, only degraded and less safe solutions can be considered.

A possible solution is a patient smart card [15], [17], [18], associated with the attribution to the patient of a secret pin code with 8 characters by the hospital, when he/she is admitted. This possibility implies the existence of a hospital information system equipped with powerful data-processing devices, filtering the access, of the firewall type. Whatever the technical solution possible today or in the future, it does not seem desirable to give a direct access to the system of management of the files to all the people, even authenticated. It will be preferable to envisage a request procedure for access, including the research of the file and the extraction of the communicable documents authorized by the law. Obviously, the original medical record which is the mean to bring evidence in case of litigations must be protected of any kind of attempt to unauthorized modifications. This approach, in which a special access file is created, could happen much faster than the time delay allowed in some European countries; for instance in the UK 40 days are allowed to comply with a Subject Access request and only 8 days in France. This approach also, permits to reach a basic level safety which is not currently assured in the majority of the healthcare systems Moreover, with this solution, PMR information can always be emailed out to the patient providing facilities have been established for its encryption.

4. Technology Against Ethic and Law: the Liability Limits

Even if we succeed to solve the problem of a secure access of the patient to his medical record with a strong identification and preventing any kind of modification of the original record, two main dangers still exist.

The first lays in the fact that this "automatic" access process is not accompanied of any medical explanation and even less medical warning about the contents that the patient will read. It is not sure that the implementation of such a routine direct access of the patient to his medical record automatic extracted from the database is a very satisfying solution from a medical point of view. The medical records may content some information which obviously are likely to cause serious psychological harm to the patient and mandatory require to be presented by a medical practitioner. If a patient get suicide after an access to his medical record because the information contained in it are unbearable or have been misunderstood by him, the liability of the hospital or of the medical practitioner could be involved from a legal point of view or at least from an ethical or deontological point of view. Obviously to desperate patients and to lead them to suicide do not complete the definition of the practice of a skill and diligent healthcare professional.

In some others situations, the contains of the medical record required also to be consciously review before to be delivered to patients. It may contains some information which are not duly updated or which were only hypothesis which have never been confirmed. In some others cases, some information recorded in it can make reference to third persons who, for example, have provided information on the patient and the name of these must be erased before giving the record to the patient. Wrong information which may be at the origin of damage or the breach of confidentiality concerning a third person may also easily involve the liability of the hospital or of the practitioner. Therefore, even if an automatic extraction of the medical record from the database at the patient's demand may appears satisfying on a technical and on a computer security point of view, it does not fulfill the quality requirements for healthcare information security and no transmission must be allowed without the consent of the medical practitioner who takes care of the patient or his representative. It is his own liability which is involved and thus his formal agreement to the transmission is required which may implies that the transmitted document should be electronically signed by him.

The second point lays on the use of the medical record by the patient. Considering that patients are responsible adults we will not consider the eventual unexpected effects for them of the communication of their medical record to their insurance or bank which have required it, officially or unofficially. From the medical or hospital point of view, the main problem could come from a modification of the medical record by the patient himself to erase some information which prevent him from having some advantages. If such modification was possible, imagine what could happen if a patient erased that he is epileptic in order to be allowed to conduct some engine. In case of litigations, it would be also necessary to take into account that the medical practitioner may also have modified the medical record by adding the missing information when the medical practitioner is informed about the problem.

Therefore, in order to avoid these difficulties, the medical record transmitted to the patients must be electronically signed by the practitioner to be sure that he has given is agreement and to be sure that no unfair modification has been introduced in it. Here also, the recognition of the legal value of the electronic signature permits a controlled electronic transmission of the medical record to the patient. Taking this into account, the use of a PMR is something interesting because it will allow the patient to mask any kind of information he does not want anybody to read. In this case, it seems important and fair play that the patient informed the reader – and above all if the reader is his/her medical practitioner – that this document is a PMR and not a MR and that some information may have been masked. The electronic signature of the MR by a medical practitioner could be the a proof that it is a MR (not a PMR).

Conclusion

Today, the direct access of the patients to their computerized medical files is not a threat for the medical information safety. However the multiplication of the requests for direct access, the increasing computerization of the medical records and the diffusion of Internet in the whole population will lead to envisage an access by using technical automatic and scientific way. It will require a strict unique identifier and identity checks using cryptographic techniques such as those planned for the electronic signature, which will ensure the protection of the confidentiality and the integrity of the files and the authentication of the requests sender and the access follow up. The electronic medical record must also been electronically signed by the practitioner in order to get evidence he has given his agreement, take the liability for that and also in order to avoid any kind of post-transmission falsification. This solution will have a very high legal value since the Directive 1999/93/EC of the European Parliament and of the Council of 13 December 1999 on a community framework for electronic signatures has defined in article 5 the legal effects of electronic signatures. Member States shall ensure that an electronic signature is not denied legal effectiveness and admissibility as evidence in legal proceedings solely on the grounds that it is in electronic form, ,or not based upon a qualified certificate issued by an accredited certification-service-provider, or not created by a secure signature-creation device.

Currently, the idea of every citizen having electronic signatures available appears positively Utopian but this is the implication of much of the work that is going on world-wide in e-Government, e-Health and e-Shopping and the same was thought about smart cards before they became generally available and useful when the banks issued them!

Acknowledgements

This research was supported by The French National Agency for Research (ANR).

References

[1]   Quantin C, Cohen O, Riandey B, Allaert FA. The French proposal for a health identification number. MIE 2006, Stud Health Technol Inform 2006;124:201-6.

[2]   Committee on Maintaining Privacy and Security in Health Care Applications of the National Infrastructure. For the record: Protecting electronic health information. Washington, DC: National Academy Press. 1997. Available from: http:/www.nap.edu/readingroom/books/ftr/52e6.html

[3]   Hui-Mei Cheao, Shih-Hsiung Twu & Chin-Ming Hsu. A patient-identity security mechanism for electronic medical records during transit and at rest.Medical Informatics and the Internet in Medicine. September 2005; 30(3): 227 – 240.

[4]   Quantin C., Allaert F-A., Gouyon B., Cohen O. – Proposal for the creation of a European healthcare identifier. MIE Genève 2005. Stud Health Technol Inform. 2005; 116 : 4-54.

[5]   Cohen O, Mermet MA, Demongeot J. HC Forum® : a web site based on an international human cytogenetic database. Nucleic Acids Research 2001;29:305-307.

[6]   Quantin C., Bouzelat H., Allaert F.A., Benhamiche A.M., Faivre J., Dusserre L. How to ensure data security of an epidemiological follow-up : quality assessment of an anonymous record linkage procedure, International Journal of Medical Informatics. 1998; 49:117-122.

[7]   Quantin C, Binquet C, Bourquard K, Pattisina R, Gouyon-Cornet B, Ferdynus C, Gouyon JB, Allaert FA. Which are the best identifiers for record linkage? Medical Informatics and the Internet Medicine, 2004;29 (3-4):221-227.

[8]   Quantin C, Binquet C, Allaert FA, Cornet B, Pattisina R, Le Teuff G, Ferdynus C, Gouyon JB. Decision analysis for the assessment of a record linkage procedure: application to a perinatal network. Methods of Information in Medicine, 2005;44:72-79.

[9]   Grannis SJ, Overhage JM, Mc Donamd C. Analysis of identifier performance using a deterministic linkage algorithm. Proceeding AMIA Symposium 2002:305-9.

[10] Jaro M. Probabilistic linkage of large public health data files. Stat Med 1995;14:491-8.

[11] Falkoe E, Rasmussen KB, Maclure M, Schroll H. Statistical linkage of treatment to diagnosis for research and monitoring of practice patterns. Methods Informatic Medicine, 2004;43:282-6.

[12] Cornet B, Gouyon JB, Binquet C, Sagot P, Ferdynus C, Métral P, Quantin C. Using discharge abstracts as a bool to assess a regional perinatal network. Revue Epidemiologie et Santé Publique 2001; 49:583-93.

[13] Bartu A, Freeman NC, Gawthorne GS, Codde JP, D'arcy C, Holman J. Mortality in a cohort of opiate and amphetamine users in Perth, Western Australia. Society for the Study of Addiction, 2004;99:53-60.

[14] Wang X. Cryptanalysis of SHA-1 Hash Function, cryptographic hash workshop national institute of standards and technology, October 31, 2005.

[15] Roger France FH, De Clercq E, Bangels SM. Purposes of health indentofocation cards in Belgium – EFMI, European Federation for Medical Informatics, IOS Press, 2005, Connecting Medical Informatics and Bio-Informatics.

[16] CEN Password standard, ENV 12251

[17] Pharow P, Blobel B. eHealth Competence Center, Regensburg, Germany. peter.pharow@ehealth-cc.de Benefits and weaknesses of health cards used in health information systems. Stud Health Technol Inform. 2006;124:320-5.
[18] Pharow P, Blobel B. Fraunhofer Institute for Integrated Circuits IIS, Erlangen, Germany. Security infrastructure requirements for electronic health cards communication. Stud Health Technol Inform. 2005;116:403-8.

Medical and Care Compunetics 4
L. Bos and B. Blobel (Eds.)
IOS Press, 2007

Semantic Interoperability between Clinical and Public Health Information Systems for Improving Public Health Services

Diego M. LOPEZ [1] and Bernd G.M.E. BLOBEL
eHealth Competence Center Regensburg, University of Regensburg Medical Center,
Germany

Abstract. Improving public health services requires comprehensively integrating all services including medical, social, community, and public health ones. Therefore, developing integrated health information services has to start considering business process, rules and information semantics of involved domains. The paper proposes a business and information architecture for the specification of a future-proof national integrated system, concretely the requirements for semantic integration between public health surveillance and clinical information systems. The architecture is a semantically interoperable approach because it describes business process, rules and information semantics based on national policy documents and expressed in a standard language such us the Unified Modeling Language UML. Having the enterprise and information models formalized, semantically interoperable Health IT components/services development is supported.

Keywords: Public Health, Services Integration, Semantic Interoperability, Business Modeling, UML.

1. Introduction

Improving efficiency and quality for health systems including social care, prevention, homecare and lifestyle in an aging society with increasing demands for innovative and better health services, can only be met by comprehensively integrating all services including medical, social, community, and public health ones. This challenge has an significant effect on supporting health information systems.

Probably the most common scenario to describe the integration between public health and clinical information systems is the data communication from clinical (health) information systems to outbreak detection systems. Event notification is improved (more timely and complete information), when diseases are directly collected from the clinical settings. However, this is not the only possible interaction; interoperability means collaboration and both, the Public Health System, as the Clinical Care system, can benefit from that information interchange.

Public health agencies can benefit by improving public health services (promotion and prevention) which can be planned based on more detailed clinical information,

---

[1] Corresponding Author: Diego M. Lopez, MSc, eHealth Competence Center, University of Regensburg Medical Center. Franz-Josef-Strauss-Allee 11, D-93053, Regensburg, Germany; Email: diego.lopez@ehealth-cc.de

better case management by direct feedback can be provided to health care providers, access to clinical information for epidemiological studies, etc. Health care providers can benefit by obtaining more complete information to improve diagnosis and treatment e.g. epidemiological information, public health guidelines and protocols, promotion and prevention programs, alerts for public health services, etc., and reduced effort in mandatory notification processes. A detailed analysis of potential benefits of public health and health information exchange is discussed in [1].

Unfortunately, to accomplish health information systems integration is not an easy task. Furthermore, difficulties in integration go beyond technological issues. Historically, clinical health and public health services have for the most part been delivered by separate organizational components that have evolved rather autonomously [2]. Clinical and public health systems belong to different domains, each one with different business process, concepts, and rules. In order to deal with the challenge of facilitating effective information interchange (semantic interoperability) between existent/ future clinical and public health information systems, information systems development have to start analyzing enterprise (business) requirements for integration.

In the paper, the some approaches for integration between Public Health and Clinical information systems are analyzed and a business and information model for realizing semantic interoperability between them is proposed. The feasibility of the architecture for designing semantically interoperable services and components is discussed in some detail.

2. Interoperability Approaches in Public Health Information Systems

The National Health Information Infrastructure (NHII), an ongoing initiative to provide a knowledge-based network of interoperable health information systems [3], is a clear example of a comprehensive approach for interoperability between Clinical and Public Health Information systems. The interaction is defined at a high level of abstraction in the NHII's three dimensions model, as shown in figure 1. The Population Health dimension encompasses specific population-based health data and resources such us surveillance information and planning, evaluation and policy documents. This dimension interacts with the Health Care Providers dimension (Clinical Information Systems) through vital statistics, registries, socioeconomic conditions, etc, and with the Personal Health dimension thought inspections reports, health education and other health promotion actions. Information systems in the Population Health dimension are principally managed by the Centers for Diseases Control and Prevention (CDC) in the context of the Public Health Information Network (PHIN) initiative.

PHIN is a national initiative to implement a multi-organizational business and technical architecture for the integration of public health information systems. In order to characterize the necessary integration with Clinical Information Systems, PHIN defines as one of its nine core functions and specifications [5]: "The Use of Electronic Clinical Data for Event Detection". This function involves the reception; management and processing of electronic data from clinical care sites and laboratories, for the purpose of conduct public health surveillance. PHIN specifies a set of HL7 messages to transmit data from clinical sources and provides tools such us PHIN Message System for messages transport and NEDSS Base System (NBS) for disease surveillance. Vocabulary standards are also provided by identifying relevant portions of existent terminologies (e.g. the Logical Observation Identifiers Names and Codes LOINC and the Systematized Nomenclature of Medicine SNOMED). Tools such as the Vocabulary Access and Distribution System (VADS), based on the HL7 Common Terminology Server (CTS), have been recently created to facilitate and encourage standard vocabulary usage. Despite the provided standards and tools to facilitate semantic interoperability, CDC has recently decided that for the moment, all National Notifiable Disease messages will be submitted to CDC in HL7 V2.5 format. This means a restricted approach towards technical interoperability.

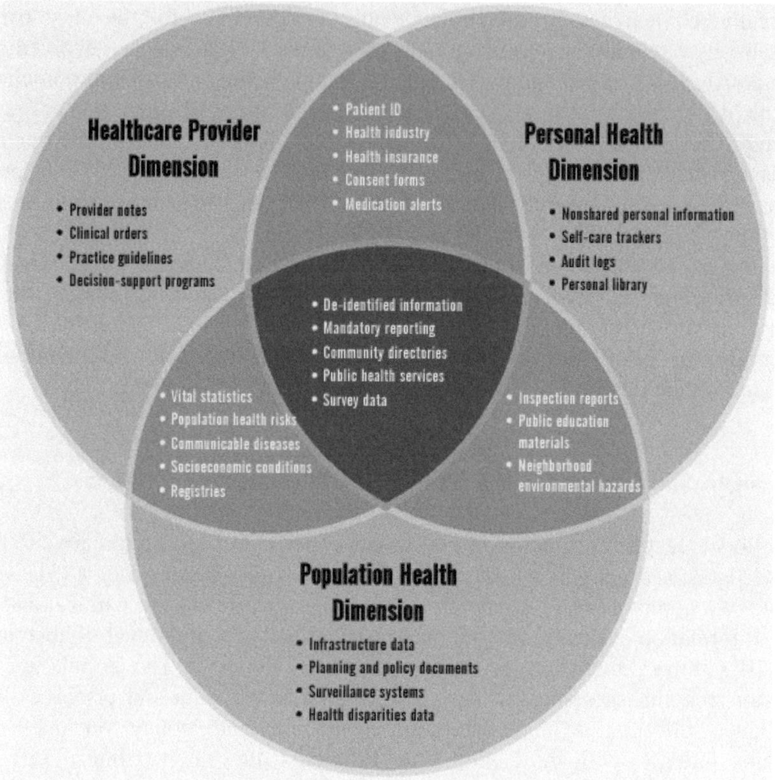

Figure 1. The USA National Health Information Infrastructure dimensions [4].

In Colombia, several computer-based information systems have been used for supporting the National Surveillance System (SIVIGILA), however all those systems are diverse in functionality, structure and technologies [6]. Recently, the National Health Institute (Instituto Nacional de Salud, INS) as governmental dependency in charge of SIVIGILA planning, development and implementation, developed a computer-based information system (named SIVIGILA2006) which is being distributed among the public health offices in the country. A new version of the system has been released (SIVIGILA2007) which support the collection of mandatory notifiable diseases (e.g. malaria, measles, hepatitis, yellow fever and 47 other diseases). None of the aforementioned developments considers the requirements for semantic interoperability, however.

3. Specifying Semantic Interoperability between Clinical and Public Health Information Systems

The requirement analysis, design, implementation, evaluation, use, and maintenance of semantically interoperable HIS must follow a standardized development process. HIS-DF [7] is an architecture development framework for sustainable, semantically interoperable HIS and components. Based on the Rational Unified Process Framework [8], HIS-DF provides a reference knowledge base of tasks, performers (roles), work products (artifacts), and guidance necessary for the architectural analysis within healthcare software development projects. HIS-DF supports the development of HIS by using Unified Modeling Language (UML) models organized as separated but interrelated viewpoints describing different aspects of the system.

HIS-DF is used as the methodology for developing the specification of integration between Public Health and a Clinical Information Systems. The proposed architecture is composed of a set of models that all together; describe the business and informational aspects of the two interrelated domains. HIS-DF Business Viewpoint describes the purpose, scope, and policies of the interrelated domains (public and clinical ones) supported on the RUP Business Use Cases Model and Business Analysis Models. HIS-DF Information Viewpoint is centered on the semantics of health information to be interchanged, being supported by the RUP Analysis model.

4. The Business Architecture

4.1. The Business Use Case Model

The integration architecture described in this paper is based on the requirements of the Colombian National Health Information System (Sistema Integrado de Información en Salud – SIIS [9]). The aim of the SIIS is to support the management of any kind of health information (administrative, clinical, public health) in a centralized way. The architecture is restricted to the semantic integration of the National System for Public Health Surveillance (SIVIGILA) with the Clinical Health Information Systems of the different Health Care services Providers (Instituciones Prestadoras de Salud IPS) in the country.

Figure 2 describes de Business Use case Model for the proposed integration architecture. The two interrelated organizations, SIVIGILA and IPS, are each one represented as a package containing their main Business Use Cases (business processes). The business processes are derived from national health system policy documents, allowing a generic business description. The models are created using UML Uses Cases Diagrams.

By definition, SIVIGILA consists of health care institutions, protocols, norms and resources organized with the objective of supporting the systematic and ongoing collection (Event Collection Use Case), analysis and interpretation (Data Analysis Use Case), delivery (Data Notification Use Case) of health events necessary to support health promotion and prevention programs (Decision Making Support Use Case). The organizations in charge of SIVIGILA are the Public Health Authorities at the different levels of the Health System: the Ministry of Health (Ministerio de Protección Social), concretely the National Public Health Office; the Territorial Public Health Authorities (decentralized system) such us local, municipal and regional offices; and associated intuitions such as the National Institute of Health (Instituto Nacional de Salud). The external users of the system (actors) are Pan-American Health Organization, Health Services Administrators, IPS -which constitutes the interface with Clinical Information Systems-, and any other organization interested in public health information for decision making. SIVIGILA supports the notification of any kind of public health event (epidemiological, risk factors, conditions, services delivery).

IPS are public and private institutions (hospitals, clinics, laboratories, primary care establishments, doctor's offices) offering individual health care services including diagnosis, treatment, control, rehabilitation and even supporting promotion and prevention programs. The actors are: the citizens (users), Ministry of Health, Health Services Administrators, and Territorial Public Health Authorities.

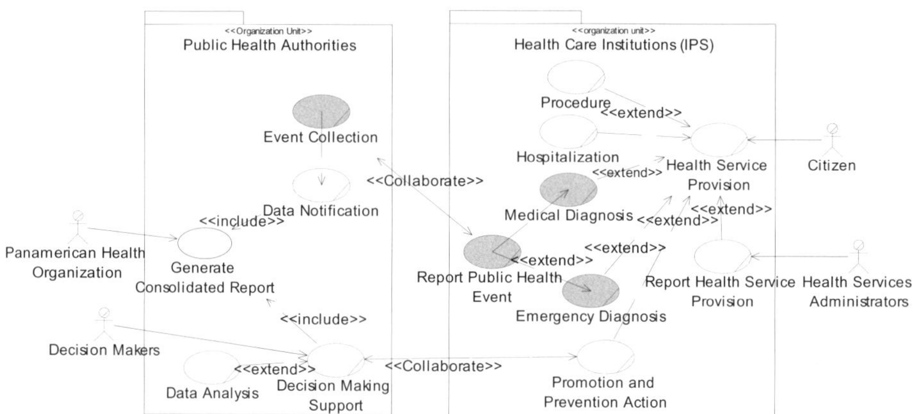

Figure 2. The Architecture Use Cases Model

Figure 2 identifies the Business Use Cases for each cooperating organization. The interaction of the Public Health and Clinical domains is prescribed by the direct collaboration between the pairs of use cases: Event Collection and Report Public Health Event, and Decision Making support and Promotion and Prevention Action. Due to complexity of the business processes, the business architecture is restricted to the collaboration among the Event Collection Use Case with the Report Public Health Event. The notification of events is limited to the reporting of communicable diseases.

4.2. Business Analysis Model

The Business Analysis Model provides details on the Business Use Cases, by defining the process's participants (Business Workers, Business Entities), the most important events (Business Events), the collaboration among participants (Business Use Cases Realizations) and the business policies (Business Rules).

The UML Sequence Diagram in Figure 3 represents the collaboration among entities within the Business Use Cases Report Public Health Event and Medical Diagnosis. The collaboration starts when the Medical Doctor suspects the presence of a communicable disease. He revises the Public Health protocol allocating the correspondent data for that event, and confirming the case. Immediately after, the Doctor registers de diagnosis in both, the Patient Medical Record and The Provided Services register. Finally, he sends a notification of the event to the Surveillance

Responsible in the IPS, who creates an Event Report according to the reporting forms established in SIVIGILA. The report is finally send to the Public Health Authority in the jurisdiction.

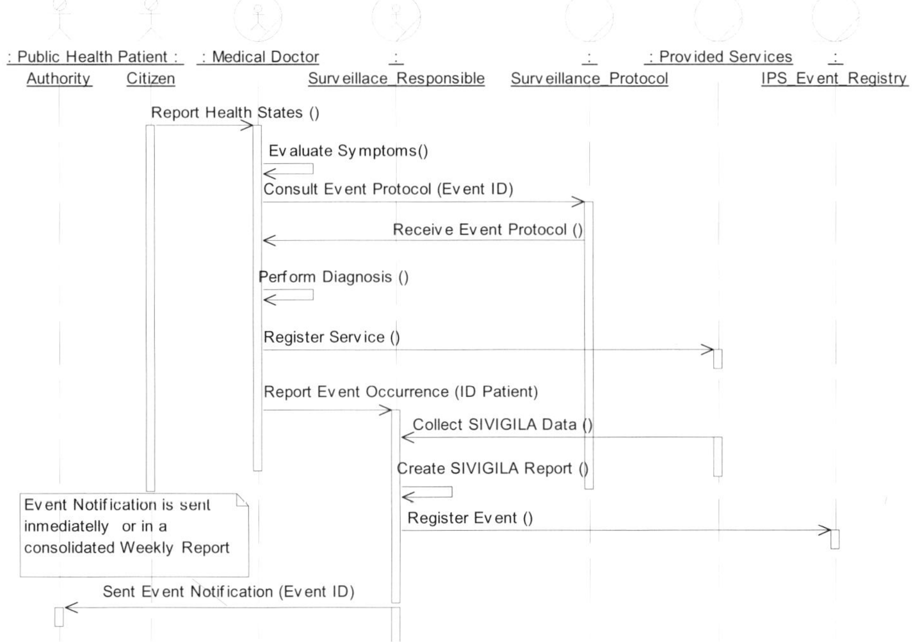

Figure 3. Use Case Realization for Report Public Health Event

The sequence Diagram in Figure 4 represents the collaboration among entities within the Business Use Cases Event Collection. After the Event Collection Responsible has received an Event Notification Message, he confirms that the same event has not been reported before and registers it in the Sivigila Event Registry.

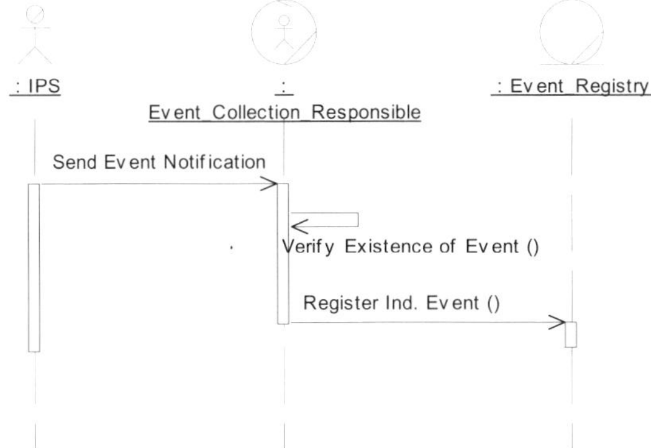

Figure 4. Use Case Realization for Event Collection

Business Rules for the Use Case Report Public Health Event

According to the Policies defined in the National Normative for SIVIGILA [10], IPS are obliged to:

1. Identify and confirm any public heath event according to the public health protocol for each case.
2. Report an Event immediately after its occurrence, in case of events classified as of immediate reporting.
3. Report weekly those Events classified as of Periodical Notification.
4. Send a consolidated report every week to the Public Health Authority in its jurisdiction.
5. Provide a local repository of Cases.
6. Guarantee the confidentiality, quality, accuracy and suitability of information.

Business Rules for the Use Case Public Health Event Collection

Correspondently, Public Health Authorities are obliged to:

1. Guarantee the human resources, infrastructure and technical resources for the Event collection.
2. Have a local repository of Cases.
3. Guarantee the confidentiality, quality, accuracy and suitability of information.

Most of the rules are already specified in the Use Cases and Sequence Diagrams. Some others such confidentiality, quality, suitability are quality requirements are specified in other system models developed in the following stages of the development process.

5. The Information Architecture

5.1. The Analysis Model

The RUP proposes the use of Class Diagrams and its correspondent Glossary to describe the information semantics.

The information Model from the IPS System is primary expressed by the Provided Services Business Entity. The structure of such information is represented in the Class Diagram in figure 5 and is based on a national normative that specifies the information that needs to be reported by IPS to the Health Care Administrators (Public and Private Health Insurance Companies) about the services they offer [11]. The Principal Class is Health Service which models a health service offered by the IPS. The types of services offered as presented as specializations of the Health Service Class: Medical Appointment, Procedure, Hospitalization and Emergency Treatment. The Health Service is associated to a patient (Class Person). Other classes in the model represent demographic data for the class Patient.

Respectively, the Business Entities Event Registry and Surveillance Protocol, characterize the information model for the SIVILA System. The UML Class Diagram is shown in figure 6. The principal Class in the model is Event which describes the data defined for a communicable disease, according to the national policy for communicable diseases structure and flow information [12]. The event is associated to the IPS which reports it, a Patient who is affected by that event and Place of occurrence. The class Epidemiological Week represents the seven-day period within the disease outbreak is notified. The Panamerican-Health Organization (PAHO) divides the 365 days of the calendar year into epidemiological weeks, for the sake of diseases surveillance reporting.

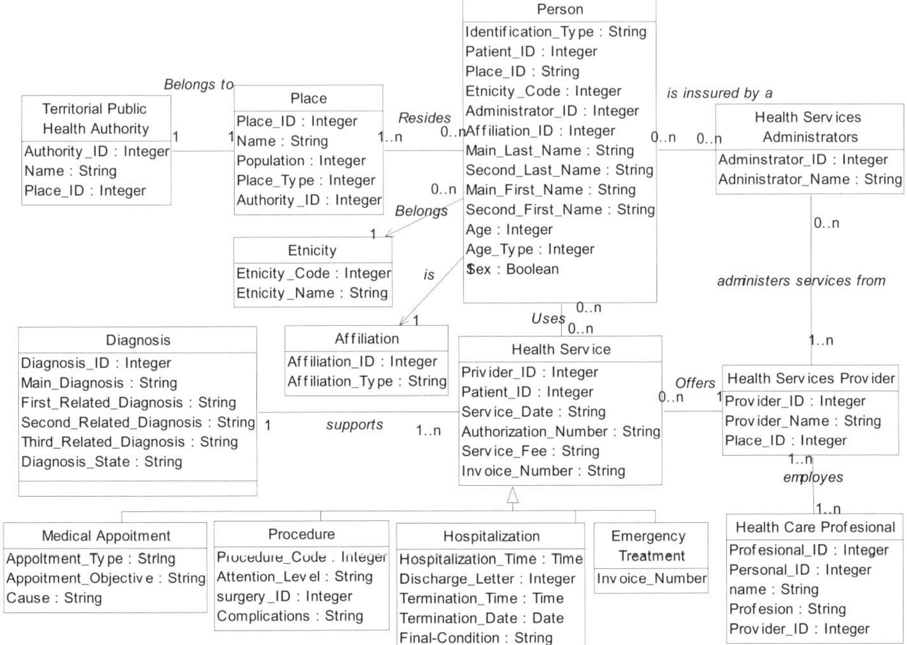

Figure 5. IPS Information Model

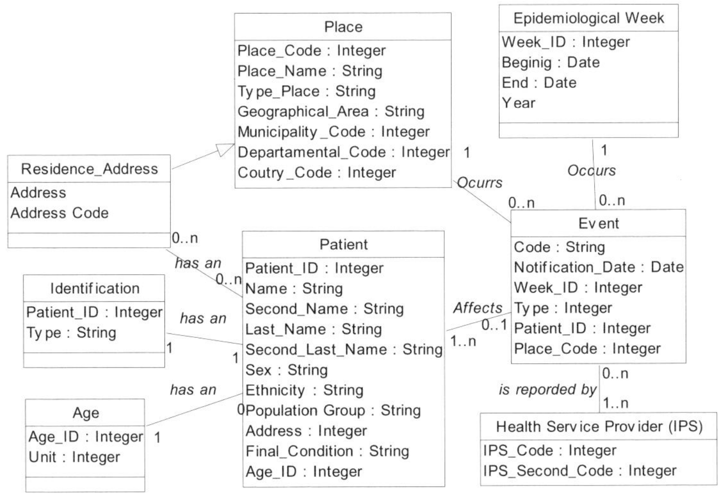

Figure 6. SIVIGILA Information Model

6. Using the Specifications for Developing Semantically Interoperable services and components

The definition of a business architecture capturing the business essence, but ignoring the ICT perspective, is essential to understand and describe semantic integration. The proposed business architecture clearly defines the business process, business and rules of the two interrelated domains overcoming the aforementioned difficulties in integration. Besides, based on the Business Architecture, the semantics of the information is defined in the Information Architecture. These two architectural views are the bases for describing any semantically interoperable solution (IT application, services or components) which in terms of the HIS-DF methodology constitutes the computational architecture.

The Computational Architecture is very dependent on the interoperability model defined in the HIS requirements. It can be as simple as an integration component which performs a direct schema matching between the Clinical and Public Health Information models, or a more flexible solution where interoperable services are designed, based on standardized domain ontologies or reference information models e.g. HL7 Reference Information model (RIM). Figure 6 represents both interoperability models. Notice that despite the ontology-based Integration Services is more open, flexible, scalable; the level of semantic mapping is still dependent on the semantically consistent description of the schemas described for each interacting system. The semantics are defined by the information models as previously explained in the information architecture.

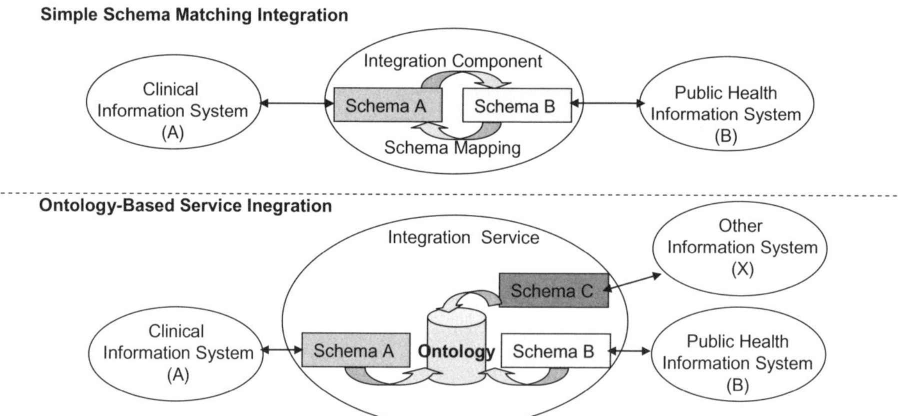

Figure 7. Interoperability models for the computational architecture, after [13].

Table 1, an example simple of schema matching for realizing integration between SIVIGILA and IPS Information Models, describes the mapping from the IPS Information Classes towards the Class Event in the SIVIGILA Information model. The Event.Code Attribute matches to one of the four types of diagnosis defined in the Diagnosis Class of the IPS Information model, thus allowing the direct event capture from the Provided Services register in the IPS. Other Attributes in the Class Event are captured from the Classes HealthService and HealthServicesProvider. The Attribute Event.Week does not need a match in the IPS Model because it is locally defined according to the Epidemiological Calendar defined by PAHO.

The mapping can be further used in the development of an Integration component to automate the Event reporting process by directly extracting the Event data from the Services Provided registers.

Table 1. Extract of SIVIGILA and IPS Information Models Matching.

Class Event SIVIGILA	Classes in IPS
Event.Code	Diagnosis.Main_Diagnosis OR Diagnosis.First_Related_Diagnosis OR Diagnosis. Second_Related_Diagnosis OR Diagnosis. Third_Related_Diagnosis
Event.Notification_Date	HealthService.Service_Date
Event.Week_ID	Does not apply
Event.Patient_ID	HealthService.Patient_ID
Event.Place_Code	HealthServicesProvider.Place_ID

7. Discussion and Conclusion

Semantically interoperable health information systems have to be able to effectively share information. Therefore, knowledge representation regarding used domain concepts, terms, and relationships must be harmonized. The proposed Business and Informational Architecture formalizes the Clinical and Public Health Information sharing, in the context of the Colombian National Integrated System.

The proposed architecture is normalized because it is based on national policy documents, constraining business process, rules and information semantics. Also the semantics of information is expressed in a standard language that is UML. Having formalized the representation of business process, concepts and rules, it is easier for stakeholders (Business Actors, Users, Systems Analyst, Developers, etc.) to "talk" a common language, avoiding semantic misunderstandings.

UML diagrams (e.g. Class Diagrams, Sequence Diagrams) have limitations for modeling knowledge, however. Combining natural and graphical languages, UML provides complete syntaxes but lacks of strict semantically control, many times causing ambiguities. As a complementary approach, The OCL language is a formal specification that allows describing additional constraints that normally are expressed in UML diagrams in natural language. In addition, more complex formal languages can be used to describe the semantics of information facilitating intelligent semantic interoperability (e.g. First Order Logics FOL, Resource Description Framework RDF; Web Ontology Language OWL). However, the more formal the specification, the more difficult for domain experts (e.g. health professionals) and even average system modelers to get involved in specification design. A good approach to maintain a compromise between the level of formalization of models, and the use of domain knowledge is to harmonize UML diagrams with domain reference models, terminologies and vocabulary. HIS-DF provides the development framework for such approach, including reference domain knowledge (e.g. HL7 Information Models) in the architecture design.

It was also demonstrated how the architecture is the basis for designing semantically interoperable services and components. After understanding the business process and the information semantics; the HIS service architecture can be further developed. For the Colombian IIS scenario, a Computational Integration model based on schema mapping was described. This is the more simple approach for the semantic integration of SIVIGILA and IPS, due to the fact that the business process and rules are governed by a single institution, the Colombian Ministry of Health. This prevents components/services providers and integrators for semantic misinterpretations, because they can refer to national policy documents to resolve semantic inconsistencies.

8. Acknowledgments

This work has been supported by the Bavarian Research Foundation; project ARCO-HIS: Applied Research & Cooperation on Architectures for Health Information Systems and Components, and the University of Cauca under contract number 136 October 2003.

9. References

[1]   G.A. Decatur, Public Health Informatics Institute. Public Health Opportunities in Health Information Exchange, Public Health Informatics Institute, 2005.

[2]   M. St-Pierre, D. Reinharz, J.B. Gauthier, Organizing the public health-clinical health interface: theoretical bases, Med Health Care Philos 9(1) (2006) 97-106

[3]   NHII. The National Health Information Infrastructure. http://aspe.hhs.gov/sp/nhii/ Last accessed January 2007.

[4]   A Strategy for Building the National Health Information Infrastructure, Report and Recommendations from the National Committee on Vital and Health Statistics, Washington D. C, 2001.

[5]   PHIN. The Public Health Information Network Functions and Specifications. http://www.cdc.gov/phin/architecture/index.html. Last accessed January 2007.

[6]   H. Rodriguez, C. Rueda. Sistema de Vigilancia en Salud Pública: Propuesta Conceptual y Tecnológica. Organización Panamericana de la Salud y Ministerio de la Protección Social. Technical Report, Bogota, 2005.

[7]   D.M López, B Blobel, A Development Framework for Semantically Interoperable Health Information Systems, Submitted to the Internationally Journal of Medical Informatics (ISSN 1386-5056), 2007.

[8]   The Rational Unified Process. http://www-306.ibm.com/software/awdtools/rup/ Last accessed January 2007.

[9]   Resolución 2542 de 1998. Sistema Integral de Información para el Sistema General de Seguridad Social en Salud – SIIS, Ministerio de la Protección Social, República de Colombia, 1998.

[10]   Decreto 3518 de 2006. Sistema de Vigilancia en Salud Pública, Ministerio de la Protección Social, República de Colombia, 2006.

[11] Resolución 3374 de 2000. Datos Básicos que deben reporter los prestadores de servicios de salud y las administradoras de planes de beneficios, Ministerio de la Protección Social. República de Colombia, 2000.

[12] Sivigila 2007. Subsistema de Información para la Vigilancia de Enfermedades Transmisibles, Flujo y Estructura de Archivos Planos, Instituto Nacional de Salud, República de Colombia, 2007.

[13] G. Vetere M. Lenzerini. Models for semantic interoperability in service-oriented architectures. IBM Systems Journal, 44(4) (2005) 887 – 903.

Medical and Care Compunetics 4
L. Bos and B. Blobel (Eds.)
IOS Press, 2007

Ten Theses on Clinical Ontologies

Stefan Schulz [1] and Holger Stenzhorn
Department of Medical Informatics, Freiburg University Hospital, Germany

Abstract: We present ten principles for clinical ontologies that describe the authors' opinion about what should be understood by the notion of clinical ontologies and what not. In contrast to clinical terminology systems, clinical ontologies are considered to be semantic reference systems and for that – first of all – strive to account for the properties of the domain entities themselves and their proper formal definitions – rather than just linking clinical terms together.

Keywords: Clinical Ontologies, Knowledge Representation

Introduction

Issues concerning the representation of knowledge in clinical contexts have been intensively discussed in the Medical Informatics community over the last two decades [1]. The challenge to provide semantic reference has thus been met by a variety of different systems of classifications, terminologies and ontologies, covering the broad range of clinical disciplines and also outreaching to the realm of molecular medicine and genomics. The impressive growth of the Unified Medical Language system (UMLS) [2] and the development of the Open Biomedical Ontologies (OBO) [3] give particular witness to this effort. However, most of these terminologies and ontologies have been created in purely application- and purpose-driven contexts and are therefore not geared towards semantic interoperability. The latter, however, constitutes a pressing requirement to the integrated care paradigm where patient data should be easily interchangeable across institutional boundaries.

This lack of interoperability is – in our opinion – at least partly due to a lack of agreement on what terminology systems are actually supposed to encode. So far, there is only a vague understanding on what the notions of "terms", "classes" and "concepts" are really referring to in current terminology systems.

Only during the last couple of years, a more principled discussion about some of the more fundamental issues has been under way, mainly driven by philosophers and computer scientists. Although this discussion has brought about some controversy, it has fertilized and ameliorated the way biomedical terminology systems have been conceived, built, maintained and used.

The main purpose of this paper is now to focus on the role of biomedical ontologies as representational artifacts being a special kind of terminology systems. Aware of the difficulties, the use of the notions "ontology" and "terminology system" can cause (for either, different and contradicting definitions can be found in literature

---

[1] Corresponding Author: Stefan Schulz, Department of Medical Informatics, Freiburg University Hospital, Stefan-Meier-Str. 26, 79104 Freiburg, Germany. Email: stschulz@uni-freiburg.de

[4]), this paper tries to streamline and clarify the notion of "ontology" in the context of integrated clinical care.

Ten Principles

The nature, purposes and limitations of clinical ontologies are presented here as a sequence of ten principle. They represent the current view of the authors and are being formulated to stimulate a clarifying discussion. They neither claim to represent a consensus among medical informaticians or terminologists, nor do they constitute a fully consistent system of thinking.

I. Terminology systems provide semantic reference

It is generally accepted that terminology systems (in a broad sense, cf. [5]) should provide some kind of semantic reference. This means that they support the relation of term meanings. Terms are the entities of language in a given domain, they may be simple or complex words, as well as multi-word strings. Terminology systems relate terms that share the same meaning (synonymy), broader and narrower, as well as related meanings. It should be emphasized here that terminologies are term-centered, i.e. that terms constitute their basic elements.

II. Ontologies are semantic type hierarchies to support organizing domain entities

Among the numerous definitions of what an ontology constitutes, the following definition is preferred for our context: Ontologies are representational artifacts whose representational units are intended to designate classes or types in reality and to relate them to each other [6]. It is important to highlight here that the single entities represented in an ontology are not terms. Nor are concrete objects, i.e. individuals (instances, particulars) represented in the ontology proper. However, one of the main purposes of ontology is to provide a means to classify exactly those entities by defining and organizing their semantic type.

The main classification principle of ontologies is the taxonomic order. Taxonomies relate types with their superordinate types. This hierarchy-forming relation is generally named *is_a*. As an example, the type "artery" is a superordinate one of "carotid artery" and the latter stands in turn to "common carotid artery" in a supertype relationship. Note that *is_a* must not be mistaken for the relation *instance_of*, which relates a concrete object to its type. Although it usual to state in natural language that "Tibble *is a* cat.", the individual entity with the name "Tibble" is related to the entity type cat by the relation *instance_of* (and hence the sentence would be "Tibble *is an instance* of the type cat.").

Fig. 1 on the next page depicts the relations between entities, their types and their denoting terms.

III. Ontologies represent universal truths

One of the major misconceptions about ontologies is that they are directly suited to represent large parts of clinical and scientific knowledge, i.e. the symptoms of a disease, the probability of a certain risk or the side effects of some drugs. But on the contrary, this is not the case: (Formal) ontologies should only represent what is assumed to be universally true, i.e. that it always the case that an artery is a blood vessel or that human blood contains erythrocytes.

Formally, ontologies provide and combine universal statements about all instances of a given type such as:

- All Xs are Ys
- For all Xs, there is some Z that…

For example, all instances of the type carotid artery are instances of the type artery. Or, for all instances of the type common carotid there is some instance of the type aorta which it is connected to. So it becomes obvious that ontologies are not the right place to represent probabilistic, vague or uncertain knowledge. An important corollary of these universality assumptions is the well-known principle of inheritance. Each property defined for some type in an ontology is inherited by all of its subtypes, as well as of its instances (and the instances of the subtypes).

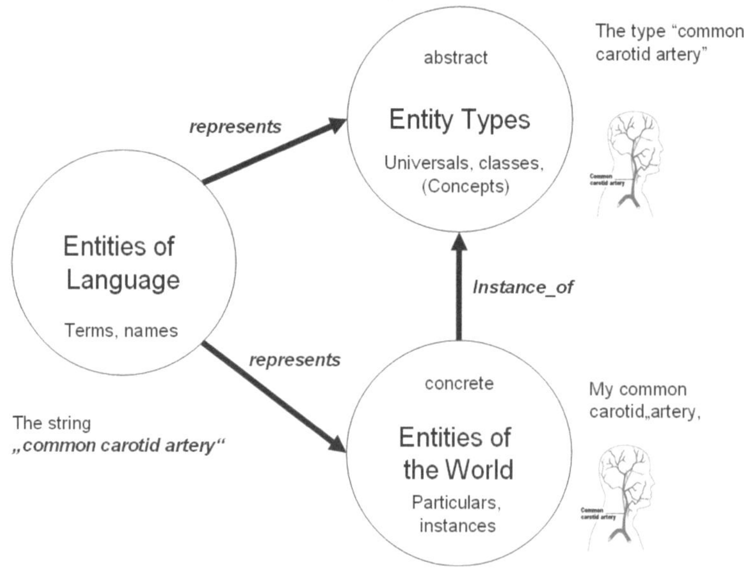

Figure 1. World entities, their types and terms denoting them

Wherever this principle does not seem to hold there is evidence of a major misunderstanding of what an ontology is supposed to be. For instance, one could add a prevalence value to disease type such as "0.5%" to the disease type "Schizophrenia". It is obvious that the same value cannot be inherited by its subtype "Bipolar Schizophrenia". But this is not an exception to the inheritance rule. The error is rather to consider prevalence as an inherent property of a disease. In contradistinction, prevalence is a property of a population with regard to a disease but not of the disease proper.

IV. Ontology types extend to classes of world entities

Types in ontologies are often referred to as classes. But as Fig. 1 depicts, classes are indeed different from types: A class is the collection of all entities in the world that instantiate a certain type. But therefore, classes and types are actually closely related. The class of entities is also considered to be the extension of a given type. In contrast to mathematical sets, classes can vary in respect to their members across time. For example, the class of E.coli (i.e. the extension of the type E.coli) remains the same although it constantly gains and loses instances. Due to the direct dependence between classes and types, usually the just described distinction between the two is not made in practical ontology engineering.

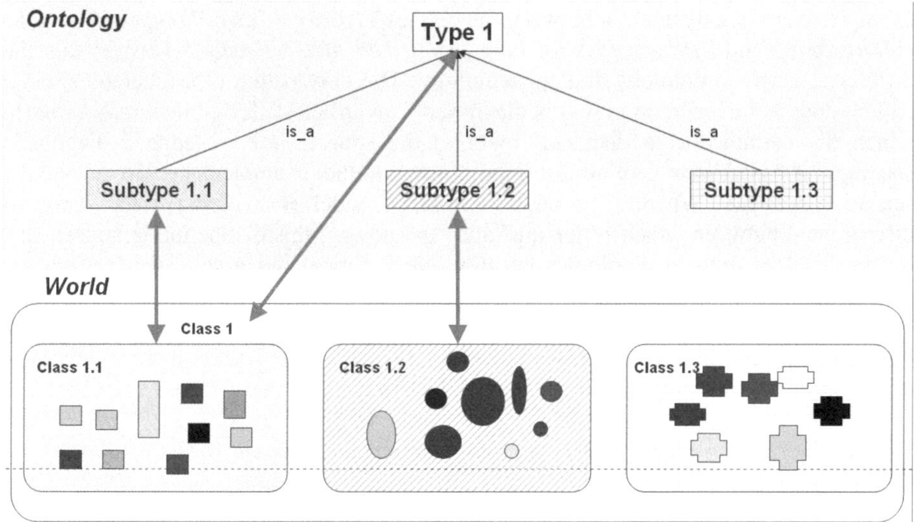

Figure 2. Types (above), Classes (below), Instances (rectangles, ellipses, polygons)

V. Ontologies organize individual entities – not concepts

Whereas the use of the notions "type" and "class" is more recent in medical informatics, the notion of "concept" has a much longer tradition. The problem with the latter is that it is applied in several different senses [7]. On the one hand "concept" is meant to stand for "entities of thought" which is mostly considered to represent word meanings, such as discussed in the first section and is, therefore, characteristic for language-centered terminology systems. On the other hand it is also used as a synonym of what has been introduced above as "type". Finally, from a computer science point of view, "concept" often stands for unary predicates in knowledge representation languages such as OWL-DL [8]. For the sake of clarity we avoid the use of the word "concept" when referring to ontologies in the sense we have defined them.

VI. Ontologies represent what is – information models represent what we know about

The task of representing clinical facts requires that the following two aspects are kept strictly separated.

1. Universal truths about entities of the world as referred to by domain terms
2. Known facts about concrete clinical cases.

Whereas the first task corresponds to what is understood by ontologies, the second one is to be embarked upon by information models. It involves not only the facts as they are in the world but also the knowledge about these facts. In terminology systems as currently used, these epistemological aspects are often mixed up [9]. In ICD 10, for example, there is a distinction between the classes *"Tuberculosis of lung, confirmed by culture only"* and *"Tuberculosis of lung, confirmed histologically"*. This reveals the difference between ontology and epistemology: The very nature of a tuberculosis in a patient does not depend on how it is diagnosed. Nevertheless, for clinical reasoning (in which the certainty of a diagnosis matters) the source of knowledge a diagnostic statement is based upon is of utmost importance. Another example is how to encode the sex of a patient. Whereas in an information model it makes perfect sense to discriminate between "male", "female" and "unknown", this distinction is nonsensical on the level of clinical ontologies because every patient has a sex, which might be known or unknown but obviously does not change according to the fact of it being known or unknown. The relation between clinical information models and ontologies has recently received an increased attention in the context of clinical archetypes, openEHR, HL-7 Version 3 and SNOMED CT [10].

VII. Practical requirements may justify controlled deviations from the "true path"

In many cases, user requirements for clinical application ontologies can make it difficult to fully follow the "pure doctrine" of ontology design, since the restriction to universal truth obviates the representation of many shared assumptions that are important in a clinical context. For instance, it may be required to classify certain health related states as risk factors for diseases. If we declare "Hypertension" as a "Risk factor for aneurysm rupture" in an ontology using an *is_a* link, we certainly go beyond the representation of universal truths, since not every hypertension causes a myocardial infarction, and "Risk factor" is rather a role ascribed by humans than a universal type. Mistaking roles for subtype relations, also called is_a overloading is a common error in ontology design [11]. For practical reasons such a routine may be, however, justified. Nevertheless it is recommended that such assertions be strictly separated from the ontology proper. In the @neurist ontology [12] this dichotomy has been made explicit by introducing a separate branch with the root node "Particular in context", as depicted in **Figure 3**.

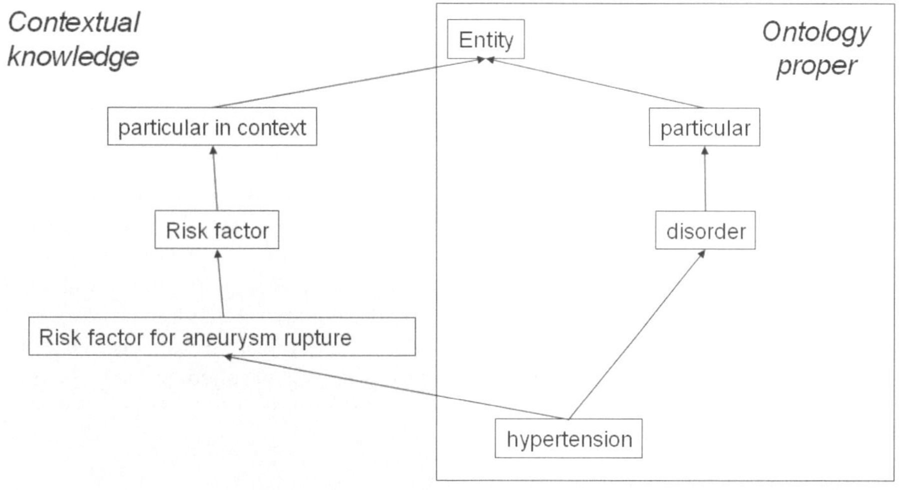

Figure 3. Epistemological knowledge as separate branch in the @neurist ontology

VIII. Ontologies need to be linked to dictionaries

Ontologies in a strict sense (i.e. as understood as taxonomies of types) do not incorporate any lexical or terminological information at all. Still the naming of the ontology nodes should be self-explanatory and employ terms commonly used in the domain. However ambiguous formulations that regularly exist in the domain should be avoided. Furthermore, special characters should be avoided and the naming conventions of the underlying language must be followed. This means that ontology labels are not to be mistaken for actual terms (even if they are named "terms" in several ontologies). Since each node can have one name only, synonyms cannot (and should not) be managed at this level. So it is necessary to provide a link between an ontology and a dictionary where each dictionary entry corresponds to a domain term and is linked to one (in the case of polysemous terms, to two or more) nodes in the ontology. Synonyms are linked to the same node. Such a dictionary is a separate data structure and it is not an integral part of the ontology itself.

IX. Ontology users need not to see the whole "engine"

From the user perspective, the internal structure of an ontology can easily lead to confusion and misunderstandings. As users are used to browse simple hierarchical trees from top to bottom, they may be overwhelmed by the complexity of the structural relations between all the types of the ontology. They may also get puzzled by the terms characterizing the upper level, such as "dependent continuant", "quality region" or "fiat object part" as provided by upper level ontologies such as BFO [13,14] or DOLCE [15]. Still, such upper ontologies are necessary for the organization of the ontology into well-defined categories, necessary for enforcing consistency of its content. However, these categories do not correspond to terms commonly used in the domain and could therefore – at a first sight – deemed superfluous by ontology users. It is therefore neither necessary nor desirable that the whole internal "machinery" be visible for ontology users (i.e. system developers and domain experts that link to ontologies when creating clinical information models, entry forms, etc.). They should only see those parts of the ontology they need for their respective work and be provided with customized user interface to support them with their tasks.

X. Ontologies should provide tailored terminology services

The concept of terminology server / service has become popular in the nineties where specifications and use cases have been formulated [16,17,18]. Under the new viewpoint of clinical ontologies this concept should be taken up and adapted to the current requirements. End users should benefit from tailored ontology based terminology services without the need to any access to the actual ontology (cf. the last section). End users just create and select terms. The terminology service in turn then takes care of linking these terms to the ontology and of the provision of controlled terms to the user (cf. **Figure 4**).

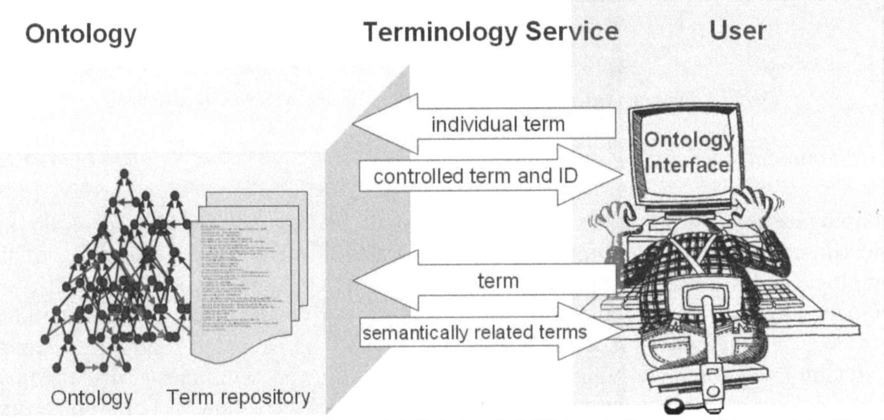

Figure 4. Terminology services mediating between the ontology and the end user

Conclusion

In this paper we presented ten principles which we believe can clarify what (formal) clinical ontologies are, what they are not and how they should be used. These principles should be applied to any artifact using formal means for representing world entities in the domain of interest, thus providing a logically and philosophically founded basis for the meaning of clinical terms. This principle should be applied especially to SNOMED Clinical Terms (CT) [19] as an emerging terminology covering whole range of clinical medicine. SNOMED CT has still a long way to go in order to fulfill common ontological standards [20]. To this end the ten principles presented here could be useful cornerstones and guidelines.

Acknowledgements

This work was carried out in the framework of the @neurIST Integrated Project, which is co-financed by the European Commission through the contract No. IST-027703 (http://www.aneurist.org).

References

1. J. J. Cimino. Desiderata for controlled medical vocabularies in the twenty-first century. Methods of Information in Medicine, 37(4/5):394–403, 1998.
2. UMLS. Unified Medical Language System. Bethesda, MD: National Library of Medicine, 2007.
3. Open Biological Ontologies (OBO) [http://obo.sourceforge.net], 2007. Last accessed March 6th, 2007.
4. W. Kuśnierczyk. Nontological Engineering. FOIS 2006 – Proceedings of the 4th Intl Conf on Formal Ontology in Information Systems; 2006. p. 39-50.
5. R. Cornet R, N. F. De Keizer, A. Abu-Hanna. A Framework for Characterizing Terminological Systems. Methods of Information in Medicine, 2006; 45: 253-266.
6. S. Schulz and I. Johansson. Continua in biological systems. The Monist, 2007, accepted for publication.
7. B. Smith, "Beyond Concepts, or: Ontology as Reality Representation", In: A. C. Varzi and L. Vieu, editors, Formal Ontology in Information Systems. Proceedings of the 3rd International. Amsterdam: IOS Press, 2004, 73–84.
8. I. Horrocks, P. F. Patel-Schneider and F. van Harmelen, "From SHIQ and RDF to OWL: The making of a Web Ontology Language", Journal of Web Semantics, 1(1), 7–26, 2003.
9. O: Bodenreider, B: Smith, and A: Burgun. The ontology-epistemology divide: A case study in medical terminology. In Achille C. Varzi and Laure Vieu, editors, *Formal Ontology in Information Systems. Proceedings of the 3rd International Conference - FOIS 2004*, pages 185–195. Amsterdam etc.: IOS Press, 2004 .
10. A. Rector, R. Qamar, T. Marley. Binding Ontologies & Coding Systems to Electronic Health Records and Messages. In: Bodenreider O, editor. Formal Biomedical Knowledge Representation (KR-MED 2006) CEUR; 2006. p. 11-19.
11. N. Guarino and C. A. Welty. An overview of ONTOCLEAN. In Steffen Staab and Rudi Studer, editors, Handbook on Ontologies, International Handbooks on Information Systems, pages 151–171. Berlin: Springer, 2004.
12. S. Hanser, M. Boeker, K. Kumpf, P. Bijlenga, S. Schulz. Design of an Ontology on Cerebral Aneurysms: Representing the Conceptual Space of the @neurIST Project. Medinfo 2007 Congress, 20-24 August 2007, Brisbane, Australia. Accepted for publication.
13. P. Grenon and B. Smith. SNAP and SPAN. Towards dynamic spatial ontology. Spatial Cognition and Computation, 4:69–103, 2004.
14. P. Grenon, B. Smith, and L. Goldberg. Biodynamic ontology: applying BFO in the biomedical domain. In D. Pisanelli, editor, Studies in health technology and informatics, Vol. 102, pages 20–38, 2004.
15. A. Gangemi, N. Guarino, C. Masolo, and A. Oltramari. Sweetening ontologies with DOLCE. In A. Gómez-Pérez and V. R. Benjamins, editors, Proceedings of the 13th International Conference – EKAW 2002, volume 2473 of Lecture Notes in Artificial Intelligence, pages 166–181. Berlin: Springer, 2002.
16. A. L. Rector, W. D. Solomon, W. A. Nowlan, and T. Rush. A terminology server for medical language and medical information systems. Methods of Information in Medicine, 34(1/2):147–157, 1995.
17. C. G. Chute, P. L. Elkin, D. D. Sheretz, and M. S. Tuttle. Desiderata for a clinical terminology server. In N. M. Lorenzi, editor, AMIA'99 – Proceedings of the 1999 Annual Symposium of the American Medical Informatics Association. Transforming Health Care through Informatics: Cornerstones for a New Information Management Paradigm, pages 42–46. Washington, D.C., November 6-10, 1999. Philadelphia, PA: Hanley & Belfus, 1999.
18. J. Ingenerf and T. Diedrich. Notwendigkeit und Funktionalität eines Terminologieservers in der Medizin. Künstliche Intelligenz, 11(3):6–14, 1997.
19. SNOMED Clinical Terms. Northfield, IL: College of American Pathologists, 2007.
20. S. Schulz, B. Suntisrivaraporn, F. Baader. SNOMED CT's Problem List: Ontologists' and Logicians' Therapy Suggestions. Medinfo 2007 Congress, 20-24 August 2007, Brisbane, Australia. Accepted for publication.

Medical and Care Compunetics 4
L. Bos and B. Blobel (Eds.)
IOS Press, 2007

The Aspects of Safety in Future Care Settings

Peter PHAROW [a,1], Bernd G.M.E. BLOBEL [a] and Mario SAVASTANO [b]

[a] *eHealth Competence Center, University of Regensburg Medical Center, Germany*
[b] *National Research Council of Italy, Naples, Italy*

Abstract. Communication and cooperation processes in the growing healthcare and welfare domain require a well-defined set of security services provided by a standards-based interoperable security infrastructure. Any communication and collaboration procedures require a verifiable purpose. Without such a purpose for communicating with each other, there's no need to communicate at all. But security is not the only aspect that needs to carefully be investigated. More and more, aspects of safety, privacy, and quality get importance while discussing about future-proof health information systems and health networks – regardless whether local, regional and national ones or even pan-European networks. The patient needs to be moved into the center of each care process. During the course of the current paradigm change from an organization centered via a process-related to a person-centered healthcare and welfare system approach, different new technologies need to be applied in order to meet the new challenges arising from both legal and technical circumstances. International organizations like WHO, UNESCO and the European Parliament increasingly aim at enhancing the safety aspect in future care settings, and so do many projects and studies. Beside typical information and communication devices, extended use of modern IT technology in healthcare and welfare includes large medical devices like, e.g., CT, X-ray and MR but also very tiny devices like sensors worn or implemented in a person's clothing. Safety gets on top of the nations priority list for several reasons. The paper aims at identifying some of these reasons along with possible solutions on how to increase patient's awareness, confidence, and acceptance in future care settings.

Keywords. Security, Safety, Quality, Harmonization, Standardization, Policy

Introduction

Undoubtedly, an inevitable prerequisite for focusing on a high quality and efficient care performance in this 21st century is the establishment of well-developed and well-accepted job sharing models accompanied by extended collaboration and cooperation between all partners within the healthcare and welfare domain – both medical and non-medical ones. This paradigm is therefore called the "shared care" principle. Any communication and collaboration needs to be provided in a trustworthy and secure way based on an established information and communication technology (ICT) with an

---

[1] Corresponding Author: Peter Pharow, University of Regensburg Medical Center, eHealth Competence Center, Franz-Josef-Strauß-Allee 11, 93053 Regensburg, DE. Email: peter.pharow@ehealth-cc.de.

underlying reliable and liable extended security infrastructure providing all required technical and administrative (non-technical) services.

The combination of trustworthiness and reliability is closely related to the concepts of communication security and application security as depicted in figure 1 below. So security is therefore very important for future care concepts, but it is just one of the parameters all modern information systems need to deal with. Others are quality, safety, and privacy as well as ethical, social and societal conditions [1].

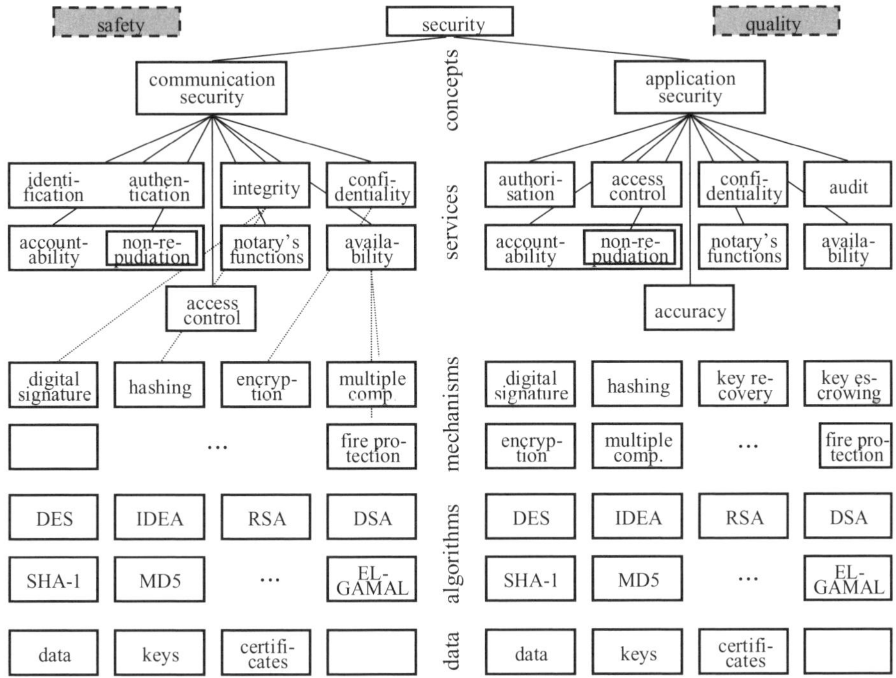

Figure 1. Concept-Service-Mechanism-Algorithm-Data Dependencies (after [1])

This paper intends to specifically deal with the paradigm change towards a personalized health services provision and its related safety and security measures. Different organizations world-wide go for enhanced and advanced consideration of different safety aspects especially from the patient's point of view. Another area to be discussed is the technology of devices. Regardless whether very large devices like CT, MI, or MR on the one hand or rather small (micro- and even nano-) devices like very tiny sensors: safety needs to be seen from different viewpoints: patient safety concerns physical, psychological and mental safety, mechanical safety, electrical safety, etc. Political and societal organizations consider safety of citizens and patients a core competency of their activities as their main goal is moving the patient into the center of healthcare and welfare workflow processes and procedures. Scientific organizations and associations like IMIA [2] and EFMI [3] address safety aspects in their various working groups. Last but not least, standards developing organizations (SDO) like ISO

TC 251 [4], CEN TC 251 [5], IEC [6], ITU [7], and ETSI [8] -just to name a few of them- have identified safety as one of the top priorities for their future work as well. A more detailed description of some of the mentioned categories as well as related -and partly implemented- standards and solutions can be found in [1], [9].

1. The Current Healthcare Paradigm Change and its Consequences

Collaboration is the very basis for any communication. Without a need to cooperate with other partners, there's no need at all to communicate any data. Knowledge allows getting information from data. Sending and receiving data is therefore just the first step. Understanding the message in a correct manner requires a certain level of interoperability between the communicating partners. Interoperability itself implies a number of different concepts, e.g. functional interoperability and internetworking, semantic interoperability and application gateways. Health information integration (eHealth) has established a demand for interoperability between clinical and healthcare stakeholders, systems and processes or workflows. Domain-specific communication and interoperability standards are well established meanwhile, but have to be supplied for extended trans-domain use.

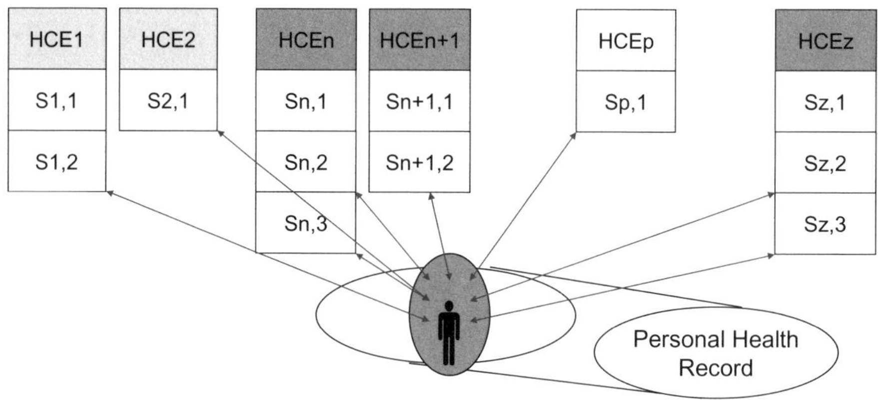

Figure 2. The Personal Health (pHealth) Paradigm (after [11])

The advanced concept of Personal Health (pHealth, see figure 2) is considered to even extend eHealth by the inclusion of devices like smart sensors, body-worn mobile systems and situation-specific activation of applications and human health professionals, thus providing personalized ubiquitous health services. Body Area Networks (BAN) and micro-systems are building blocks of future personalized health telematics infrastructures that extend existing interoperability concepts [10], [12].

Using devices in an extended way increases the demands towards safety. In this way, safety is not just a technical term any longer but gets into domains like ethics and psychology. Guaranteeing patients and citizens as well as health professionals not to get lost in a world of electrical and electronic devices regardless whether big or small requires even new health policies. The European Commission, e.g., aims at taking specific safety and quality measures into account for the years to come.

2. European Initiatives and Concepts for Health Safety and Quality

After a serious of preparatory measures starting in the 1980s, the European Commission launched an initiative: "eEurope 2002 - An Information Society for All" back in 1999 [13]. Intended to accelerate positive changes in the European Union, eEurope 2002 aimed to provide equal access to digital systems and services for all of Europe's citizens, to promote computer literacy and, crucially, to create a partnership environment between users and providers of systems, based on trust and enterprise. Its ultimate objective was therefore to bring everyone in Europe -every citizen, every school and every company- on-line as quickly as possible.

Building on the success of eEurope 2002, an Action Plan for eEurope 2005 was launched in June 2002 [14]. Its objective was to provide a favorable environment for the creation of new services and new jobs, to boost productivity, to modernize public services, and to give everyone the opportunity to participate in the global information society. The result was intended to "make the EU the most competitive and dynamic knowledge-based economy" with improved employment and social cohesion by the end of year 2010.

The eEurope 2005 Action Plan proposed policy measures to bring about modern safe and secure on-line public services. Concerning e-Health it further proposed actions on Electronic Health Cards, Health Information Networks and on-line Health Services. The European Committee for Standardization CEN [5] was expected to consider the respective standardization requirements to support all these different actions. The International Standardization Organization ISO [4] has undertaken very similar standardization activities.

A healthy living and working environment for all European citizens in an inclusive society is still the overriding goal of the European Union. To further improve individual health and well-being, access to reliable high quality and safe services, quality assurance and benchmarking, public health measures and surveillance, and knowledge generation and decision support, connected health systems -that is, fully interoperable technical solutions and intensive collaboration of health and care providers- are fundamental prerequisites. It is these connected health systems that will underpin better health services organization and delivery, and improve citizens' awareness of how to prevent disease and preserve good health.

The European eHealth Action Plan, adopted in April 2004, provides a mid-term roadmap for the development of interoperable healthcare systems in and across Member States [15]. To make further progress towards health systems and services connected at local, regional, national and pan-European level further concrete steps are urgently needed. This is necessary to avoid implementation of costly isolated and stand-alone solutions that necessitates large investments in order to render them interoperable. Priority topics must be pursued rigorously in order to reach the goals of the eHealth Action Plan, and to ensure the competitiveness of the European healthcare industry in a global market situation by moving towards a single eHealth market in Europe, while respecting Member States' responsibilities in delivery and organization of their national healthcare systems.

Steps are set out to reach these goals for the benefit of Europe, its citizens and its societies, thus supporting the longer-term objectives of the Lisbon strategy. In the short term, the result of this process will be a set of guidelines on European eHealth Interoperability. In the medium term, implementation sites (large scale pilots) will be designed. In the long term, an agreed process for implementation of interoperable solutions in Member States and throughout the Union will be set up. A coordinated effort by Member States representatives and all stakeholders -citizens, health professionals, and relevant organizations- accompanied by a wide consultation of interested parties, is necessary in order to agree on such a set of guidelines. This initiative will enable easy and fast access to a citizen's electronic health record or a targeted extract from it (e.g. a patient summary, medication data, or emergency data), from any place, and at any necessary time, in Europe and even beyond.

3. Framework on Connected Health: Quality and Safety for European Citizens

Interoperability itself is not just a technical matter. It has a set of legal, ethical, economic, social, medical, organizational, and cultural aspects. To comprehensively approach eHealth interoperability, all these aspects need to be addressed. It could be argued that, under certain conditions, the technical requisites for eHealth interoperability may be the ones that can be more easily fulfilled in this complex equation [9], [16]. But eHealth is considered a much wider approach.

In September 2006, a report was therefore published written with input from both the i2010 sub-group on eHealth and the eHealth stakeholders' group [17], [18]. The report focuses on the overriding theme of eHealth interoperability: eHealth systems must be interoperable to facilitate and foster the collaboration of health professionals and healthcare establishments (HCE) as well as between health professionals and their patients. To achieve this, national/regional representatives and stakeholders must closely cooperate in order to resolve the various associated legal, organizational and policy issues.

Member States are directing their health safety policies to subscribe increasingly to the paradigm of citizen-centered and patient-centered services. This implies several activities that are: to gather, analyze and disseminate relevant quality information for policy-making; support the need to improve patient safety along the full continuum of care; support healthcare professionals in their daily work and provide citizens with tools that enable them to become both well-informed and self-assured patients. All this will be aided by the provision of optimal medical services independent of their location within the European Union. Privacy is the basis of all these services [19].

To achieve that vision, health, social care and other providers must no longer work in isolation, but need to collaborate as a team, if necessary beyond their national and linguistic borders; information and communication technologies can facilitate this cooperation. It is vital that parties can have access to, and share, securely up-to-date information on a citizen's health status, data which they can correctly understand and act on. Without an appropriate information and communication technologies-based infrastructure this goal can't be reached. Full interoperability is the key to success not only in the field of safety.

The main reasons for accelerating the introduction of interoperable eHealth solutions in a collaborative and coordinated way in Europe are the increasing mobility of European citizens, the aging population and the empowerment of citizens, the continuity of care and the creation of a bigger, European-wide market for many health applications and technologies. This will lead to the increased opportunity for provision of new services, new jobs, and new technologies [17].

Developed with major input from experts of both the i2010 sub-group on eHealth and the eHealth stakeholders' group, the report on European eHealth interoperability contributes to enhancing the continuation of care and ensuring that the flow of information between primary care, secondary care, and tertiary care is promoted, on behalf of better patient care, safety and quality of life as well as better or new citizen-oriented services. A systematic approach, that establishes a collaborative network among all health professionals and organizations, will be extremely beneficial for achieving the proposed goals [17], [18], [19], [20].

Health technologies should also be used to reinforce the information tools available to citizens, helping them for example to inform themselves better about health issues, particularly preventative health measures and safety procedures.

The European eHealth Action Plan of April 2004 provides a mid-term roadmap for the development of these interoperable eHealth solutions in and across Member States. To progress towards interconnected and collaborative eHealth services at the regional, national and pan-European level, further concrete and structured steps are needed.

The report outlines priority issues which must be pursued rigorously to reach all health systems goals like "improving patient safety, encouraging well-informed citizens and patients on health matters, and creating high-quality health systems and services" and, at the same time, face international competition in the eHealth sector. It focuses on the overriding theme of comprehensive eHealth interoperability: eHealth solutions must be interoperable to facilitate and foster the collaboration of health professionals and healthcare organizations; the various stakeholders must cooperate and involve themselves to resolve legal, organizational and policy barriers.

Member States have realized that implementing eHealth interoperability is a long-term process requiring a sustained commitment with respect to political involvement and resources. Achieving interoperability not only for increasing safety in healthcare and welfare workflow is seen as a goal that can be achieved only gradually "application by application" and is often envisioned in a ten-year framework.

The report recommends necessary steps to reach those goals for the benefit of Europe, its citizens and its societies, thereby supporting long-term objectives. These cover the domains of political, social, and regulatory issues; appropriate processes and structures to achieve eHealth interoperability; technical standardization; semantic interoperability; and certification and authentication processes. The result of this process will be a series of guidelines set on eHealth interoperability, as well as an agreed process to uniquely implement these guidelines in the various Member States and at the Union level.

4. Technical Means for Ensuring Safety

In analyzing the various safety aspects which will certainly characterize future care settings, some issues concerning the electronic identity management technologies including anonymization and pseudonymization should not be neglected since, according to the vision of many experts, they are expected to play a role of growing importance role in the healthcare sector. Human beings have, generally, one single identity in the so-called real world but can, and will for sure have many identities in the electronic universe. Some services require a proved identity whereas others may even work in an anonymized or pseudonymized manner. The decision upon the required level of security will be based on policies.

4.1. Identity Management Procedures

Identity Management has been defined as how a person, interacting with an information system, defines what is known and not known about him/her to others using the system and how this relates to the information known or not known to the persons maintaining the system. In others words: identity is mutually defined instead of one-way [21]. New technologies of electronic identity management appear, the most prominent and innovative ones are biometrics and RFID (Radio Frequency IDentifiers).

4.2. Biometric Technologies and their Safety Aspects

As health information technology started to become in many countries a national political imperative, it was realized by many stakeholders that biometric technologies could represent a valid support. Initially used for enforcing simple time and attendance applications, biometric technologies are becoming more popular in the context of normal activities of healthcare establishments. For example, in the phase of applying and accepting the patients in the hospitals, fingerprint-based systems may prevent the fraudulent use of health insurance cards and again, once the patient has been accepted in the hospital premises, a biometric authentication may make it clear to health professionals that there has been no misidentification of the patient before surgery or other procedures.

Current biometric applications in the healthcare sector generally are based on fingerprint scanning, hand geometry and iris recognition devices. Anyway, the strong impulse of the research on face recognition) e.g. by issuing electronic passports with biometric algorithms) could lead to new applications based on this technology, in a medium to short time period to new applications correlated to this technology.

It is widely accepted that the "user's acceptance" represents of the main factors which may facilitate the diffusion of biometrics and, whit reference to this aspect, considering the peculiarities of the hospitals' context, some issues pertaining user acceptance should be taken into the right account.

A relevant factor influencing user acceptance is the possible concerns for medical implications in using biometric devices and, in particular, the fear about possible contaminations and potential damages of the eye.

Hand geometry and fingerprint recognition require a physical contact with the sensor and therefore some users fear that germs would pass from one individual to another since the sensor is often used consecutively. Touching the sensor is the same as touching a public doorknob or money and the same hygiene practices should apply but. in the light of the increasing awareness for Hospital Acquired Infections (HAI) the countermeasures proposed to reduce the threat, in the future, could potentially interest also the biometric devices.

In the past years the safety of the iris recognition process has been assessed by specific studies concerning the compliance with international eye safety standards, including ANSI/EISNA RP27.1-96 (Photobiological Safety of Lamps and Lighting Systems) and IEC 60825-1.2-2001. For the sake of clarity, the safety assessments available concern specific models and can't be applied to other devices. In this logic context it should be wise that every iris recognition unit could report a certification of compliance to the specific safety standards.

4.3. RFID Technologies and their Safety Aspects

As said, RFID stands for Radio Frequency IDentification and refers to information systems consisting of RFID chips exchanging data with an RFID reader at radio frequencies. RFID devices are currently used to identify persons (passports, employee ID cards/tokens, pay systems), objects (cargo, retail, devices) and animals (livestock, pets). In health care systems they, most commonly, are associated with tracking goods and persons.

The use of RFID is sometimes correlated to possible physical threats, like the omnipresence of Electromagnetic Fields (EMF) resulting from RFID tags and readers in work and private environments. EMF effects on biological systems are of electric and thermal nature (mainly stimulation of the central or peripheral nervous system or temperature rise), but there is currently very few evidence of adverse health effects for low-level exposure to EMF except for certain groups (e.g. pacemaker holders) [22].

The situation is very controversial and some EC projects have analyzed several aspects of Environmental Hazards from Low Energy EMF. In particular, a report [23] showed that EMFs can damage DNA cells in laboratory conditions.

The report was cited in the Opening Declaration of the RFID Consultations Workshop 3: "Security, Data Protection & Privacy, Health & Safety Issues" held in Brussels, Belgium in 2006, and the conclusions were that although the results cannot be readily transferred to human beings, the report, urged the European governments to ensure further multidisciplinary EMF research in order to take care that the solution of the presently existing problem of uncertainty about a possible health risk for the citizens due to EMF exposure will not be postponed in the far future [24].

5. Safety Standardization

Aspects of privacy and health-related safety (patient safety) play a very important role in healthcare and welfare as medical (clinical) and patient-related administrative data are among the most sensitive data categories ever. Security standards, normative references, specifications and reports include, e.g., algorithms and service descriptions whereas privacy and safety standards are more related, but are not limited, to policies and administrative procedures.

5.1. Standards for Electrical and Mechanical Safety

As the expected paradigm shift from eHealth to pHealth aims at widely making use of advanced sensor and micro-devices technology, systems supporting pHealth need to focus on designing, developing, implementing, evaluating and validating sensor-based medical systems for diagnosis and treatment as well as monitoring of certain disorders.

As sensors and devices of any type appear close to human beings, several behavioral aspects need to be taken into consideration. Beside ethical and social aspects, it is especially the safety of the electrical medical equipment that counts. Several standards developing organizations (SDO), especially IEC, have taken care of respective safety standards [6]. Table 1 gives an overview of some of the relevant work. In the following, an example of one of the standards will be given.

Table 1. Examples of Safety Standards on Medical Electrical Equipment

IEC 60513 Ed. 2.0 b:1994	Fundamental aspects of safety standards for medical electrical equipment
IEC 60601-1 Ed. 3.0 b:2005	Medical electrical equipment - Part 1: General requirements for basic safety and essential performance
IEC 60601-1-1 Ed. 2.0 b:2000	Medical electrical equipment - Part 1-1: General requirements for safety - Collateral standard: Safety requirements for medical electrical systems
IEC 60601-1-6 Ed. 1.0 b:2004	Medical electrical equipment - Part 1-6: General requirements for safety - Collateral standard: Usability
IEC 60601-2-25 Ed. 1.0 b:1993	Medical electrical equipment - Part 2-25: Particular requirements for the safety of electrocardiographs
IEC 60601-2-49 Ed. 1.0 b:2006	Medical electrical equipment - Part 2-49: Particular requirements for the safety of multifunction patient monitoring equipment
IEC 62354 Ed. 1.0 b:2005	General testing procedures for medical electrical equipment
ISO 16142	Medical devices - Guidance on the selection of standards in support of recognized essential principles of safety and performance of medical devices

IEC 60601 is a standard that rules medical electrical equipment. Part 1-6 is called "General requirements for safety - Collateral standard: Usability". Medical practice is increasingly using medical electrical equipment for observation and treatment of patients as errors caused by inadequate medical electrical equipment usability have become an increasing cause for concern. The usability engineering process is intended to achieve reasonable usability, which in turn is intended to minimize use errors and to minimize use associated risks. Some, but not all, forms of incorrect use are amenable to control by the manufacturer. The usability engineering process is part of the process of risk control. This Collateral Standard describes a usability engineering process, and provides guidance on how to implement and execute it to provide medical electrical equipment safety. It addresses normal use and use errors but excludes abnormal use.

5.2. Standards for Medical Safety and Health Product Safety

In addition to the purely technical safety standards and specifications issued, e.g., by ETSI and IEC, other safety policies and documents rule more health-related aspects. Among those are medical safety and health product safety. The latter is related to both devices and software. The respective standards are therefore manifold. The following list contains relevant medical safety standards and respective specifications mainly focused on medical safety aspects. Following that table, an example standard will be explained in more detail.

Table 2: Medical Safety Standards Overview

CEN CR 13694	CEN Report: Health Informatics - Safety and security related software quality standards for healthcare (SSQS)
CEN TR 15299	Health informatics - Safety procedures for identification of patients and related objects
CEN TS 15260	Health informatics - Categorization of risks from health informatics products
ISO DTS 25238	Health Informatics - Classification of safety risks from health informatics products
ISO TR 21730:2005	Health informatics - Use of mobile wireless communication and computing technology in healthcare facilities - Recommendations for the management of unintentional electromagnetic interference with medical devices

As an example, the technical report CEN TR 15299 defines a framework for the definition of safety critical objects in the healthcare process and the related safety critical data according to modeling methodologies, as well as for the definition of the rules of interaction among safety critical objects in the process, and the acquisition and processing of safety critical data by health informatics systems. Finally, this standard defines a possible roadmap for a stepwise approach for an effective standardization activity in the area of patient safety, including the main health sub-processes that involve the hospitalized patient as: Laboratory Medicine and Pathology, Bio-imaging, Drug Therapy Management, Blood Transfusion Management, Surgery Management. Such sub-processes can be considered, from a process modeling perspective, a case-mix that covers most of the process requirements of patient safety for the hospitalized patient and an appropriate starting point for the health processes that involve non-hospitalized patients.

6. Conclusions

All countries are currently faced with the challenge to increase efficiency and quality of healthcare, independent of constraints in time, location and resources of principals involved. This challenge must be met by developed countries and countries in transition alike, despite of demographic changes towards aging population, increasing expectations on quality of life and lifestyle, growing demands for health services, rising costs for diagnostic and therapeutic procedures and decreasing insurance funds. A solution out of this dilemma is seen in specialization and de-centralization combined with extended communication and collaboration, called shared care paradigm.

Collaboration and co-operation in this context is meant in a pan-European context. This results in a paradigm change from organization-centered to process-controlled care. The concept is widely known as eHealth.

Collaboration and cooperation in a European context must be based on a legal framework and the underlying technical solutions, e.g. a security infrastructure along with access rules and identity mechanisms (e.g. cards, tokens, biometrics, etc.) guaranteeing the highest level of patient safety. Physical, mechanical and electrical safety alike needs to be addressed herewith. European directives help providing this framework. The European Member States need to adopt and adapt European Directives making them national law within a short period of time. From this perspective, a European safety services framework for eHealth and pHealth can be based on existing and emerging fundamental directives and technologies of which some are described in this paper. Countries like The Netherlands, Spain, Germany, France, and Belgium have already updated their national legislation accordingly. Other countries, especially the newly affiliated ones, need to undergo this process rather soon.

The very basis for a reliable, trustworthy, liable, safe and secure eHealth services is the fast and consequent adoption and adaptation of the existing European legal and technical framework by all European Member States. In addition to the aspects and challenges discussed above, other directives, standards, norms, specifications, and reports are to be considered as well [25], [26]. Based on experience made by several Member States and other countries alike, the European Union currently undergoes a process of political, economic, and cultural enlargement. Healthcare and welfare in general and aspects of patient and citizens safety in particular are among the top priorities of all nations – no doubt about that. Because unlike virtually any other domains, the healthcare and welfare sector can easily be characterized by just one single statement: Safety First!

Acknowledgement

The authors are in debt to the European Commission for the funding of several European research projects (e.g. BioHealth") as well as to other regional, national and international partners and organizations (e.g. ISO TC 215 WG 4, CEN TC 251 WG III, ETSI, HL7 as well as DIN and GMDS Germany) for their support and their kind co-operation during the course of the aforementioned projects, activities, and beyond.

References

[1] Blobel B. Analysis, Design and Implementation of Secure and Interoperable Distributed Health Information Systems. Series Studies in Health Technology and Informatics, Vol. 89. Amsterdam: IOS Press, 2002
[2] International Medical Informatics Association – IMIA. http://www.imia.org
[3] European Federation for Medical Informatics – EFMI. http://www.efmi.org
[4] International Standardization Organization, TC Health Informatics - ISO TC 215. http://www.iso.org
[5] European Standardization Committee CEN, TC Health Informatics - CEN TC 251. http://www.centc251.org
[6] International Electrotechnical Commission IEC. http://www.iec.ch
[7] International Telecommunication Union ITU. http://www.itu.int
[8] European Telecommunication Standardization Institute – ETSI. http://www.etsi.org

[9]   Pharow P, Blobel B: Public Key Infrastructures for Health. In: Blobel B, Pharow P (Edrs.) Advanced Health Telematics and Telemedicine. The Magdeburg Expert Summit Textbook. Series Studies in Health Technology and Informatics, Vol. 96. IOS Press, Amsterdam (2003).

[10]   Norgall T, Blobel B, Pharow P: Personal Health – The Future Care Paradigm. In: Bos L, Roa L, Kanagasingam Y, O'Connell B, Marsh A, Blobel B (Edrs.) Medical and Care Compunetics 3. Proceedings of ICMCC 2006. Series Studies in Health Technology and Informatics, Vol. 121. IOS Press, Amsterdam (2006).

[11]   Blobel B, Norgall T: Von "e-Health" zu "Personal Health" - Strukturen und Dienste. CeBIT 2005, Medizintag der Fraunhofer-Institute.

[12]   Blobel B, Pharow P: Paradigm Change towards Personal Health. In: Medical Informatics in Enlarged Europe. Proceedings of STC 2007, Brijuni Island, Croatia, May 30th – June 1st, 2007.

[13]   eEurope 2002 – Increased Internet Connectivity - A Cheaper, Faster and Secure Internet. COM (2001) 140. http://europa.eu/scadplus/leg/en/lvb/l24226a.htm

[14]   eEurope 2005 – An Information Society for All. eEurope 2005 Action Plan. COM (2002) 263. http://europa.eu/scadplus/leg/en/lvb/l24226.htm

[15]   e-Health Action Plan on health services and information delivered and exchanged through the internet and related technologies. http://www.epha.org/a/1211

[16]   Blobel B, Pharow P (Edrs.) Advanced Health Telematics and Telemedicine. The Magdeburg Expert Summit Textbook. Series Studies in Health Technology and Informatics, Vol. 96. IOS Press, Amsterdam (2003).

[17]   i2010 – A European Information Society for Growth and Employment. A European Commission's Strategic Policy Framework. http://ec.europa.eu/information_society/eeurope/i2010/index_en.htm

[18]   European Commission Report on "Connected Health: Quality and Safety for European Citizens. http://www.ehealthnews.eu/content/view/202/27/

[19]   Directive 97/66/EC of the European Parliament and of the Council of 15 December 1997 concerning the processing of personal data and the protection of privacy in the telecommunications sector

[20]   Electronic Commerce Directive of the E. C. COM (1998) 586 final, O.J. 1999/30/04. http://www.opsi.gov.uk/si/si2002/20022013.htm

[21]   European Technology Assessment Group ETAG. Case Study on RFID and Identity Management in Everyday Life. http://www.itas.fzk.de/eng/etag/document/hoco06a.pdf

[22]   European Commission. RFID Consultation Website "Towards an RFID Policy for Europe. www.rfidconsultation.eu/workshops/21/225.html

[23]   Report on Environmental Hazards from Low Energy EMF. Brussels, Belgium, 2006. http://ec.europa.eu/research/quality-of-life/ka4/pdf/report_reflex_en.pdf

[24]   RFID Consultations Workshop 3: "Security, Data Protection & Privacy, Health & Safety Issues" 2006. http://www.rfidconsultation.eu/docs/ficheiros/RFID_WS_3_16052006_GS_opening_0.pdf

[25]   ISO FDIS 17090 Health Informatics -- Public Key Infrastructure: Part 1: Overview of digital certificate service; Part 2: Certificate profiles; Part 3: Policy management of certification authority. ISO 2006. http://www.iso.org/iso/en/CombinedQueryResult.CombinedQueryResult?queryString=17090

[26]   ISO/IEC 9594-8 | International Telecommunication Union: ITU-T Recommendation X.509 (1997 E): Information Technology – Open Systems Interconnection – The Directory: Authentication Framework, 6-1997.

Medical and Care Compunetics 4
L. Bos and B. Blobel (Eds.)
IOS Press, 2007

Security and Privacy Issues of Personal Health

Bernd BLOBEL[1] and Peter PHAROW
*eHealth Competence Center, University of Regensburg Medical Center, Regensburg,
Germany*

Abstract. While health systems in developed countries and increasingly also in developing countries are moving from organisation-centred to person-centred health service delivery, the supporting communication and information technology is faced with new risks regarding security and privacy of stakeholders involved. The comprehensively distributed environment puts special burden on guaranteeing communication security services, but even more on guaranteeing application security services dealing with privilege management, access control and audit regarding social implication and connected sensitivity of personal information recorded, processed, communicated and stored in an even internationally distributed environment.

Keywords. Personal Health; Security; Privacy; Policy; Privilege management; Access control

1. Introduction

All developed countries are faced with the challenge for guaranteeing quality and efficiency of healthcare independent of constraints in time, location or resources. Advanced programmes define the transition from organisation-centred to person-centred care. Serving a citizen before becoming a patient by prevention and monitoring or supporting homecare for a citizen before getting an inpatient is called Personal Health. This includes care delivery from different providers always considering the real status of the individual in question including the current living conditions, preferences, interests, etc. Such personal care settings require extended communication and co-operation of all principals involved in the person's care. The term "Principal" has been introduced by the Object Management Group (OMG) defining any actor in an information network such as persons, organisations, systems, applications, devices or components [1]. Such approach reflects the challenge of Personal Health.

2. Challenge of Personal Health

The Personal Health paradigm allows for communication between principals independent of time and location. Actions include questions and answers, transfer of

---

[1] Corresponding Author: Bernd Blobel, PhD, Associate Professor, eHealth Competence Center, University of Regensburg, Franz-Josef-Strauss-Allee 11, D-93053 Regensburg, Germany; Email: bernd,blobel@klinik.uni-regensburg.de; URL: www.ehealth-cc.de

recommendations but also the exchange of images for assessing a situation. The described services are based on the mobile computing paradigm. Furthermore, Personal Health enables interventions independent of time, location, resources, etc. The underlying paradigm is that of pervasive computing. As no person is equal another, the way for optimally diagnosing his/her status as well as the optimal service for meeting requirements or wishes are individual. This personalisation concerns both processes and methodologies or concepts applied. As a consequence, particularly organisation-centred processes but also common clinical guidelines do not fit. Therefore, care settings, procedures, diagnostics and therapeutics have to be adapted to the person and his/her environment and current conditions. This includes also information systems applications. The paradigm for providing self-organising and adaptive information systems is named autonomous computing. Combining the three aforementioned paradigms for advanced eHealth supports ubiquitous care based on the ubiquitous computing paradigm. Personal Health delivered for supporting a permanently changing environment, its requirements and principals involved but also underlying policies, independent of location, time, resources, puts important challenges regarding the information systems' architecture as well as the security, privacy, safety and quality requirements of systems and processes.

3. Advanced Information Systems Architectures for Personal Health

For meeting the requirements for open, flexible, portable, semantically interoperable, knowledge-based, service-oriented and business-oriented, legally compliant, user-accepted, and trustworthy health information systems, the Generic Component Model (GCM) has been developed [2].

3.1. The Generic Component Model

The GCM allows for requirement analysis, system design, implementation, and deployment following a Unified Process [3]. It considers information systems including devices, organisations, and any other principal in three dimensions: the domain the system supports including other interrelated domains; the composition and decomposition of the system's components; and the view on the system. According to ISO 10746 Open Distributed Processing [4], five viewpoints have been defined representing computation-independent business aspects, information aspects, computational viewpoints for aggregating concepts towards reasonable functions and services but also the engineering viewpoint of implementation as well as the technology view reflecting user aspects, training, etc. The GCM with the interpretation of a security-relevant business view meta-instance is shown in Figure 1.

Within a single domain, a system can be described by components representing basic concepts which can be aggregated to different aggregation levels ranging from basic services and functions, relations networks up to the concepts of a domain business the system aims at serving. The specialisation represented through domains as well as the aforementioned different aggregation levels can be derived by constraint modelling. The concepts and the aggregation rules representing the domain knowledge have to be formally described using meta-languages such as XML or -even better- the UML standards family. This allows for describing structure and function of a system architecture including its specialisation for autonomous system design.

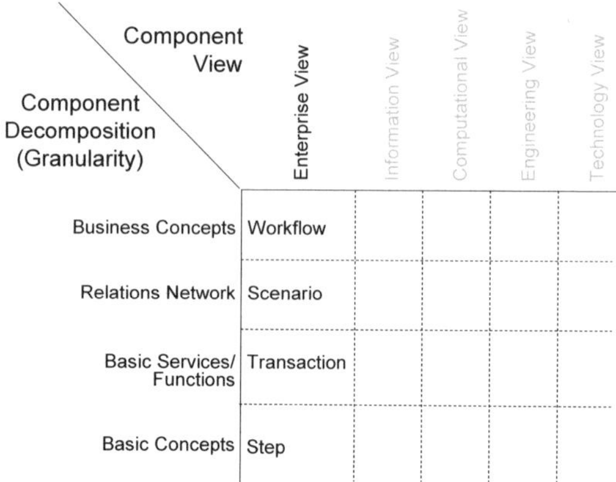

Figure 1. The Generic Component Model

3.2. The Layered Security Model

Another model for analysing security, safety, and quality requirements as well as for designing trustworthy systems solutions is the Layered Security Model (LSM), shown in Figure 2 [5]. This model considers security, safety, and quality analogue to the domain perspective defining service concepts and services needed being based on mechanisms, which are implemented using algorithms applied to data. Similar to GCM, the Layered Security Model provides the representation of a real system by a formal model. Contrary to the GCM, LSM does not describe a system's structure and behaviour but the services in question.

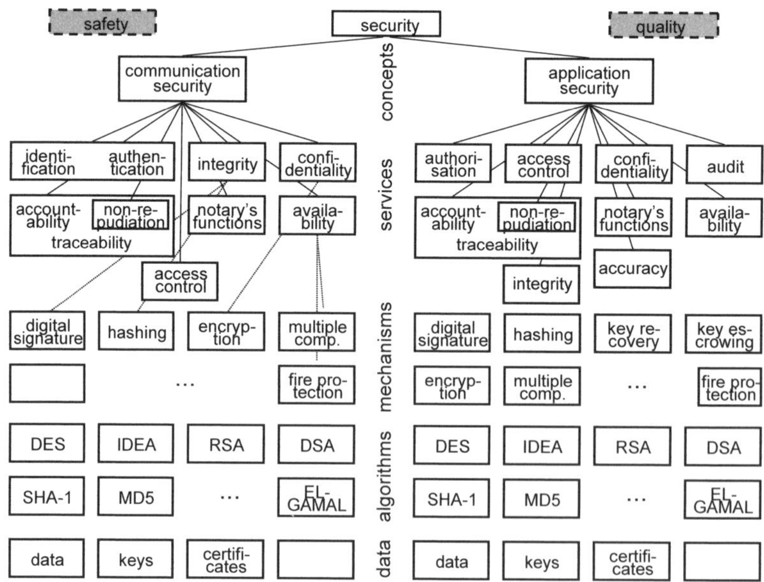

Figure 2. Layered Security Model

Because not considering the component structure of any system, LSM does not go below services and ignores service aggregations.

4. Security Requirements and Services

At the concept layer, LCM distinguishes between communication security and application security.

4.1. Communication and Application Security

Communication security deals with identification and authentication of communicating principals, access control allocated to the requested principal, integrity, confidentiality, availability, and accountability for as well as traceability of communicated information. Application security services concern authorisation of principals privileged to access the other party for performing certain functions. In that context, access to data and functions as well as availability, integrity, and accountability for as well as traceability of data recorded, entered, processed, and stored at the principals site. Communication and application security services are supported by notary's functions thereby bridging between the legal and the technological domain. Special security services to be considered are, e.g. audit and Trusted Third Party (TTP) services. While different domains deploy the same or at least similar communication security services, application security services are policy-driven and therefore domain-specific. So, existing communication security services from domains like banking or government can be re-used in Personal Health environments. Application security services are very specific, however. For this reason, the paper will mainly address application security services in Personal Health.

4.2. Security Policy

Security policy is a complex of legal, organisational, functional, medical, social, ethical and technical aspects, which must be considered in the context of data protection and data security. Security policy defines the framework, rights and duties of principals involved but also consequences and penalties in the case of disregard of the fixings taken. Therefore, security policies have be considered for every single security services, calling those services policy-driven.

Table 1. Common TTP policy

Legal Domain	Technological Domain
Based on the Electronic signature directive	Based on the EESSI electronic signature standard
Legal coherence with European rules	Technical coherence with European (international) standards
Legal coherence with national rules, i.e. legal interoperability	Technical coherence with standards, i.e. technical interoperability

From the GCM's perspective, a security policy is a complex system establishing services and processes. As a consequence, a security policy has to be analysed, designed, implemented and deployed like any other system, following the GCM architectural approach. As any other system alike, the addressed domain and their interrelated domains have to be modelled. More details will be discussed in Section 5. Table 1 presents the interrelationships between the legal and technological domain in the TTP security policy context.

4.3. Special Requirements and Solutions for Secure Personal Health

Ambient intelligence, supported by networked information and communication technologies, provides ubiquitous computing enabling ubiquitous health services. Totally connected and networking daily life promises unimagined opportunities but means also additional risks regarding data security and privacy.

Personal Health does not only put the citizen in the centre. It increases also the person's autonomy and responsibility. This empowerment has to be supported by the industry proving trustworthy and user-friendly health information systems. On the other hand, the government has to implement the legal and administrative environment for Personal Health as part of the eSociety establishing a security culture.

In Personal Health settings, communication and co-operation have to be established in a dynamically changing network of users and systems, provided services and running processes, underlying policies, applied technical security protocols (part of policy according to the policy definition), etc. In such settings, a pre-definition of workflow, system environments, and organisational security services such as security management, cannot be established. Therefore, security services must be embedded in the chosen architectural approach by binding the security service to the domain-specific service at component level performing the rule-based aggregation in the GCM. By this way, the required flexibility and adaptability of security services can be provided.

5. Modelling Security Services and Processes

For analysing, designing, implementing and using security services, security systems have to be formally modelled as appropriate representation of the complex and interrelated reality. As any other complex system, many different domains have to be considered which are presented by exploiting corresponding domain experts' knowledge expressed using domain-specific language and vocabulary. This knowledge describes concepts and processes which have to be combined with other domains and implemented in real information and communication technologies.

The challenge consists of the expression of policies reflecting aspects of legal, organisational, ethical, social, functional, and technological domains. The domain knowledge must be transferred into formal models which are represented using meta-languages. Such consideration is not in common so far. Therefore, knowledge for modelling security services and re-usable security components is rarely available.

5.1. Considered Models

For managing application security services in Personal Health settings, two basic class types must be dealt with: Entities and Acts. In this paper, acts and services have not been distinguished.

Entities can be specialised to principals, policies, documents and roles. Specialisations of an act relevant in the paper's context are, e.g., policy management, principal management, privilege management, authentication, authorisation, access control management and audit.

The acts mentioned are needed to enable the described security services. A series of static and dynamic models must be introduced to describe the entities and to define, how activities will be performed. Following models have to be considered in Personal Health application security:

- Domain Model,
- Delegation Model,
- Control Model,
- Document Model,
- Policy Model,
- Role Model,
- Information Distance Model,
- Authorisation Model,
- Access Control Models.

Details of the aforementioned models are discussed, e.g., in [6]. In this paper, only some models will be considered.

5.2. Policy Model

Figure 3 shows the policy class model hierarchy defined in ISO 22600.

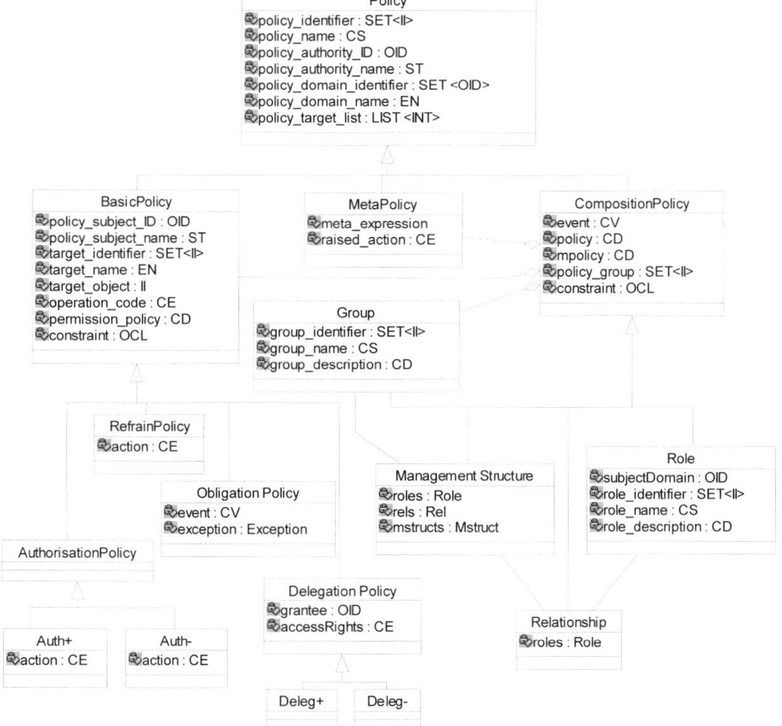

Figure 3. Security Policy Base-Class Diagram

As all other models, also the policy model must comply with the GCM architectural approach. For this purpose, it has to allow for separation in different domains as well as for composition (generalisation) and de-composition (specialisation), so enabling fine-grained embedded security services.

Based on the expression mode for aggregating policy concepts to policies, there are different ways of representing policy. The best approach covering both structural and functional (behavioural) aspects is the policy representation in UML (Unified Modeling Language) (Figure 3) including the Object Constraint Language (OCL) constraint definitions. Both languages have been developed by OMG; they are adapted by ISO meanwhile. There are many alternatives for expressing concepts and rule using constraint languages, however.

A special policy with tangible consequences for Personal Health is the person's or patient's consent. The responsibility bound to the citizen's role of a decider depends on the informational basis for such decisions. Therefore, any consent has to be an informed one.

5.3. Other Constraint Representations

According to the Generic Component Model, healthcare and its supporting information systems is dealing with other domains beside medicine and biology. In that context, finance, technology, legislation, security, etc. have to be mentioned. Regarding the latter one, legal and policy concepts have to be modelled. A policy covers all implications on health and health information systems such as legal, social, organisational, psychological, functional, and technical ones.

Managing security policy may include some or all of the following steps: writing, reviewing, testing, approving, issuing, combining, analysing, modifying, withdrawing, retrieving and enforcing policy. The complete Policy applicable to a particular Decision Request may be composed by a number of individual Rules or Policies. For instance, in a personal privacy application, the owner of the personal information may define certain aspects of disclosure policy whereas the enterprise that is the custodian of the information may define certain other aspects. In order to render an Authorization Decision, it must be possible to combine the two separate policies to form the single policy applicable to the request.

OASIS' Security Assertion Markup Language (SAML) defines security services assigned to entities in a header-body-reference structure using XML. For formally modelling policies and ruling access control, the Extended Access Control Markup Language (XACML) has been developed by OASIS with the XML meta-language. Other examples are Web Service Description Language (WSDL), Business Process Execution Language (BPEL), Web Services Policy Language (WSPL), or Domain-Independent Web Services Policy Assertion Language (DIPAL). An overview about application security modelling approaches is given in [7].

5.4. Role Model

Rights and duties based on policies also considering context information and current conditions have to be assigned to principals involved in Personal Health. As already mentioned, this includes systems, applications, or devices. Authorisation by managing the binding of every principal to possible functional steps, occurring pieces of information, all possible contextual information as well as conditions happening would cause an administrative overload. Therefore, principals are grouped according to common properties in relations to other principals, according to the context and conditions to perform. The resulting class is called role of the principal. Many roles can be assigned to one single principal. Information object are grouped according to their sensitivity forming sensitivity classes or information classifications.

Roles may be assigned to any principal. Roles are associated to entities (actors) and to activities (acts) alike. For managing relationships between the entities mediated by an activity, two different roles have to be defined: structural roles at the entity's side and functional roles at the act's side. The assignment to structural roles is rather static, whereas the assignment to functional roles is highly dynamic. Structural roles specify relations between entities in the sense of competence (RIM roles) often reflecting organisational or structural relations (hierarchies). They correspond with HL7 RIM Role. Functional roles are bound to an act. Functional roles can be assigned to be performed during an act. They correspond to the HL7 RIM participation. Meanwhile, the models and definitions for privilege management and access control (PMAC) on the one hand as well as for functional and structural roles on the other hand -all presented in this paper- became ISO standards meanwhile: ISO 22600 and ISO 21298, respectively.

International harmonisation of structural roles is very tricky due to their legal relations. Because of different opinions and regulations, harmonisation of complex workflows might be difficult as well. The chance for international harmonisation grows with the granularity of functional roles up to their basic concepts. Therefore, communication and co-operation between principals across organisational, regional or even national borders can be properly managed at the functional role level.

Regarding the healthcare business process, generic functional roles can be defined in levels of authorisations and access rights in the following generic way re-using slightly changed definitions established in the Australian HealthConnect Project [8], cross-referenced against other works:

- Subject of care (normally the patient),
- Subject of care agent (parent, guardian, carer, or other legal representative),
- Responsible (personal) healthcare professional (the healthcare professional with the closest relationship to the patient, often his GP),
- Privileged healthcare professional
  - o Nominated by the subject of care,
  - o Nominated by the healthcare facility of care (there is a nomination by regulation, practice, etc.),
- Healthcare professional (involved in providing direct care to the patient),
- Health-related professional (indirectly involved in patient care, teaching, research, etc.),
- Administrator (and any other parties supporting service provision to the patient).

The list fixes the set of functional roles applied to manage creation, access, processing, and communication of health information. Another way for grouping functional roles according to the relation to the information created, recorded, entered, processed, stored, and communicated could be: Composer, Committer, Certifier, Authoriser, Subject of information, Information provider. A third alternative for functional roles' structure related to information and its use complying with the

European Data Protection Directive [9] and elated ISO CD 22857 "Health Informatics – Guidelines on data protection to facilitate trans-border flows of personal health information" [10] has been introduced through the Information Distance Model [11].

5.5. Access Control in Personal Health

Because conditions, context, regulations, resulting authorisations etc. change, the process of binding them to roles, workflows, and accessed objects leads to extended lists of roles. Therefore, all components of an access control schema need to be bound to corresponding policies resulting in a policy-driven, role-based one as demonstrated in Figure 4.

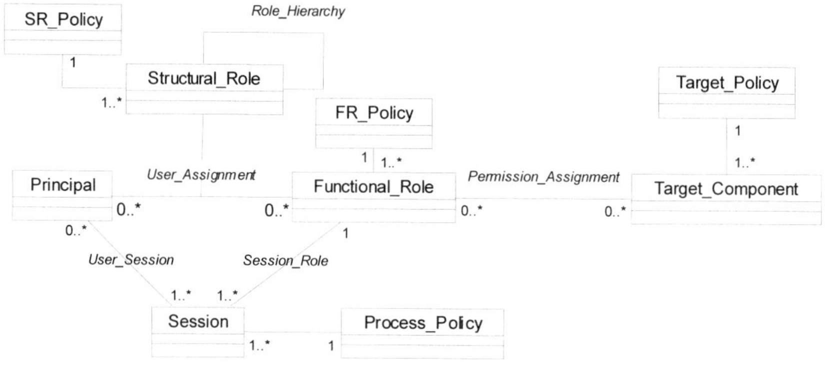

Figure 4. Role-Based Access Control Schema

6. Results and Discussion

For enhancing efficiency and quality of healthcare, health systems are changing from being organisation-centred towards Personal Health. This care paradigm includes homecare and prevention therefore additionally addressing citizens before becoming patients. Personal Health, information and services have to be provided independent of time, location, and resources. Therefore, it represents the advanced eHealth paradigm.

Personal Health settings imply permanently changing, numerically bigger provider communities from different domains which collaborate under flexible conditions, altering policies, and adaptive processes for delivering dedicated services. This is bound to highly compartmented processes with extensive communication and co-operation between all kinds of principals. Person monitoring and homecare are essential components of this approach.

Such environment requires extraordinary security and privacy services. Communication security services have to be provided according to the state-of-the-art. The even bigger challenge concerns the application security services, amongst them authorisation, privilege management and access control but comprehensive audits to guarantee the lawfulness of processes and services.

Pivotal point of Personal Health is the citizen served. On the one hand, this implies a growing responsibility of persons for their health as well as for communication and co-operation activities. On the other hand, it leads to a citizen/patient empowerment.

Such environment must be supported by the vendors and providers through the development of user-friendly and trustworthy eHealth solutions. The government has to provide an appropriate legal and organisational framework. Finally, education and training are basically for playing the role dedicated to the different parties involved in the business. Summarising, a security culture has to be developed. Legally this mean to present data security and privacy as prerequisites for guaranteeing civil and human rights in an on-line world. As an economic challenge, information security must be presented as opportunity and virtue. From social perspective, individual users must realise that their home systems are critical within the security chain. Therefore, diversity, openness, and interoperability have to be supported as integral security components [12].

The maturity of solutions for ubiquitous health, such as mobile services, pervasive computing and intervention as well as self-organising system design and implementation based on autonomous computing, is differently developed. Pervasive technologies are growing, while autonomous computing remains a challenge. Nevertheless, bioinformatics and genomics for individual diagnosis and therapy, but also biomedical engineering enabling telemedicine by sensors and actuators are evolving.

Acknowledgement

The authors are indebted to the colleagues from HL7, ISO TC 215 and CEN TC 251 for kind support.

References

[1]　Object Management Group: http://www.omg.org
[2]　Blobel B: *Analysis, Design and Implementation of Secure and Interoperable Distributed Health Information Systems.* Series Studies in Health Technology and Informatics, Vol. 89. IOS Press, Amsterdam 2002
[3]　Lopez DM, Blobel B (2006) Realising Semantic Interoperability by Using the Unified Process. European Notes in Medical Informatics, Vol. II, 2 (2006) pp. 316-321.
[4]　ISO/IEC 10746 Information technology – Open Distributed Processing – Reference Model
[5]　Blobel B, Roger-France F: A Systematic Approach for Analysis and Design of Secure Health Information Systems. *Int. J. Med. Inf.* **62** (2001) 3, pp. 51-78, http://dx.doi.org/10.1016/S1386-5056(01)00147-2
[6]　Blobel B, Nordberg R, Davis JM, Pharow P (2006) Modelling privilege management and access control. International Journal of Medical Informatics **75**, 8 (2006) pp. 597-623.
[7]　Blobel B (2007) Formally Modelling Application Security Services. Internal research document, eHCC Regensburg.
[8]　Australian Government, Department of Health and Aging: The Australian HealthConnect Project, http://www.health.gov.au
[9]　Council of Europe: Directive 95/46/EC, On the Protection of Individuals with Regard to the Processing of Personal Data and on the Free Movement of such Data (OJ L281/31-50, 24 October 1995). Strasbourg1995, http://www.cdt.org/privacy/eudirective/EU_Directive_.html
[10]　ISO CD 22857 Health informatics – Guidelines on data protection to facilitate trans-border flows of personal health information
[11]　Yamamoto K, Ishikawa K, Miyaji M, Nakamura Y, Nishi S, Sasaki T, Tsuji K, Watanabe R: The Awareness of Security Issues among Hospitals in Japan. IMIA Conference: *Caring for Health Information Safety, Security and Secrecy*, November 13-16, Heemskerk, The Netherlands1993
[12]　COM(2006) 251 A strategy for a Secure Information Society – "Dialogue, partnership and empowerment".

Medical and Care Compunetics 4
L. Bos and B. Blobel (Eds.)
IOS Press, 2007

HL7 Conformance:
How to do Proper Messaging

Frank OEMIG [a,1] and Bernd G.M.E. BLOBEL [b]
[a] *Agfa HealthCare / GWI Medica GmbH, Bonn, Germany*
[b] *eHealth Competence Center, University of Regensburg Medical Center, Germany*

Abstract. Communication and cooperation between different applications is mediated by interfaces following corresponding standards. The interpretation of standards, the understanding of requirements and specification of solutions is very different within the vendor community. In a shared care environment based on extended inter-organizational inter-relationships, this interoperability has to be provided at semantic and service-oriented level. For that purpose, harmonized reference models, agreed terminologies, ontologies and concept representations as well as a unified development and deployment process have to be standardized. The latter also includes testing and certification procedures. The paper shortly introduces in the semantic interoperability approach provided by HL7.

Keywords. Health telematics; Communication standard; HL7; Semantic interoperability; Conformance

1. Introduction

The health systems of all industrial countries are faced with the challenge of improving quality and efficiency of health delivery. The way for meeting these requirements is the introduction of shared care, which is bound to extended communication and cooperation between all healthcare establishments and their information systems. Such communication and collaboration can be provided at different levels of interoperability as shown in the next section. If communication focuses on message exchange, collaboration highly depends on the semantic understanding of the messages. The standard itself allows for a wide variety of options, which are used in many different ways.

This paper investigates HL7 from the aspect of advanced interoperability for implemented interfaces.

2. The HL7 Communication Standard

Following, the primary members of HL7 communication standard and the objective towards conformance will be shortly discussed. For more information see [1-4].

---

[1] Corresponding Author: Frank Oemig, Dipl.-Inf., Agfa Healthcare, GWI Medica GmbH, Konrad-Zuse-Platz 1-3, D-53227 Bonn, Germany, E-mail: Frank.Oemig@agfa.com, URL: http://www.agfa.com

2.1. General Principles

The advent of an increasing number of computer systems in combination with complex applications from different vendors raised the challenge to connect those systems. This can be done at different levels of interoperability: At the lowest level, mechanical plugs including the voltage and the signals used have been harmonized. We are talking of technical interoperability. At the next level, the data exchanged have been standardized providing data level interoperability. Nevertheless, different terminologies might be used. Therefore, at the next level, terminology must be agreed upon. For realizing a common understanding, the semantics of terms must be harmonized providing semantic interoperability. At the highest level, concepts and context of information exchanged are harmonized including the realized services based on that information. We call this highest level service oriented interoperability.

HL7, an ANSI accredited standards development organization with close liaison to ISO TC 215 Health Informatics, specifies communication contents and exchange formats on the application layer. In the ISO communication model for Open System Interconnection (OSI), this layer is the seventh, which led to the name Health Level Seven Communication Standard (HL7). It is important that the communication solution is independent from the software used as well as from the underlying hardware and the chosen network. Thus, the user has the freedom to realize a solution best suited to his needs or "best of breed".

The HL7 communication standard was especially developed for the health care environment of hospitals and enables meanwhile communication between almost all institutions and fields of healthcare and public health as well. With HL7, all important communication tasks of a hospital can be handled and the efficiency of the communication process is decidedly improved.

2.2. HL7 Version 2.x

The best known and widely implemented communication standard for healthcare is the HL7 v2.x family. This standard has been developed the pragmatic way as a spin-off of ASTM [10] without an explicit data and design model. This gap can be filled by reverse engineering [5], the result of which is demonstrated in figure 1.

Such an approach helps to understand the standard and to enhance its usability by:
1. creating a more consistent standard, which identifies and supports the re-use of data elements,
2. making the two dimensional parsing architecture on message and field level explicit, and
3. taking advantage from this specification in form of a well structured implementation.

The last, but most important point ("conformance") will be discussed shortly.

By a consensus process, new requirements are added to newer versions. Each vendor can offer a proposal to add new messages, segments and fields, which are normally added in a backward compatible way. Unfortunately, these elements are intended to solve specific needs, mostly for a relative small group of vendors, so that these elements are optional by their nature. The standard ([1]) provides some guidance in chapter 2 on how the HL7 optionality must be implemented without loosing interoperability (table 1): deployment of a conformance process.

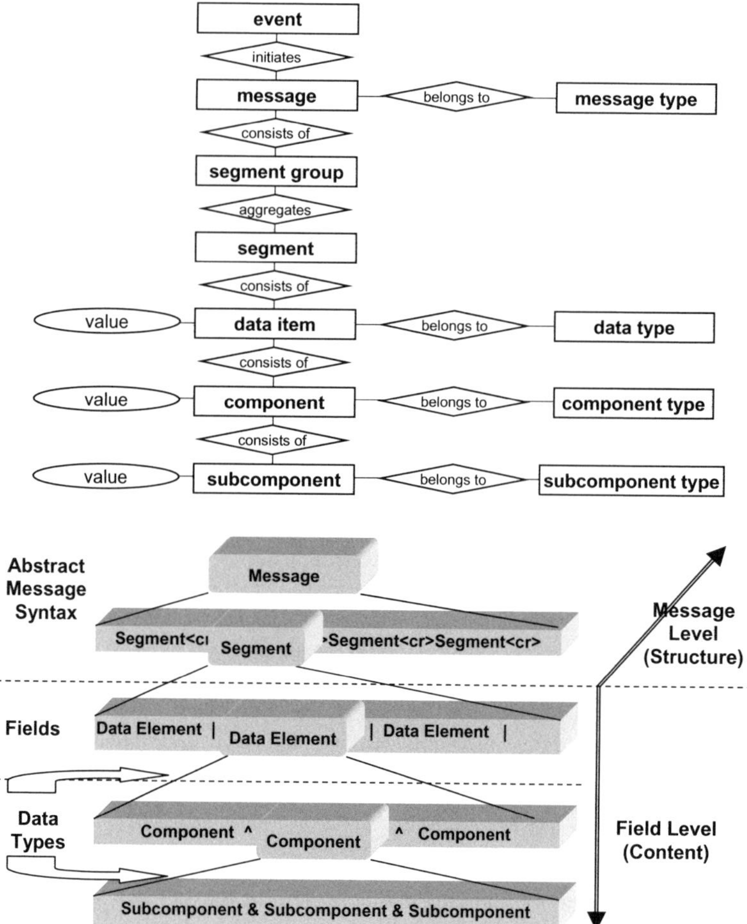

Figure 1. Message Component Model and Parsing Architecture of HL7 version 2.x [4]

The standard itself distinguishes between "HL7 optionality" and "Conformance Usage", i.e. between two distinct set of codes (the "E" in the codes represents "but may be empty"). These two sets have a close relationship, however (see also table 3).

Unfortunately, table 1 is not sufficient, i.e. not every combination with respect to profile hierarchies is expressed explicitly. The arrows in figure 2 demonstrate how a specific optionality can be constrained from one profile type to a more restrictive one (solid arrows). This process is a repetitive one, i.e. a constrainable profile can be used as a basis for another constrainable profile. (The dashed arrows in this figure represent the substitution of conditional elements.) Whenever an element has been made required, it can never be loosed again. This process of iterative refinement stops once all optionality is eliminated.

Table 1. HL7 Optionality and Usage Codes

HL7 Optionality	Allowed Conformance Usage	Comment
R – Required	R	
O – Optional	R, RE, O, C, CE, X	O is only permitted for constrainable profiles
C – Conditional	C, CE, R	
X – Not Supported	X	
B – Backward Compatibility	R, RE, O, C, CE, X	O is only permitted for constrainable definitions
W – Withdrawn	R, RE, O, C, CE, X	

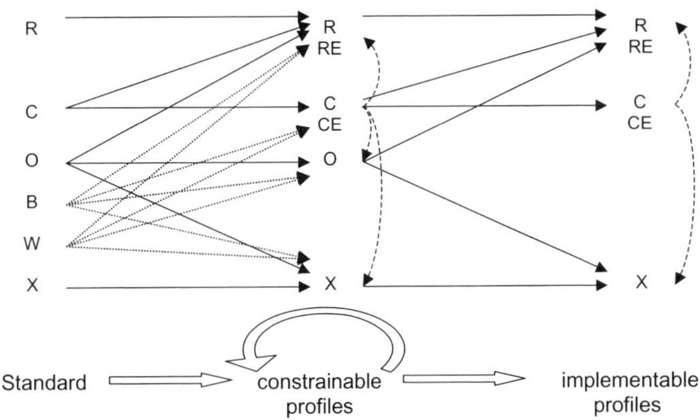

Figure 2. Permitted Optionality/Usage Code Transition

In the end, the used codes in table 2 combine two different aspects for elements:

- whether they must be supported when implementing
- whether they must convey information during transmission in form of a message

Table 2. Support Properties of Elements

	R	RE	C	CE	O	X
support	yes	yes				no
support under certain conditions			yes	yes		no
information	yes					no

As listed, some cases are not clearly specified, so that an interface engine does not know how to react to specific circumstances. The only way out is a well documented, exact and complete specification known as "implementable profile". Table 3 provides an overview in which kind of profiles the appropriate codes may be used.

Table 3: Subsets of Optionality/Usage Codes

	R	RE	C	CE	O	B	W	X
standard (optionality)	√	?	√	?	√	√	√	√
conformance profiles	√	√	√	√	√	-	-	√
implementable profiles	√	√	√	√	-	-	-	√

2.3. HL7 Version 3

HL7 Version 3 provides more than a new version in the course of development of the standard. HL7 has established a new methodology for creating models as well as the process that supports the inference from one model to another.

2.3.1. HL7 Version 3 Basics

This new and comprehensive development methodology or unified process is called HL7 Development Framework (HDF). It covers the whole life cycle of standard specification from development through adaptation and maintenance up to implementation, use and testing of messages by the means of object-oriented analysis and design as well as formal modeling.

Within a hidden migration process towards a service paradigm, the **Reference Information Model** (RIM) is the underlying meta-model, which has been step by step generalized to only a few generic core classes: **Entity**, i.e. the physical information object or better the actor of the domain; **Role** played by this entity and therefore assigning it the competence for **Participation** in specific **Acts** as the subject of the message; and **Role Link** to manage interactions between entities in their corresponding roles as well as **Act Relationship** chaining different acts.

These six core classes are used to model different health domains by constraining and instantiating their specializations and establishing the appropriate associations between those classes.

Beginning with a verbal description of scenarios – the so-called storyboards – a graphical representation facilitating UML Use Case Diagrams is created. This activity is supported by the help of state diagrams or transition diagrams.

For developing domain-specific messages therefore, the classes needed according to the information requirements must be selected and their attributes have to be updated, i.e. non-required attributes must be cancelled and missing attributes must be added resulting in a **Domain Message Information Model** (D-MIM). For defining relationships between different entities as well as chains of activities, the corresponding core classes or their specialization have to be cloned from the RIM, at the same time updating the attributes properly.

While creating models for different domains, it became obvious very early that the same assembly of classes has been specified or used more often. If those models of characteristic objects and their relations can be standardized, a set of **Common Message Element Types** (CMETs) can be established, which are re-usable in different domains and help to build modules for implementation.

The next step in this process is the definition of messages by extracting the required subset of classes out of the parent model resulting in **Refined Message Information Models** (R-MIMs). Walking through this graph with its clones leads to a serialized representation. Latest during this step, the binding of the different vocabularies must be provided. Using a HL7-internally developed schema generator, the **Hierarchical Message Description** (HMD) of the related message structure is finally transferred into an equivalent XML schema definition.

2.3.2. Application Roles

Requirements and conditions of interoperating applications related to their data and functionality have to be clearly defined in order to assure communication between them. Besides defining mandatory data, this includes also the specification of messages and trigger events needed. That specification of functional and data-related requirements and conditions of applications is called Application Roles. Today, such a set of application roles is not normative and has to be mutually negotiated.

The current definition treats an application role as a bracket to define a set of transactions/interactions, which must be comprehensively supported.

2.3.3. Specialization vs. Standardization

HL7's version 3 strategy of model-based message definition reduces optionality by modeling and defining every message according to its specific requirements and conditions. Even if these messages are based on the same domain model, the direct results and consequences are that most of the components in a specific message are not optional any more, but the amount of similar but specific messages has been increased. In other words, uncertainty has been replaced by a vast complexity of the standard, which has to be reduced via mutual agreements based on a formal process. This provides additional burden to the required and also claimed interoperability. The solution can be provided by following principles:

- Reference to a globally acknowledged Reference Information Model;
- Specification of an accepted and binding vocabulary (value set) for all reference components as well as all domain concepts (knowledge concepts) defined in the framework of RIM, all DMIMs, RMIMs, etc.;

- Development of Application Roles for characterizing the participation in message interchange;
- Definition of requirements profiles, which lead to Conformance Statements.

2.3.4. Refinement and Localization

The failure in defining a globally accepted data model and the resulting migration to the RIM as well as the definition of the aforementioned components (from D-MIMs up to CMETs) as a multi-model approach [6] allows for an easy replacement of those modules by local (realm-specific) ones, which are more constrained than the original ones or extended by locally required data.

The resulting XML schemas for validating messages are not normative and vary in numerous ways resulting in difficulties for cross-realm-communication.

2.3.5. Required vs. Mandatory

Within a message instance, certain attributes must be present and must convey a non-null value. These elements are called "mandatory". This is especially true for structural attributes which, are essential to understand the meaning and context of a message. A mandatory element shall also be required!

On the other side, a required element must be present in a message, but it can contain a null value.

3. Conformance

Conformance testing is normally conducted at the suppliers' premises using their hardware. During the test the system is operated entirely by the suppliers. Suppliers need to provide an operator, who should be familiar with all aspects of the system. Each observation is discussed and noted during testing, and a summary report is provided on completion of testing for reference or action as appropriate.

3.1. Conformance Statements

For providing interoperability in a very complex and divergent world, interesting solutions have been developed. Mostly known is DICOM (Digital Imaging and Communication in Medicine, [7]), which is the globally established image communication standard. Contrary to HL7, DICOM realizes interoperability not only at the level of message exchange independent of the level of semantic interpretation, but also at the level of service-oriented interoperability. That linking of communicated data and functions has been defined as Service Object Pairs (SOP) for different modalities within a client-server environment. By that way, an optimal coding (assuring the same interpretation of the message at the originator side and the receiver side) has been guaranteed. The needed equivalence of SOPs, client and server properties, protocols, presentation instructions, etc, is defined by Conformance Statements. Two communicating applications have to meet the corresponding mutual Conformance Statements.

HL7 Version 3 is using an analogue way of defining Conformance Statements. References to a global RIM and a binding vocabulary, messages between two interoperable applications have to follow the corresponding Application Roles as sender and receiver including the assigned responsibilities.

In that context, the current specification of Clinical Templates as well as the work on CDA Level 2 are especially important.

3.2. Conformance Criteria and Guidance Documents

A precondition for establishing a certification process is the existence of implementation manuals (here: message profiles), which exactly describe what must be implemented. On the other hand, these documents are the source of truth describing the properties a certification has to verify [8].

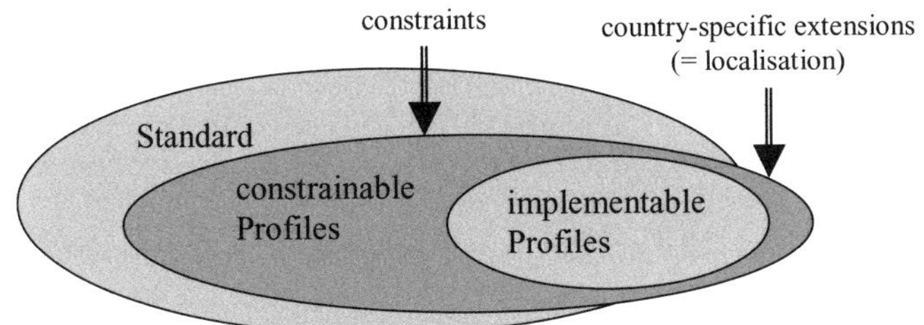

Figure 3. Conformant Implementation of Standards

Normally, such an implementation manual restricts the freedom a vendor has by constraints (figure 3). But sometimes, it is also necessary to enrich the specification by country-specific requirements, also called local extensions.

3.3. Test Procedures

Two different approaches exist to verify that messages conform to a specification. First of all, life testing against other applications in the way it is done by IHE ("Integrating the healthcare enterprise") during a connect-a-thon [9]. The primary goal is to demonstrate that interfaces are working. Corrections to an interface engine are allowed.

Another possibility is to certify that a message conforms to a specification provided in form of an implementable profile. This specification must be a valid constraint on a constrainable profile according to the rules described above. Within this check, a vendor has to demonstrate that the created/consumed messages follow his specification.

In total it is clear that both ways of checking are orthogonal and complementary, but not competitive, i.e. vendor as well as costumer have a clear understanding of the implemented and working functionality.

3.4. Certification

If conformance is achieved, i.e. tested and demonstrated, this must be doubtless documented, i.e. certified.

The purpose of certification is the indisputably binding of an object to another object with specific properties. For that reason, certification authorities have to be accredited following an accreditation process. Therefore, the first step of establishing a certification schema is to define the process and the issues being certified. This is closely related to terminology issues, legal aspects and organizational/behavioral challenges.

There are many ways for guaranteeing specific behavior of objects, components or systems. One is to define the process of specifying and implementing specific items. The process will be certified. This is the way ISO 9000 is guaranteeing quality and conformance of processes and resulting products. Another way is to specify a product and to check whether this specification is implemented in that product. The third approach is the definition of properties to be hold in a product. After testing and evaluating the product, the certification provided by an authority documents that the product meets the claims.

Summarizing the certification process, the following steps have to be realized:

- The **definition** of both the underlying specification as well as the conformance statement is the basis of any further activity.
- Next, the specification must be **implemented**.
- Independently, the institution executing the certification must be **accredited**.
- The vendor seeking certification **offers** his documentation and **installs** his product for testing purposes.
- The first part of the process is the **evaluation** of the conformance statement against the specification. If this holds, the **test** can start during which the independent institution tries to find gaps and/or errors in the implemented product.
- Finally, the result of this process has to be documented in form of a **Certification**/Labeling.

Certificates have the same properties as any other "legally" binding documents.

4. Conclusions

The different HL7 communication standard families have evolved during the years. They have established a methodology to support the development of message interfaces. Beside the used terminology and vocabulary it is pretty much important to understand the basics in form of supportive elements. In order to check and verify the correct processing of conveyed information, a detailed and complete documentation in form of a conformance statement is required. For a user – here: a healthcare establishment – it would be very helpful that these conformance statements are published either on the vendor's website or in a central registry. The latter exists for the HL7 v2.x family on www.hl7.org, but right now it only contains two example profiles. Can this be treated as the vendor's indignation to create interoperable solutions?

In the ever increasing world of communication it becomes obvious that clear guidelines are the basis for a successful communication. They help to ensure the quality needed.

5. References

[1]   Health Level Seven, Inc.: http://www.hl7.org
[2]   Heitmann KU, Blobel B, Dudeck J: *HL7 Communication Standard in medicine. Short introduction and information.* Köln: Verlag Alexander Mönch, 1999. (completely revised and extended edition)

[3]   Hinchley A: Understanding Version 3 – A primer on the HL7 Version 3 Communication Standard. Köln: Verlag Alexander Mönch, 2003

[4]   Blobel B: Analysis, Design and Implementation of Secure and Interoperable Distributed Health Information Systems. Series Studies in Health Technology and Informatics, Amsterdam: Vol. 89. IOS Press, 2002

[5]   Oemig F, Dudeck J.W.: Problems in developing a comprehensive HL7 database, AMIA Fall Symposium 1996, 841

[6]   Oemig F, Blobel B: Does HL7 Go towards an Architecture Standard? In: Engelbrecht R, Geissbuhler A, Lovis Ch, Mihalas G (Edrs.): Connecting Medical Informatics and Bio-Informatics. Proceedings of MIE 2005, 761-766, IOS Press, Amsterdam, Berlin, Oxford, Tokyo, Washington DC.

[7]   DICOM: Digital Imaging and Communication in Medicine, 2003, http://www.rsna.org

[8]   Oemig F: The HL7 Comprehensive Database, http://www.oemig.de/HL7

[9]   IHE, Integrating the Healthcare Enterprise, http://www.ihe-europe.org

[10]   ASTM, http://ww.astm.org

Round Table on the Responsibility Shift
from Doctor to Patient

Medical and Care Compunetics 4
L. Bos and B. Blobel (Eds.)
IOS Press, 2007

WHO Recommendation on Record Access (Draft)

1. AIM:

To ensure that patient record access (RA) is incorporated in WHO development plans.

2. WHAT

RA is the process whereby a user of a health service has the power to access their personal health record (PHR). The PHR means any health record holding information pertaining exclusively to that person. The PHR can be held centrally, when all health records, including community, GP and hospital, are held in a central store; or they can be distributed, stored in different places. RA thus means that a person can see all or part of the health information held about them.

Full RA means that citizens and their selected family, friends and carers can see and use all information, for instance, their full primary care record. A full primary care record would typically include a summary of their main health problems, letters to and from their clinical team, medication details, allergies, immunizations, investigation results.

Citizens should have active access to add personal information, like use of over the counter drugs or results from home monitoring devices.

3. WHY SHOULD CITIZENS HAVE ACCESS TO THEIR RECORDS?

3.1. Ethical reasons:

3.1.1 People increasingly have a right to see information held about them that is not damaging to national security. In some countries, access to health information is constrained by concerns for damage to the person and exposure of third parties. [1]

3.1.2 RA puts more emphasis on citizens and clinicians to use all of the rich material within the record. This use of the truth and its consequences leads to a more proactive and purposeful partnership of health creation and care.

Although it is extremely rare for clinicians to lie, it is not uncommon to be less than clear about the logic and the reasons for a particular course of action. For instance, if patients can read that an investigation has been carried out in order to exclude cancer, then it also becomes important that the clinician explains this at the outset when ordering the test.

3.2. Direct benefit to health

3.2.1 RA supports patients in being more informed about their health, disease and care pathways. We know that informed patients have both better outcomes and use health services less

3.2.2 RA can enhance this process by linking health information and advice to the record. For instance, problem titles can be automatically linked to information about that problem. There can be links also to national self-help groups, national guidelines for good practice and decision aids.[2]

Record access improves communication between national programmes, local care providers and patients and citizens. It allows the automatic updating and sharing of health and disease management plans between citizens', patients and carers. Care pathways, health behaviour and health plans that took twenty or thirty years or centuries to change could now change with record access in weeks or months.

3.2.3 RA seems to enhance compliance in patients with heart failure.

3.2.4 RA improves health promotion behaviour. There is some evidence that smoking quit rates are higher in patients who have RA.

3.2.5 RA helps patients keep track of fragmented care[3]. This can be a serious problem in many health services. Many patients, especially the elderly, are treated for multiple problems by various carers and institutions. Results may get lost, coordination can be poor. If a patient has access to their information, particularly by having access to their primary care record where most of this information is stored in summary form, they can take charge of failed linkages, if they so wish.

Record access may therefore also stimulate improvements in care across interfaces.

Record access allows patients to use valuable information about themselves to their own advantage. Expensive tests and results can be re-used and shared as and where the patient wishes to share them.

3.2.6 RA will establish portability of the PHR, also across national boundaries.

3.2.7 Poor health and behavior causes illness and illness causes disease. RA can stimulate behavioural changes in citizens. [4]

3.2.8 RA educates patients and their selected families and friends. Adults and children with health and disease learning needs need to take on new roles as participants in health creation and disease management. Knowledge and understanding are delivered to citizens and patients through the PHR. Care, monitoring of health and disease and implementation of procedures can be shared or delegated to citizens and patients using the shared record.

3.3. RA empowers patients

3.3.1 Patients with RA feel more in control.[5]

3.3.2 RA helps patients can find information out for themselves. For instance, through test results, care pathways or letters about them. Support information must be linked to these items, to enhance patients' understanding, involvement and commitment.

3.3.3 With RA, patients can have access to information about good medical practice, tailored to their personal health needs. For instance, by linking their health problems as viewed in their record electronically to information such as national good practice guidelines, diabetic patients can see if their blood sugar and blood pressure fall within good practice boundaries.

3.3.4. RA supports shared decision-making. The record can support this in many ways. Just having access to what your clinicians are saying about you, access to investigation results with interpretation, access to letters enables patients to take greater part in their care and health creation. In addition, if there are links to specific decision aids, patients are more likely to take decisions that change their management. [6]

3.3.5 RA helps patients understand their consultation better. Research suggests that patients who leave a consultation with a clinician unclear about what has been said can understand it more clearly by reading afterwards what the clinician has written.

3.3.6 RA helps carers and advocates support patients better. So long as permission has been freely given, carers can understand the patient's condition better and be up to date with their management. In this way, patients with dementia or mental health problems, for instance, can participate more in their care. [7]

3.3.7 RA will encourage citizens to add personal issues to the EPR, such as their use of over the counter drugs.

3.3.8 RA will promote the use of monitoring devices, as the results will be part of the EPR.

3.4. Improved record keeping

3.4.1 RA enables patients to correct their records. The commonest errors in UK records are demographic. RA allows patients to point out or indicate errors in their records and enables them to request for correction.[8]

3.5. Benefits to the health service

3.5.1 Patient with RA may need fewer appointments. Research suggests that, if patients have seen the information in their records that they need, they do not make unnecessary appointments.[9]

3.5.2 Patients with RA may take less time in consultations. Research suggests that patients only raise those issues that they have not been able to resolve by looking at their records. Of course, explanations of data that remain unclear may also result in longer consultations. Overall, evidence suggests that RA is time-neutral. [10]

4. COMPLEX ISSUES

These can be addressed by appropriate administrative and technical approaches
4.1. Access to their records by children and their parents
4.2. Third party information
4.3. Language
4.4. Patients with psychiatric problems
4.5. Litigation
4.6. Security and authentication
4.7. Insurance companies and solicitors trawling through records for business.

5. ACTIONS FOR THE WHO

5.1 The WHO should recognize the significance benefits accrued by full RA to the personal health record.

5.2 The WHO should promote RA as a key aspect of care.

5.3 The WHO should ensure that health services around the world enable patients to see their full personal health record if they want to. The administrative, cultural and technical infrastructure to support RA should be encouraged.

5.4 The WHO should support research into RA and how it can be best harnessed for patient care.

Signatories

Dr Brian Fisher MBBCh MSc, GP
Wells Park Practice
1 Wells Park Rd
UK-London SE26 6JQ
brian.fisher403@ntlworld.com

Dr Richard Fitton, GP
Hadfield Medical Centre
82 Brosscroft, Hadfield, Glossop
UK-Derbyshire SK13 1DS
Richard.fitton1@btopenworld.com

Drs Lodewijk Bos
President ICMCC
Stationsstraat 38
NL-3511 EG Utrecht
lobos@icmcc.org

REFERENCES

[1]   Access to Medical Reports Act 1988 www.opsi.gov.uk/acts/acts1988/Ukpga_19880028_en_1.htm

[2]   www.paers.net

[3]   Richards T BMJ 2007;334:510 (10 March), doi:10.1136/bmj.39146.615081.59

[4]   Ross SE, Moore LA, Earnest MA, Wittevrongel L, Lin CT. (May 2004) Providing a web-based online medical record with electronic communication capabilities to patients with congestive heart failure: randomized trial. J Med Internet Res. 20;6(2):e14.

[5]   Winkelman WJ, Leonard KJ, Rossos PG.. 'Patient-perceived usefulness of on-line electronic medical records: Employing grounded theory in the development of information and communication technologies for use by patients living with chronic illness'. J Am Med Inform Assoc. 2005 Jan 31

[6]   www.icmcc.org

[7]   Richards T BMJ 2007;334:510 (10 March), doi:10.1136/bmj.39146.615081.59

[8]   Powell J, Fitton R, Fitton C. (2006) Sharing electronic health records: the patient view. Informatics in Primary Care 14:55-7

[9]   NHS Connecting for Health unpublished data

[10]   Op cit

Medical and Care Compunetics 4
L. Bos and B. Blobel (Eds.)
IOS Press, 2007

Author Index